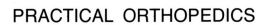

PRACTICAL ORTHOPEDICS

PRACTICAL ORTHOPEDICS

LONNIE R. MERCIER, M.D.

Clinical Instructor
Department of Orthopedic Surgery
Creighton University School of Medicine
Omaha, Nebraska

with

FRED J. PETTID, M.D.

Chairman and Associate Professor of Family Practice
Department of Family Practice
Creighton University School of Medicine
Omaha, Nebraska

YEAR BOOK MEDICAL PUBLISHERS, INC.
CHICAGO • LONDON

Library of Congress Cataloging in Publication Data

Mercier, Lonnie R.
   Practical orthopedics.

   1. Orthopedia. I. Pettid, Fred J., joint author.
II. Title. [DNLM: 1. Orthopedics. WE168 M555p]
RD731. M43   617'.3   80-15304
ISBN 0-8151-5863-7

Foreword

IT IS A PRIVILEGE to welcome this first edition. Musculoskeletal problems are among the most frequent challenges presented to the primary care physician. The National Ambulatory Medical Care Survey has found that complaints involving the upper extremities, lower extremities, and back are consistently among the ten most frequent outpatient problems encountered by practicing physicians. Our present educational system is still deficient in that many physicians who do a great deal of primary care receive inadequate exposure to these common problems during their residency programs. Since their inception, family practice training programs have placed heavy emphasis on musculoskeletal complaints and although many internal medicine residencies have added some experience in orthopedics there remains a great need for practical reference texts of this type to serve the everyday needs of the practicing family physician and other primary care physicians.

Doctors Mercier and Pettid have done an excellent job of focusing on the orthopedic problems most frequently encountered in practice. Their comments are succinct and clear. They appropriately avoid the complicated and rare problems that require referral and deal in depth with those that the primary care physician is called upon daily to diagnose and manage. This book covers the breadth of ambulatory orthopedics, extending from the management of common problems such as bursitis or back strain to the care of severe injuries such as Colles' fracture or skin grafting a fingertip injury.

I commend the policy of joint authorship used in this book. Pairing an authority in the field with an experienced family physician assures the relevance necessary to make this a valuable reference.

ROBERT E. RAKEL, M.D.

Preface

THE STIMULUS to write this book was our participation in the orthopedic training of students and residents whose primary fields of interest are those other than orthopedic surgery. We were frequently asked to recommend an appropriate text for them to study but we found that none was available that met their needs. Most orthopedic surgery books are either too detailed or not complete enough to have any practical value in general medicine. We discovered, also, that no book existed that could be used as a current, practical guide and clinical reference by practicing physicians in the daily care of their patients. This book was undertaken to meet these needs.

In presenting a useful overview of orthopedic disorders, we have tried to discuss, in some depth, those conditions that are encountered frequently in daily practice. By emphasizing certain common features of these disorders, it is hoped that the fundamental concepts can be applied in the diagnosis and treatment of other musculoskeletal conditions.

The text is divided into two general sections. The first deals with musculoskeletal disorders by anatomical region. The later chapters discuss the arthritides, infection, injuries, and other common problems of interest, including a particularly useful chapter on radiologic aspects of orthopedic disease. The reader interested in sports medicine is directed to the index, where he will find references to discussions throughout the text on treatment of patients with athletic injuries.

The practice of orthopedics is, in a sense, rehabilitative medicine. It has as its goals improvement in the level of function of the patient and the diminution of pain. We hope you will find this book helpful in meeting these goals.

It is difficult to acknowledge all of the people who have helped in the preparation of this book. We would begin, however, by paying special thanks to our wives, without whose patience and understanding this book would not have been possible. We would also like to express our gratitude to Loren Corell for the fine illustrations and to John Busse for the photographic prints. Our appreciation also goes to Nancy Chorpenning and the rest of the people at Year Book Medical Publishers for their expertise and guidance. In addition, the following people were invaluable in the preparation of the manuscript, roentgenograms, and demonstrations: Betty Newman, Clarice Kramer, Kathy Schuster, Richard Nelson, P. A., Jeanne Kane, Karen Swesey, and Jo Arthur.

LONNIE R. MERCIER
FRED J. PETTID

Contents

1 / Physical Examination

THE DIAGNOSIS OF DISORDERS of the musculoskeletal system begins with a complete history and physical examination. The history is of special significance because physical findings are often minimal. Its importance cannot be overemphasized.

HISTORY

Birth History

The history of the pediatric patient should include several important points. It should first be determined whether fetal movements were experienced by the mother during pregnancy. Absence or weakness of these movements by the fourth or fifth month of gestation may indicate neuromuscular disease in the newborn.

The type of delivery should also be noted. This is important because certain disorders, such as congenital hip dysplasia, are more common following breech delivery.

The condition of the child at birth and

TABLE 1–1.—NORMAL
MILESTONES

AGE (MO)	MILESTONE
1–2	Holds up chin
6–8	Sits alone
8–10	Stands with support
10–12	Walks with support
14	Walks without support
24	Ascends stairs one foot at a time

NOTE: There is frequently a wide variation in physical development, but if a child cannot walk unsupported by 18 months of age, a neuromuscular disorder should be suspected.

immediately after delivery should be ascertained. The presence of any jaundice, cyanosis, or difficulty with the delivery that might predispose the infant to brain damage is also recorded.

The physical and mental development of the child are then determined and any deviation from normal progress, such as premature hand preference, is noted (Table 1–1). Ambidexterity is normal up to 12 to 18 months of age, and its absence may signify unilateral injury to the upper extremity or cerebral palsy.

Family History

A review of the family history is important not only for certain obvious musculoskeletal problems, such as polydactyly, but also for those disorders that may not be so obvious, such as scoliosis and tuberculosis. Other family members may even need to be examined.

Past History

The general health of the patient is recorded, as well as any recent weight loss or gain. The patient's exact occupation should be determined and any relevant military history noted, especially if a disability rating resulted from time spent in the service. All chronic renal, metabolic, pulmonary, and previous orthopedic disorders should be assessed in view of the initial complaint.

Present Illness

The nature of the onset of symptoms, whether gradual or sudden, should be established. If an injury is involved, the exact date and place of the injury are recorded. This is frequently an important fact in determining injury liability. The chief complaint should also be evaluated in relation to any previous similar symptoms or other musculoskeletal complaints. In addition, it should be noted if the patient has had any other recent, seemingly unrelated illness or symptoms, such as fever or chills.

The exact location and nature of any pain should be determined. In addition, the following important facts are noted: (1) the relationship of the pain to normal daily activities; (2) whether the pain is worse in the morning or late in the day; (3) if coughing, sneezing, or other similar activities aggravate the pain; (4) if the pain improves with rest; and (5) whether the pain remains well localized or is radicular in nature. If the pain is radicular, it should be determined if the radiation follows any dermatome or peripheral nerve pattern. The effect of any home remedies on the pain should also be assessed.

Weakness and numbness are less common symptoms and may be extremely subjective. An attempt should be made to document them, however. The following information should be ascertained: (1) whether the weakness is generalized or involves specific muscles or muscle groups; (2) whether there is any loss of sphincter control; and (3) whether the numbness follows a dermatome, peripheral nerve, or stocking/glove pattern. The pain and numbness that follow specific dermatome nerve patterns are often very diagnostic but the numbness that follows a stocking or glove type of distribution frequently indicates psychosomatic illness. It should also be determined whether the symptoms are worse at night or during the day. The pain from carpal tunnel syndrome, for example, is characteristically most severe at night.

When deformity is the initial complaint, the following information should be obtained: (1) whether the patient or someone else first noticed the deformity; (2) whether it is increasing or decreasing; and (3) whether it is associated with any recent injury, joint swelling, or stiffness. The amount of actual disability that the deformity causes the patient is also of considerable importance.

EXAMINATION

Valuable information can frequently be gained by merely observing the gait, general posture, and stance of many patients. This is especially helpful in the child who may otherwise be difficult to examine. The height and weight of the patient are recorded and all examinations are performed with the affected area completely exposed (Fig 1–1). The patient should always be viewed in profile as well as from the front and back.

The specific affected area is then inspected and any swelling, discoloration, or areas of tenderness are noted. Palpa-

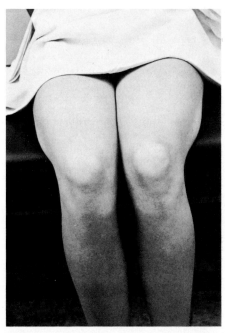

Fig 1–1. – Proper attire for knee examination. Both lower extremities are completely exposed.

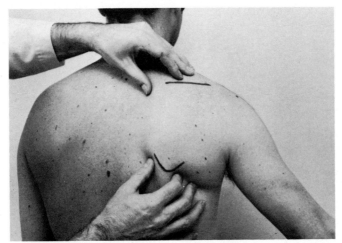

Fig 1–2.—True glenohumeral motion is measured by first stabilizing the scapula to prevent scapulothoracic motion. This is accomplished by prohibiting movement of the palpable spine and inferior angle.

tion should be gentle but persistent. Every attempt should be made to describe affected areas according to their exact anatomical location. Movements or maneuvers that exacerbate the pain are recorded. Any muscle atrophy is noted and compared with measurements of the opposite extremity. Muscle power is tested in a similar manner. Alterations in skin temperature or perspiration are also noted.

Active and passive ranges of joint motion are carefully measured and the patient is observed for any crepitus or resistance to movement. During the examination, adjacent joints may need to be stabilized in order to properly measure the affected joint (Fig 1–2).

Measurements of limb length and circumference are also made when indicated, and a complete neurologic examination is performed when neuromuscular disease is suspected.

ORTHOPEDIC TERMINOLOGY

General

Ankylosis: restriction of motion in a joint (synostosis)

Arthrodesis: surgical stiffening of a joint (fusion)

Arthroplasty: to restore motion and function to a joint

Coxa: hip bone or joint (os coxae)

Cubitus: elbow

Effusion: escape of fluid into a cavity

Genu: knee or knee joint

Hallux: great toe

Paresthesia: abnormal sensation, such as burning and tingling

Pes: foot

Radicular: spinal nerve involvement

Spondylolisthesis: slipping of a vertebra

Spondylolysis: dissolution or loosening of a vertebra

Spondylosis: disease, usually degenerative, of a vertebra

Sprain: injury to joint ligament or capsule

Strain: injury to muscle or tendon

Subluxation: incomplete dislocation

Motion

Flexion: the bending of a joint

Extension: the straightening of a joint

Abduction: movement away from the middle line (in the hand, the long finger is the middle line)

Adduction: movement toward the middle line

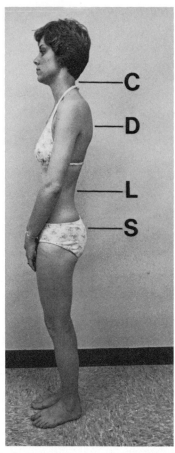

Fig 1–3.—A mild kyphosis is normally present in the dorsal (D) and sacral (S) spine. Lordosis is normally present in the cervical (C) and lumbar (L) spine.

Pronation: to rotate the forearm in such a way that the palm looks backward when the arm is in the anatomical position

Supination: to rotate the forearm in such a way that the palm looks forward when the arm is in the anatomical position

Eversion: turning outward (in the foot, valgus, eversion, and pronation are frequently synonymous)

Inversion: turning inward (in the foot, varus, inversion, and supination are frequently synonymous)

Deformity

Kyphosis: curvature of the spine with convexity posterior (Fig 1–3)

Lordosis: curvature of the spine with convexity anterior

Scoliosis: abnormal lateral curvature of the spine

Equinus: plantar flexion of the foot

Calcaneus: dorsiflexion of the foot

Planus: flat; abnormally low arch

Cavus: hollow; abnormally high arch

Varus: the distal part angulates toward the midline of the body

Valgus: the distal part angulates away from the midline of the body

Recurvatum: backward bending or hyperextension (Fig 1–4)

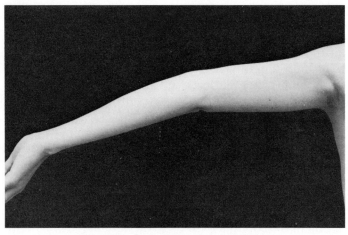

Fig 1–4.—Recurvatum of the elbow.

2 / The Cervical Spine

THE CERVICAL SPINE is exceeded only by the lumbar spine in the number of patients affected by conditions causing pain or dysfunction. These disorders vary from those that are annoying to those that may be functionally disabling. The diagnosis and treatment of these disorders are a major part of orthopedics.

ANATOMY

Seven cervical vertebrae make up the bony elements of the cervical spine. A typical cervical vertebra is similar to other vertebrae, in that it is composed of a body and a neural arch (Fig 2-1). The neural arch is composed of two pedicles that form the sides and two laminae that meet in the midline to form the roof. Projecting dorsally where the laminae meet is the spinous process, and projecting laterally from the junction of the pedicle and lamina is a transverse process on each side. Two articular processes, the superior and inferior, project upward and downward, respectively, from the junction of the pedicle and lamina on each side and articulate with similar processes on adjacent vertebrae to form the zygoapophyseal or facet joints.

The first two cervical vertebrae are atypical in that C1, the atlas, has no body (Fig 2-2). Its body is attached to C2, the axis, and forms the dens, or odontoid process. This arrangement allows for most of the rotation in the cervical spine. Strong ligaments bind C1 to C2, the most important of which is the transverse ligament. The seventh cervical vertebra, vertebra prominens, is also somewhat atypical in that it has a long spinous process that is easily palpable beneath the skin.

Several major ligaments stabilize the cervical spine (Fig 2-3). The anterior and posterior longitudinal ligaments are applied to the respective surfaces of the vertebral bodies. Where the posterior longitudinal ligament crosses the disc, it tends to be somewhat weak laterally, thus forming a point where disc herniation may occur. Some gliding motion is allowed to occur between vertebrae by relatively weak capsular ligaments that bind together each articular joint. The ligamentum flavum, or yellow ligament, is situated between adjacent laminae, and in the cervical spine, extremely strong ligaments—the nuchal ligament and interspinous ligaments—provide posterior support.

The vertebrae are separated from each other by the intervertebral discs, which constitute approximately one fourth of the length of the vertebral column. Each

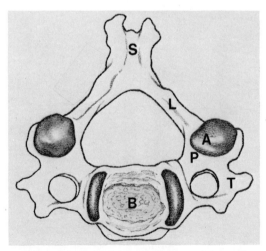

Fig 2-1.—A typical cervical vertebra: *S* = spinous process; *L* = lamina; *A* = articular facet; *P* = pedicle; *T* = transverse process; *B* = body.

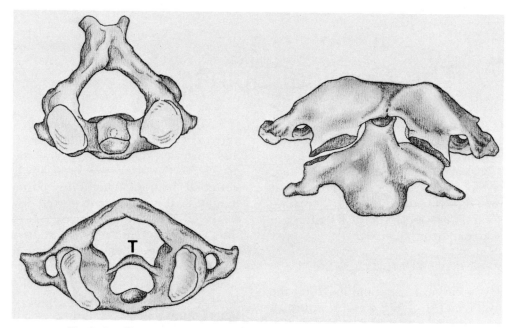

Fig 2–2. – The axis *(top),* atlas *(bottom),* and transverse ligament *(T).*
Right, the articulation of the atlas and the axis.

disc is composed of an inner nucleus pulposus, which is mainly gelatinous, and an outer layer, the anulus fibrosis, which is mainly fibrous. The discs function to distribute stress over a wide area of the vertebrae, to absorb shock, and to allow mobility. The nucleus pulposus has a very high water content in early life, but with age this tends to diminish. With this loss of water, abnormal pressures begin to be exerted on the anulus, which leads

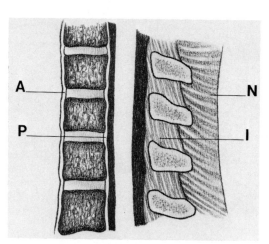

Fig 2–3. – Ligaments of the cervical spine: *A* = anterior longitudinal ligament; *P* = posterior longitudinal ligament; *N* = nuchal ligament; *I* = interspinous ligament.

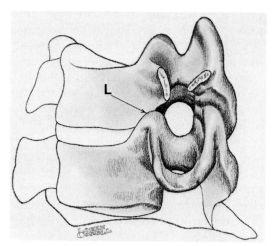

Fig 2–4. – The intervertebral foramen. Note the proximity of the joint of Luschka *(L).* (Adapted from DePalma, A. F., and Rothman, R. H.: *The Intervertebral Disc* [Philadelphia: W. B. Saunders Co., 1970].)

to pathologic changes in adjacent structures.

Eight pairs of nerve roots arise from the cervical spinal cord. Each nerve exits above the vertebra of the same number. Thus, the sixth nerve root exits at the C5-C6 disc space. Each nerve except the first two pairs leaves the spinal column by passing through an intervertebral foramen (Fig 2–4). Each foramen has as its superior and inferior boundaries the pedicles of the adjacent vertebrae. Posterolaterally, it is bounded by the apophyseal joint, and anteromedially, by the so-called joint of Luschka. In the cervical spine, this foramen is quite small and is almost entirely occupied by the nerve root. Thus, anything that compromises this space, such as disc degeneration with spur formation, will cause pressure on the nerve root.

EXAMINATION

Examination of the neck begins with observation of the posture of the head and neck in relation to the torso. Any decrease in the normal cervical lordosis is noted. The neck is gently palpated for tender areas, trigger points, and muscle spasm. The range of motion of the cervical spine is then measured and any movement that reproduces pain is noted. Flexion, extension, right and left bending,

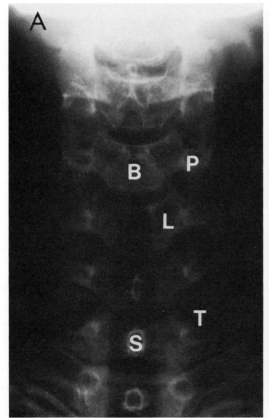
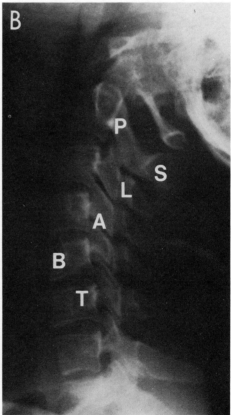

Fig 2–5.—Anteroposterior (A) and lateral (B) views of the cervical spine: S = spinous process; T = transverse process; B = body; A = articular (zygoapophyseal) facet joint; P = pedicle; L = lamina. Note the slight lordosis and even spacing of the vertebrae and discs.

and right and left rotation are all recorded. A complete neurologic examination, including muscle strength testing, is always performed. The peripheral nerves are percussed for tenderness and tested for function. In addition, the shoulders and elbows are always carefully examined, particularly if there is any radiation of the pain or numbness and tingling.

ROENTGENOGRAPHIC ANATOMY

The examination of all neck disorders should include a standard roentgenographic evaluation. The roentgenographic

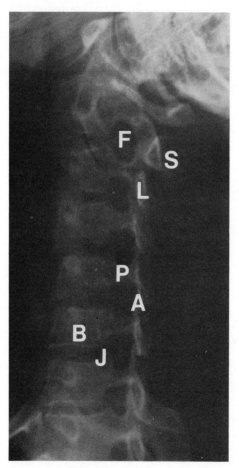

Fig 2–6.—Oblique view: *S* = spinous process; *F* = intervertebral foramen; *J* = joint of Luschka; *L* = lamina; *P* = pedicle; *A* = articular facet joint; *B* = body.

features of the cervical spine are well visualized by the following: (1) anteroposterior view (Fig 2–5), (2) lateral views in flexion and extension, (3) oblique views in both directions to visualize the intervertebral foramen (Fig 2–6), and (4) an open-mouth odontoid view to visualize the odontoid process and the relationship between C1 and C2.

CERVICAL DISC SYNDROMES

Over 90% of disc lesions in the cervical spine occur at the C5 and C6 levels, those being the most mobile segments. As disc degeneration occurs, either gradually or following acute trauma, two types of lesions result that produce very similar symptoms. The first of these is the so-called soft disc protrusion or nuclear herniation. With this lesion, a mass of nucleus pulposus begins to bulge outward, usually at the area of the greatest weakness in the anulus fibrosus (Fig 2–7). Complete extrusion of this disc material may even occur. This lesion is more common in the younger patient. With acute rupture of a cervical disc, immediate compression of the nerve root occurs, resulting in nerve root symptoms and radicular pain.

The second, more common, lesion results from chronic disc degeneration with subsequent narrowing of the disc space and alterations in the surrounding structures. This is the so-called hard disc lesion or cervical "spondylosis" and occurs primarily in the older age group. As narrowing and collapse of the disc proceeds, the vertebrae become more closely approximated, which leads to spur formation along the disc edges and at the joints of Luschka. Mild subluxation of the facet joints also occurs. All of these changes decrease the size of the intervertebral foramen, which results in pressure on the nerve root. Mild inflammation and swelling are usually present in conjunction

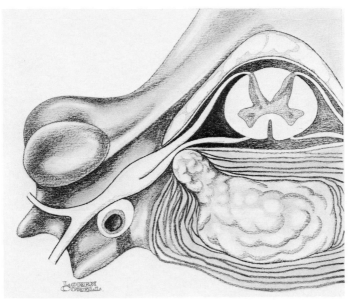

Fig 2–7.—Disc herniation causing nerve root compression. Spur formation may occur in the same area. (Adapted from DePalma, A. F., and Rothman, R. H.: *The Intervertebral Disc* [Philadelphia: W. B. Saunders Co., 1970].)

with the osteophyte formation, which further contributes to the narrowing of the foramen and nerve root compression. Large posterior osteophytes may also cause pressure on the anterior portion of the spinal cord, producing mixed symptoms of upper extremity nerve root pain and lower extremity weakness. This is commonly termed cervical spondylosis with myelopathy.

CLINICAL FEATURES

Pain associated with cervical disc disease may develop either gradually or acutely. Patients often complain of a tightness or stiffness in the neck that is made worse with activity. Morning stiffness is common, and certain movements, especially extension, exacerbate the pain. Coughing, sneezing, and straining can

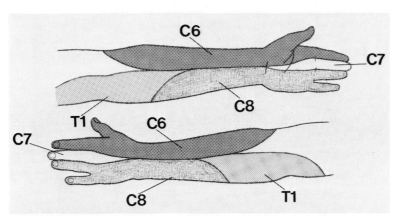

Fig 2–8.—Volar and dorsal dermatome pattern of the forearm and hand. Pain and paresthesias may radiate into these areas when the affected nerve root is compressed.

accentuate the pain, which may radiate into the shoulders and arms and along the radial aspect of the forearm (Fig 2–8). Numbness and tingling are often noted in these same areas, and referred pain, which does not follow a dermatome pattern, is common along the medial border of the scapula. Headaches are not uncommon, and dysphagia has even been reported secondary to large anterior osteophytes.

Examination frequently reveals a decreased range of motion. Pain on hyperextension and local tenderness in the cervical spine are often observed. Trigger-point tenderness is commonly noted in the area of referred pain in the interscapular region. Pressure against the top of the head may reproduce the pain in the arm (Fig 2–9). Some sensory changes are occasionally seen along the specific dermatome, but the sensory examination is frequently not very helpful. Motor weak-

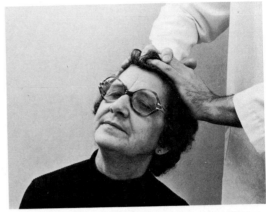

Fig 2–9.—Vertex compression test. Reproduction of neck and arm pain may be observed.

ness and reflex changes are frequently noted (Table 2–1).

Spondylosis in the cervical spine may occasionally produce symptoms referable to the lower extremities (cervical spondylotic myelopathy). These symp-

TABLE 2–1.—CLINICAL FEATURES OF COMMON CERVICAL
DISC SYNDROMES

DISC	PAIN	SENSORY CHANGE	MOTOR WEAKNESS, ATROPHY	REFLEX CHANGE
C4–C5 (C5 root)	Base of neck, shoulder, anterolateral aspect of arm	Hyperesthesia in deltoid region	Deltoid, biceps	Biceps
C5–C6 (C6 root)	Neck, shoulder, medial border of scapula, lateral aspect of arm, dorsum of forearm	Dorsolateral aspect of thumb and index finger	Biceps, extensor pollicis, longus	Biceps
C6–C7 (C7 root)	Neck, shoulder, medial border of scapula, lateral aspect of arm, dorsum of forearm	Index, middle fingers, dorsum of hand	Triceps	Triceps

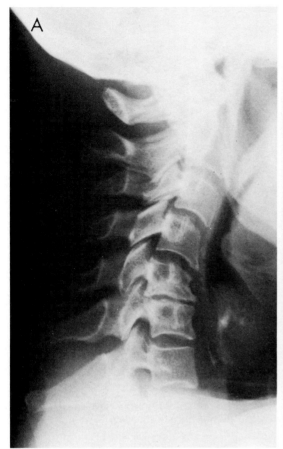

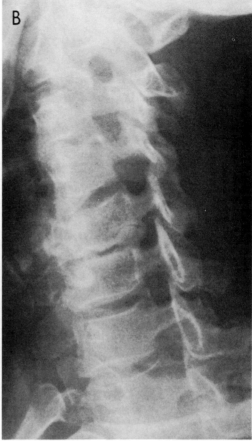

Fig 2–10. — Lateral **(A)** and oblique **(B)** roentgenograms showing degenerative disc disease at the C5–C6 level. Note the osteophyte formation and narrowing of the intervertebral foramen.

toms occur as a result of pressure of posterior osteophytes on the anterior portion of the cervical spinal cord. The symptom complex appears as a combination of cervical root and cord symptoms. The patient may have a typical disc syndrome in the upper extremities but, in addition, gait difficulties, weakness, and spasticity may be present in the lower extremities. The lower extremity symptoms have a gradual onset at about age 50 and progress slowly.

The roentgenographic examination is usually normal in soft disc rupture. With chronic degenerative disc disease, however, loss of the height of the disc space, anterior and posterior osteophyte formation, and encroachment on the intervertebral foramen by osteophytes are noted on routine films (Fig 2–10). Myelography is helpful in localizing the lesion but is not without some morbidity and is indicated only under two circumstances: (1) if surgical intervention is contemplated, or (2) if other serious spinal abnormality is suspected. Loss of the normal root "sleeve" and indentation of the dural sac are often seen (Fig 2–11). Spinal fluid analysis

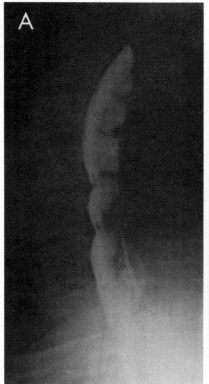

Fig 2–11.—Myelographic findings in cervical disc disease. Note the filling defects from osteophyte formation on the lateral view **(A)** and absence of the normal root sleeve *(arrows)* on the anteroposterior view **(B).**

performed at the time of myelography may show a slight increase in protein content.

Electromyography and discography are also occasionally performed in the evaluation of cervical disc disease, but the diagnosis can usually be well established on the basis of the history, physical examination, and myelogram alone.

TREATMENT

Rest is the cornerstone of therapy for cervical disc disease. In the acute disc protrusion, it permits the healing of soft parts to occur. In chronic disc disease, it allows the inflammatory reaction to subside. Rest is accomplished by various means, but absolute bed rest is the most beneficial. Various soft collars that restrict motion are also helpful (Fig 2–12).

Moist heat applied to the affected area will help relieve tenderness and muscle spasm. Aspirin, given in adequate doses for analgesia and inflammation, is probably the most effective of the anti-inflammatory drugs. Cervical traction, which may be used at home, is also beneficial (Fig 2–13). Physical therapy, in the form of diathermy, massage, and intermittent cervical traction, may also be necessary.

After the acute pain subsides, a program of gentle, graded exercises, to increase the strength and mobility of the cervical spine, are recommended (Fig 2–14). Recurrences are prevented by avoiding fatigue and poor postural habits, especially hyperextension (Fig 2–15). A

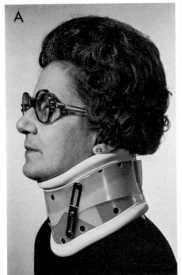
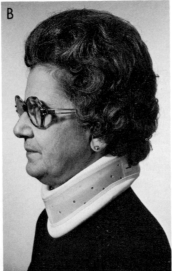
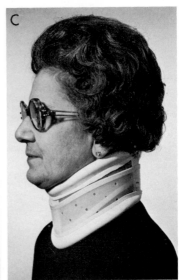

Fig 2–12.—Proper usage of the cervical collar. **A,** a collar too high places the neck in too much extension. **B,** a collar too short does not immobilize and allows too much flexion. **C,** proper height of the collar maintains the head in a slightly flexed or neutral position.

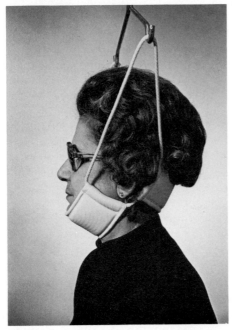

Fig 2–13.—Proper usage of cervical traction. The direction of pull should be neutral; 4 to 6 pounds of weight should be used for 20 to 30 minutes. It should be repeated three to four times daily, depending on response. The pressure should be equally distributed between the chin and the occiput.

pillow approximately 7.5 to 10 cm thick should be used for sleeping and should be placed under the neck rather than under the head. An overly thick pillow may place the head in too much flexion, while an overly thin one may allow too much extension to occur.

Most patients can be told that they will improve with time and that less than 5% of all patients with cervical disc symptoms require surgery. The time period required for improvement varies considerably among patients. They may be advised, however, that there is generally no danger in waiting and continuing conservative treatment. Surgery is reserved for those cases in which the pain and level of disability become intolerable. The procedure consists of removal of the affected disc, usually followed by arthrodesis of the two adjacent vertebrae with a bone graft (Fig 2–16). The pain usually subsides immediately after surgery, and osteophytes that have formed in the foramen and adjacent structures are usually absorbed within 9 to 18 months.

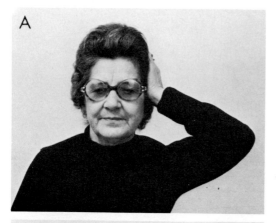

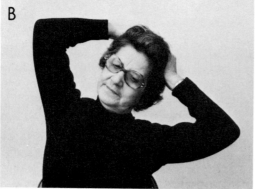

Fig 2–14.—**A,** cervical isometric exercises are performed in each direction with the neck in the neutral position. **B,** range-of-motion exercises are done by carefully rotating and bending the head in each direction several times. The motion should never be forced. These exercises are repeated three to four times daily.

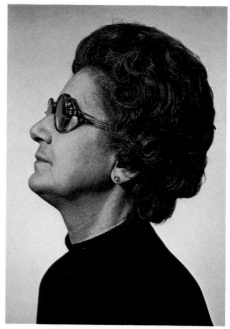

Fig 2–15.—The hyperextended "spectator" attitude that often causes neck strain and aggravates disc disease. The head and neck should be maintained in a neutral position at all times. Positions that produce sharp angulation or rotation of the head, such as sleeping on the abdomen or resting on a couch with the armrest as a "pillow," should also be avoided.

CERVICAL SPRAIN

Most soft tissue injuries of the cervical spine are the result of a hyperextension force. This is the nature of the injury most commonly sustained in the rear-end automobile collision. Rarely is there any osseous injury. Most of the force is absorbed by ligaments, muscles, and disc. Acute disc protrusion is not common but disc injury is, and serial roentgenograms taken at later dates may show significant progressive degenerative changes.

All soft structures, including muscle, anterior longitudinal ligament, esophagus, and trachea, may be severely stretched. Dysphagia and hoarseness are sometimes seen shortly after the injury. Hemorrhage and edema may be present in the prevertebral area, and the sympathetic nerve chains, which are located near the vertebral bodies, are occasionally stretched. This may produce somewhat unusual symptoms, such as nausea, tinnitus, blurred vision, and dizziness.

Chronic pain, which continues for weeks or months, is not uncommon. Degenerative changes may result from the injury at one or more levels in a previously normal cervical spine, which may lead to significant disability. Similarly, the patient with previously asymptomatic

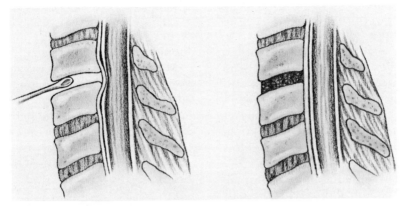

Fig 2–16. — Arthrodesis of the cervical spine.
The disc is removed and replaced with a bone graft.

degenerative disc disease may have the onset of symptoms related to a hyperextension injury.

CLINICAL FEATURES

Frequently there are very few symptoms immediately following the injury. A few hours later, however, the patient begins to notice stiffness in the neck, followed by pain and inability to move the neck normally. The pain is generalized to the neck region and may radiate to the occiput along the path of the greater occipital nerve. Shoulder, arm, and interscapular pain may be noted, and there may even be pain in the anterior chest wall. Symptoms such as nausea, tinnitus, blurred vision, and occipital headaches are not uncommon.

Examination may reveal generalized tenderness in the anterior and posterior neck musculature. Motion may be greatly limited, and extension of the spine is often quite painful. Mild torticollis may be present. The results of the neurologic examination are usually normal.

After the initial examination, if there is any reason to suspect a significant cervical spine injury, a full lateral roentgenogram of the cervical spine should be taken without moving the patient. This view should always include the body of the

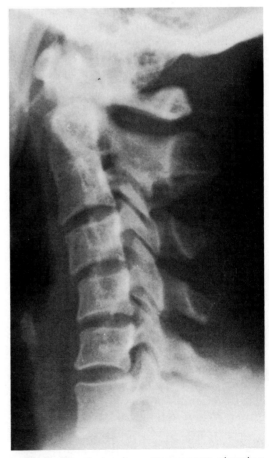

Fig 2–17. — Lateral roentgenogram showing reversal of the cervical lordosis.

seventh cervical vertebra; if it does not, the vertebra is probably being obscured by the shoulder soft tissue shadow. In this case, the shoulders should be pulled down manually and the roentgenogram repeated. If a satisfactory view of C7 still has not been obtained, then a "swimmer's" view may be performed. If no significant injury is seen on this view, then the remainder of the cervical spine films are obtained.

Usually, the initial roentgenographic examination is normal, but with the passage of time, reversal of the normal cervical lordosis may be observed (Fig 2–17). This finding is quite significant and is often seen in patients with prolonged disability. Late degenerative changes may even occur. "Loss of the normal cervical lordosis," often noted on early roentgenograms, is probably not significant. Any degenerative changes present in the cervical spine at the time of the initial injury should also be noted for both medical and medicolegal purposes.

Treatment

Rest is the most important treatment modality in the acute cervical strain. It should be continuous and should consist primarily of bed rest. A soft cervical collar holding the neck in slight flexion is worn day and night for approximately one to two weeks. Analgesics are given in amounts sufficient to relieve pain. Heat should not be used initially after the injury as it may increase swelling. Cervical traction should be avoided early in the treatment because it may stretch already stretched soft parts. Anti-inflammatory drugs given soon after the injury may be helpful in the patient who has preexisting degenerative disease of the cervical spine. When the acute pain subsides, isometric and gentle range-of-motion exercises are started and the collar is discontinued for daytime use. General measures, including a proper pillow and the avoidance of stress, should be instituted. If symptoms persist after four to six weeks, cervical traction and physical therapy may be beneficial.

Most patients will improve in four to six weeks if the initial treatment has been adequate. Less long-term disability and anxiety on the part of the patient will result if aggressive, conservative treatment is instituted, especially in the initial stage of the injury. Surgery is rarely necessary.

DISC CALCIFICATION

Calcification of the intervertebral disc is not uncommon. It frequently occurs in the dorsal spine of adults in the anulus fibrosus and is probably secondary to a degenerative process. Multiple disc calcifications also occur with ochronosis. Disc calcification is usually an incidental roentgenographic finding and generally does not produce symptoms.

In children, however, disc calcification occurs more commonly in the cervical spine, and in this age group it appears as a definite clinical entity with symptoms. The cause is unknown but it may represent a nonspecific inflammatory reaction. It is probably not infectious in nature. In contrast to the adult, it is the nucleus pulposus that calcifies.

Clinical features

The disorder has its onset about the age of 7 and usually begins with neck pain and stiffness. Localized tenderness and a decrease in the range of motion of the cervical spine are usually present. A mild torticollis may be noted. There is usually an elevation of the temperature, sedimentation rate, and WBC count.

Roentgenograms reveal the disease to primarily affect the lower discs in the cervical spine (Fig 2–18). Multiple discs may be affected and the calcification usually begins to regress with the onset of symptoms.

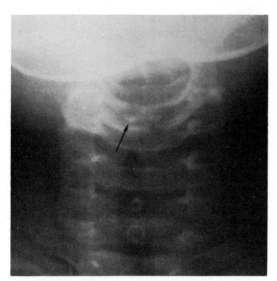

Fig 2–18. – Disc space calcification *(arrow).*

ened and contracted sternocleidomastoid muscle. If untreated, secondary changes appear in the cervical vertebrae, and marked asymmetry of the face becomes apparent. These changes frequently persist in spite of later treatment.

CLINICAL FEATURES

The diagnosis generally can be made shortly after birth. The "mass" is usually palpable, and the head is characteristically tilted toward the side of the mass and rotated in the opposite direction (Fig 2–19). Roentgenograms of the cervical spine are usually normal but should always be performed to rule out injury and congenital osseous disorders of the cervical spine.

TREATMENT

The treatment is conservative and consists of a soft collar, cervical traction, and analgesics as necessary. Antibiotics are not as a rule indicated. The patients usually become asymptomatic in one to two weeks without any sequelae.

TORTICOLLIS

Torticollis is a deformity of the neck that causes rotation and tilting of the head, usually in opposite directions. It may be present on a congenital basis or acquired as a result of trauma or disease.

Congenital Muscular Torticollis

This deformity is usually noted at birth and is much more common after breech deliveries. It results from a unilateral contracture of the sternocleidomastoid muscle. The cause is unknown but fibrosis of the muscle occurs, possibly secondary to a vascular disturbance in the muscle. A "tumor" consisting of dense fibrous tissue is often found in the muscle shortly after birth. This mass gradually subsides over the ensuing weeks, leaving a short-

TREATMENT

Conservative treatment, if instituted early, will usually result in a cure. No improvement can be expected without treatment. In mild deformities, gentle stretching exercises carried out by the mother will usually correct the problem. The exercises should be repeated several times daily. The crib should be so placed that the child must turn toward the corrected position when someone enters the room.

Surgery is reserved for late cases or those that fail to respond to conservative

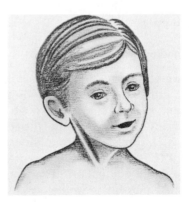

Fig 2–19. – Congenital muscular torticollis.

treatment. The procedure consists of the release of the sternocleidomastoid muscle followed by traction or casting and exercises. The results are usually good.

Torticollis Secondary to Inflammation

Torticollis may be seen in the 5- to 10-year age group following an upper respiratory tract infection or cervical lymphadenitis. A few days after the onset of the infection, a spontaneous subluxation of the atlas or a unilateral subluxation of C2 on C3 occurs. There may be a history of a minor neck injury. Typically, there is no sternocleidomastoid tightness or spasm; if any is present, it is on the long side of the neck rather than on the short side as seen in myositis and congenital muscular torticollis. Examination may reveal tenderness of the spinous process of C2 and an obvious tilting of the head. Treatment consists of cervical traction and warm, moist packs. The subluxation will usually improve and a collar is worn afterward until all symptoms subside.

An inflammatory condition sometimes referred to as "myositis" often causes tenderness of the cervical musculature. The cause is unknown, but the disorder usually follows exposure to cold air or a draft. Clinically, there is tenderness in the musculature of the cervical spine, and the head is held toward the side of the tenderness. This entity is treated with rest, moist heat, and a soft collar until symptoms subside.

Spasmodic Torticollis

Spasmodic torticollis is a term that refers to a disease entity consisting of the spontaneous onset of painful contractions of various muscles about the cervical spine including the sternocleidomastoid muscle. The cause is unknown and the disease has a gradual onset in adulthood. "Spasms" may occur in the cervical musculature, and they may be bilateral. These spasms tend to hold the head toward the affected side and are uncontrollable.

These patients have strong psychoneurotic tendencies, and there is little likelihood of spontaneous recovery. The disease is usually resistant to ordinary conservative treatment and surgical treatment is sometimes required. This consists of sectioning the spinal accessory nerves and upper cervical rhizotomies. The surgical results are only fair.

Miscellaneous Causes of Torticollis

Spinal cord tumor, neuritis of the spinal accessory nerve, cervical spine anomalies, and rheumatoid arthritis will occasionally produce torticollis. Ocular disturbances may produce the same symptoms, and any child who has gradually increasing torticollis should have a complete eye examination. Fracture or unilateral rotatory subluxation may also cause torticollis and should always be ruled out by an adequate roentgenographic examination.

BIBLIOGRAPHY

Adson, A. W., Young, H. H., and Ghormley, R. K.: Spasmodic torticollis, J. Bone Joint Surg. 28:299, 1946.

Bohlman, H. H.: Cervical spondylosis with moderate to severe myelopathy, Spine 2: 151, 1977.

Clark, E., and Robinson, P. K.: Cervical myelopathy: A complication of cervical spondylosis, Brain 79:483, 1956.

Coventry, M. B., and Harris, L. E.: Congenital muscular torticollis in infancy, J. Bone Joint Surg. 41A:815, 1959.

DePalma, A. F., and Rothman, R. H.: *The Intervertebral Disc* (Philadelphia: W. B. Saunders Co., 1970).

Eyring, E. J., Peterson, C. A., and Bjornson, D. R.: Intervertebral-disc calcification in childhood: A distinct clinical syndrome, J. Bone Joint Surg. 46A:1432, 1964.

Hohl, M.: Soft tissue injuries of the neck in automobile accidents, J. Bone Joint Surg. 56A:1675, 1974.

Robinson, R. A.: The results of anterior interbody fusion, J. Bone Joint Surg. 44A:1569, 1962.

Robinson, R. A., and Smith, G. W.: Antero-lateral cervical disc removal and interbody fusion for cervical disc syndrome, Bull. Johns Hopkins Hosp. 96:223, 1955.

Robinson, R. A., et al.: Cervical spondylotic myelopathy: Etiology and treatment concepts, Spine 2:89, 1977.

Ruge, D., and Wiltse, L. L.: *Spinal Disorders:* *Diagnosis and Treatment* (Philadelphia: Lea & Febiger, 1977).

Scoville, W. B.: Types of cervical disc lesion and their surgical approaches, J.A.M.A. 196: 105, 1966.

Sherman, W. D., et al.: Calcified cervical intervertebral discs in children, Spine 1:155, 1976.

Tachdjian, M. O.: *Pediatric Orthopedics* (Philadelphia: W. B. Saunders Co., 1972).

3 / The Cervicobrachial Region

AFFECTIONS OF THE brachial plexus are usually the result of either compression or injury. The resultant symptoms and signs are often confusing, but these disorders should always be considered in the differential diagnosis of neuropathies of the upper extremity.

ANATOMY

The brachial plexus is formed by the anterior rami of the last four cervical and first thoracic nerves (Fig 3–1). In general, the upper portion of the plexus innervates the shoulder abductors and external rotators and the elbow flexors. It also provides sensation to the shoulder and radial side of the arm. The lower portion of the plexus primarily innervates the forearm and hand muscles and provides sensation to the ulnar side of the arm, forearm, and hand. The first thoracic ramus also communicates with the first thoracic ganglion, through which sympathetic fibers are carried to the face from the spinal cord. Thus, involvement of the lower portion of the plexus by disease or injury may produce a Horner's syndrome (ptosis, miosis, enophthalmos, and anhidrosis).

The plexus passes distally between the middle and anterior scalene muscles, which attach to the first rib (Fig 3–2). Beneath the clavicle, it is joined by the subclavian artery. The subclavian vein

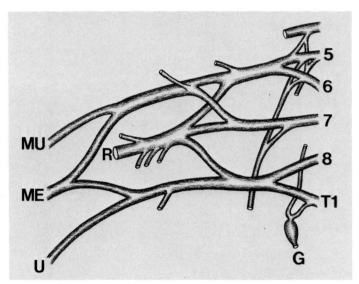

Fig 3–1.—The brachial plexus. Five rami normally combine to form three trunks, which divide to form three cords. The lower trunk (C8, T1) lies on the first rib and is most commonly involved in thoracic outlet syndromes. The posterior cord continues as the radial nerve (R). The medial cord contributes half of the median nerve and continues as the ulnar nerve (U). The lateral cord continues as the musculocutaneous (MU) nerve after contributing the other half of the median nerve (ME). G = ganglion.

20

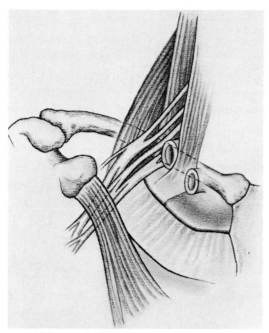

Fig 3–2.—Anatomy of the cervical brachial region. Note that the lower trunk of the brachial plexus lies on the first rib.

passes anterior to the scalenus anticus muscle. Artery, vein, and plexus then enter the axilla beneath the pectoralis minor muscle with the lower trunk of the plexus (C8, T1) lying on the first rib.

THORACIC OUTLET SYNDROMES

Thoracic outlet syndrome is a term given to four different syndromes that have in common neurovascular compression at the base of the neck. These syndromes are referred to as the cervical rib syndrome, the scalenus anticus syndrome, the costoclavicular syndrome, and the hyperabduction syndrome. These disorders all have very similar clinical features and it is often impossible to differentiate among them on this basis alone. The symptoms and signs are related to the degree of involvement of each of the various structures at the level of the first rib. Primary neural involvement may lead to pain and numbness. Arterial

involvement usually causes the extremity to feel "asleep." This symptom may have a glove type of distribution and is occasionally associated with paresis. Venous involvement may produce swelling.

Cervical Rib Syndrome

The cervical rib usually arises from the seventh cervical vertebra and is the most common cause of neurovascular compression at the base of the neck (Fig 3–3). The condition may be bilateral. The rib or its fibrous extension narrows the interval between the anterior and middle scalene muscles and produces a higher barrier that the neurovascular structures must arch over on their way into the arm. In older patients or those with muscular weakness, the shoulder may also sag more than normal, which further increases the tension on the neurovascular structures. The compression is also increased by carrying a heavy object in the hand.

The lowest components (C8, T1) of the plexus are most commonly involved be-

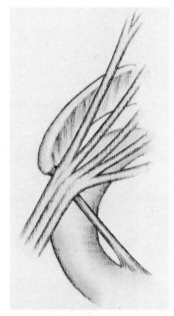

Fig 3–3.—Compression caused by a cervical rib. (Adapted from Nichols, H. M.: Clin. Orthop. 51:17–25, 1967.)

cause of their position against the rib. The symptoms therefore tend to be most noticeable in the hand and inner aspect of the forearm. Pain and paresthesias are frequently produced along the distribution of the ulnar nerve. Weakness, numbness, and clumsiness in use of the hand are common complaints. Coldness, Raynaud's phenomenon, or even gangrene may be the initial symptom.

Clinically, the cervical rib may be palpable and the brachial plexus is often tender. Weakness and atrophy of the muscles supplied by the lower trunk (interossei, hypothenar muscles) are occasionally seen. Sensation may be diminished over the ulnar aspect of the forearm, arm, and the ulnar 1½ fingers. Swelling, coldness, cyanosis, trophic skin changes, and other signs of circulatory insufficiency are occasionally observed.

Adson's test may be positive (Fig 3–4). This test takes advantage of the fact that by tensing the scalene muscles the interval between them is decreased and any existing compression is increased. The test is performed by having the patient breathe deeply, extend the neck, and turn the chin toward the affected side. When the test is positive, a decrease in the radial pulse is noted. If the test is

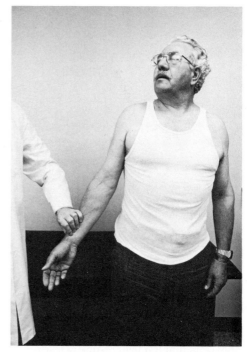

Fig 3–4. — Adson's test.

negative, it is repeated with the chin turned to the opposite side. Although a positive test is highly suggestive of compression in the interscalene region, it is sometimes positive in the normal population and is not necessarily diagnostic of

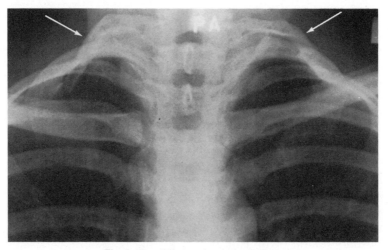

Fig 3–5. — Bilateral cervical ribs.

cervical rib or scalenus anticus syndrome.

Roentgenographic examination reveals an extra rib extending from the transverse process of the seventh cervical vertebra (Fig 3–5). The rib may be fully developed or rudimentary and it is often bilateral. Its presence does not necessarily imply that it is symptomatic, however, as it may be present in asymptomatic individuals.

Scalenus Anticus Syndrome

In the absence of a cervical rib, compression can still occur between the middle and anterior scalene muscles. This may be due to abnormal scalene muscle insertions or the presence of additional muscle slips in the interscalene interval (Fig 3–6). The clinical findings are the same as those produced by a cervical rib.

Costoclavicular Syndrome

The space between the clavicle and the first rib may be narrowed by down-

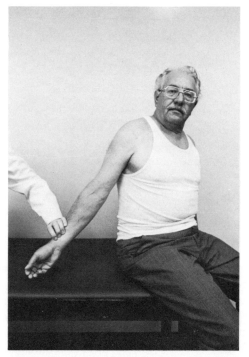

Fig 3–7.—The costoclavicular maneuver. The radial pulse may be diminished in many normal individuals.

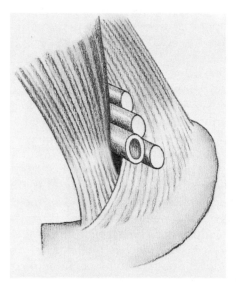

Fig 3–6.—Abnormal scalene muscle insertions that may cause compression at the cervicobrachial region. (Adapted from Telford, E. D., and Mottershead, S.: J. Bone Joint Surg. 30B:249–265, 1948.)

ward and backward pressure on the shoulders for a prolonged period of time. Abnormalities of the clavicle, such as malunion or nonunion following fracture, may contribute to the narrowing.

The syndrome is occasionally seen in individuals who are required to carry heavy packs on their shoulders. Intermittent numbness and pain in the hand and arm are the most common symptoms. They may be reproduced by the costoclavicular maneuver (Fig 3–7). In this test, the shoulders are drawn downward and backward, and any change in the radial pulse or reproduction of symptoms is noted.

Hyperabduction Syndrome

Neurovascular symptoms may also follow prolonged assumption of the position of shoulder hyperabduction. This position is often assumed during sleep and in

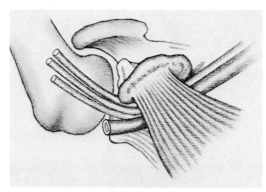

Fig 3–8.—Hyperabduction of the upper extremity that may produce neurovascular compression. (Adapted from Nichols, H. M.: Clin. Orthop. 51:17–25, 1967.)

certain occupations such as overhead painting. The neurovascular structures are compressed as they pass under the coracoid process and pectoralis minor muscle with the arm in hyperabduction (Fig 3–8). Numbness and paresthesias are common but the pain tends to be less

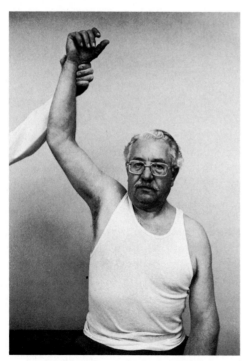

Fig 3–9.—Wright's test.

severe than that seen in the other compression syndromes. Wright's test (diminution of pulse or reproduction of symptoms on hyperabduction of the arm) may be positive (Fig 3–9).

TREATMENT

The initial treatment is conservative in all thoracic outlet syndromes except those with vascular complications. Symptomatic relief may be obtained by resting the elbow of the affected side on the arm of the chair, thereby elevating the shoulder. A sling may serve the same purpose. Physical therapy, in the form of moist heat, ultrasound, and pendulum exercises may also be helpful (chapter 4). Specific strengthening exercises for the shoulder girdle muscles are begun (Fig 3–10). Faulty posture should be corrected and positions that aggravate the condition are avoided. For the hyperabduction syndrome, avoidance of the hyperabducted position is usually the only treatment necessary. A gauze strip tied to the wrist and attached to the foot of the bed to prevent hyperabduction at night may be temporarily necessary for those patients whose symptoms occur primarily at night.

Operative treatment is considered when conservative measures fail to obtain significant relief after four to six months. Removal of the first dorsal and cervical ribs combined with release of any abnormal scalene muscle insertions is recommended for the cervical rib and scalenus anticus syndromes. First rib removal is also recommended for the costoclavicular syndrome, except when abnormalities of the clavicle are the primary causative factor. In this case, excision of the outer clavicle may be recommended. Clavicular excision, however, is cosmetically more deforming than first rib resection and is usually reserved for unusual cases. For those cases of hyper-

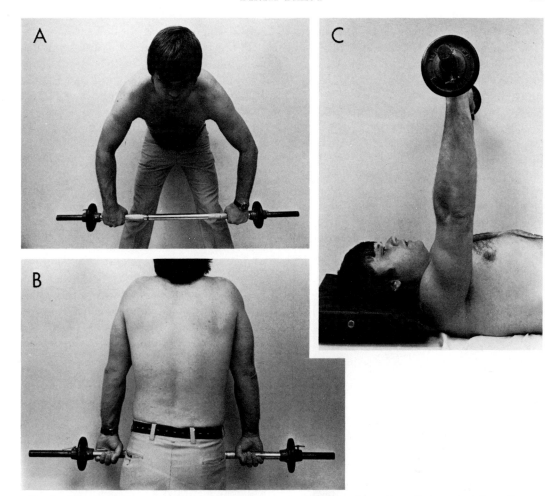

Fig 3–10.—Shoulder exercises for thoracic outlet syndrome. **A** and **B,** the trapezius is strengthened by raising and drawing the shoulders backward to bring the scapulae upward and together. **C,** to strengthen the serrati, the weight is pushed upward so that the shoulders are lifted off the table.

abduction syndrome that fail to respond to conservative treatment, first rib resection, sometimes combined with release of the pectoralis minor muscle, is usually the treatment of choice. These procedures are all combined with vascular repair when indicated.

BIRTH PALSY

Paralysis of the upper extremity at birth usually follows a difficult and prolonged delivery. The upper plexus is usually injured by lateral flexion of the neck against either a fixed head or a fixed shoulder, and the lower plexus by an injury that forces the arm upward. The damage may vary from simple stretching to complete avulsion of nerve roots.

Clinically, the involved extremity is noted to remain motionless at the side with the elbow extended. The Moro reflex is also absent on the affected side. There may be swelling above the clavicle due to hemorrhage. Tenderness to palpation is often present from a traumatic neuritis. Fractures of the clavicle or upper humerus may be present and cause a "pseudoparalysis." They should always be ruled out in cases of birth palsy. Horner's syndrome may be observed if the injury involves the thoracic root.

Recovery may occur within a few days or may take three to six months. If no recovery is seen within six months, then no further improvement can be expected. In older patients, underdevelopment of the entire upper extremity is frequently seen and the humerus is often markedly shortened. Contractures and disuse atrophy are also observed. Unawareness of the extremity, despite satisfactory motor and

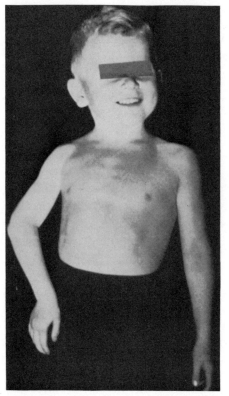

Fig 3–11.—The "waiter's-tip" position. The upper extremity is frequently shortened. (From Brashear, H. R., Jr., and Raney, R. B., Sr.: *Shands' Handbook of Orthopaedic Surgery* [9th ed.; St. Louis, C. V. Mosby Co., 1978].)

sensory recovery, may also be noted in late cases.

Three types of paralysis are seen, depending on the area of the injury: Erb-Duchenne or upper-arm paralysis, whole-arm paralysis, and Klumpke's or lower-arm paralysis.

Erb-Duchenne Paralysis

This is the most common type of obstetric paralysis. Damage to the upper roots (C5 and C6) leads to paralysis of the deltoid muscle, the external rotators of the shoulder, the elbow flexors, and the supinators of the forearm. Residual weakness of these muscles leads to the characteristic "waiter's-tip" position, in which the arm is held adducted and internally rotated, the elbow is extended, and the forearm is pronated (Fig 3–11). Wrist and finger function are usually normal.

Whole-Arm Paralysis

The limb is often completely flaccid and without motor function in this uncommon type of birth palsy. The hand tends to be dry and atrophic, and extensive sensory loss is often present.

Klumpke's Paralysis

In Klumpke's paralysis, the lower cervical and first thoracic roots are involved. This is the least common of the birth palsies. The finger and wrist flexors are denervated along with the intrinsic muscles. A clawhand deformity often results. Horner's syndrome may also be present. Sensory loss involves the affected dermatomes of the lower plexus. The upper part of the arm is frequently uninvolved.

TREATMENT AND PROGNOSIS

Treatment is designed to prevent fixed soft tissue contractures from developing so that any muscles that regain function will have a flexible joint on which to act. Gentle, repetitive, meticulous range-of-motion exercises are instituted as soon as the tenderness disappears. Intermittent pinning of the arm of the child in a position of 90° of abduction and external rotation while the infant is recumbent is sometimes combined with the range-of-motion exercises. Supportive splints for the wrist and fingers are helpful when used in conjunction with, but not instead of, a good exercise program. The "Statue of Liberty" splint or cast is not recommended as it may lead to overimmobilization and abduction contractures.

Reconstructive surgery is often beneficial for late deformities. Muscle transfers and osteotomies are utilized to restore motor function and correct malposition.

The overall prognosis for Erb's palsy is relatively good compared to Klumpke's and the whole-arm paralysis. Over 50% of upper-arm paralyses show fair to good recovery of arm function. Only about one in ten patients, however, will have complete return of normal use of the extremity.

BIBLIOGRAPHY

Brashear, H. R., Jr., and Raney, R. B., Sr.: *Shands' Handbook of Orthopaedic Surgery* (9th ed.; St. Louis: C. V. Mosby Co., 1978).

Britt, L. P.: Nonoperative treatment of thoracic outlet syndrome symptoms, Clin. Orthop. 51:45, 1967.

Eng, G. D.: Brachial plexus palsy in newborn infants, Pediatrics 48:18, 1971.

Ferguson, A. B., Jr.: *Orthopaedic Surgery in Infancy and Childhood* (3d ed.; Baltimore, Williams & Wilkins Co., 1968).

Grant, J. C. B.: *A Method of Anatomy* (6th ed.; Baltimore: Williams & Wilkins Co., 1958).

Nichols, H. M.: Anatomic structures of the thoracic outlet, Clin. Orthop. 51:17, 1967.

Tachdjian, M. O.: *Pediatric Orthopedics* (Philadelphia: W. B. Saunders Co., 1972).

Telford, E. D., and Mottershead, S.: Pressure at the cervicobrachial junction: An operative and anatomical study, J. Bone Joint Surg. 30B:249, 1948.

Wickstrom, J.: Birth injuries of the brachial plexus: Treatment of defects of the shoulder, Clin. Orthop. 23:187, 1962.

4 / The Shoulder

THE SHOULDER is a complex series of joints that provide an extraordinary range of motion. This extreme mobility is accomplished at the expense of some stability, however. This lack of stability, combined with its relatively exposed position, make it vulnerable to injury and degenerative processes.

ANATOMY

The shoulder is composed of three bones: the scapula, the clavicle, and the humerus. The scapula is a thin bone that articulates widely and closely with the posterior chest wall. It also articulates with the humerus by way of a small, shallow, glenoid cavity and with the clavicle at the acromion process. The clavicle and scapula are suspended from the cervical and thoracic vertebrae by the trapezius, levator scapulae, and rhomboid muscles.

Four articulations constitute the shoul-der joint: the glenohumeral, scapulothoracic, acromioclavicular, and sternoclavicular joints. The stability of these joints is provided by a series of ligaments and muscles (Fig 4–1).

Motion of the arm results from the coordinated efforts of several muscles. With the initiation of shoulder motion, the scapula is first stabilized. The muscles of the rotator (musculotendinous) cuff then steady the humeral head in the glenoid cavity and cause it to descend (Fig 4–2). Elevation of the arm results from a combination of scapulothoracic and glenohumeral joint movements. One third of total shoulder abduction is provided by forward and lateral movement of the scapula. The remaining two thirds occurs at the glenohumeral joint through progressively increasing activity of the deltoid and supraspinatus muscles. Thus, even in the complete absence of glenohumeral motion, scapulothoracic move-

Fig 4–1.—Bones and ligaments of the shoulder: *R* = rotator cuff; *B* = long head of the biceps; *AC* = acromioclavicular joint capsule; *CC* = coracoclavicular ligaments; *A* = acromion; *C* = coracoid process; *CA* = coracoacromial ligaments.

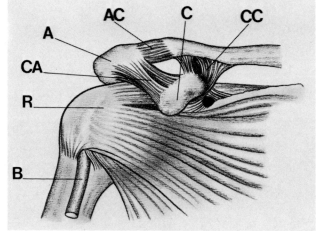

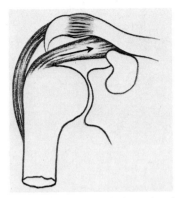

Fig 4–2.—Abduction of the shoulder. By stabilizing the humeral head in the glenoid, the superior portion of the rotator cuff prevents it from being forced into the acromion by the deltoid muscle.

ment can still abduct the arm approximately 60° to 70°.

The muscles of the rotator cuff (supraspinatus, teres minor, infraspinatus, and subscapularis) are separated from the overlying "coracoacromial arch" by two bursae, the subdeltoid and the subcoracoid (Fig 4–3). These bursae frequently communicate and are affected by lesions of the musculotendinous cuff, acromioclavicular joint, and adjacent structures.

They are frequently referred to as the subacromial bursa. Primary diseases of this bursa are rare, although secondary involvement is quite common.

EXAMINATION

The examination is performed with both shoulders widely exposed (Fig 4–4). The general contour of the shoulder is noted, as well as any atrophy or swelling. The shoulder is thoroughly palpated and any areas of tenderness are determined. These are frequently located over the acromioclavicular joint and the rotator cuff.

Active and passive ranges of motion are tested and compared with those of the opposite arm. The examiner should determine whether the scapula and humerus move together or independently. Any crepitus during the examination is also noted. Active motion is measured in abduction, forward flexion, and extension. External and internal rotation can be measured by instructing the patient to reach behind the head and then back-

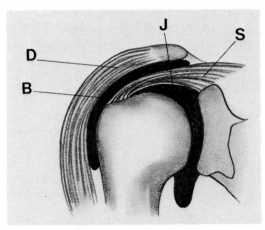

Fig 4–3.—The subacromial bursa (B) is shown between the deltoid (D) and supraspinatus (S) muscles. Deep to the rotator cuff is the glenohumeral joint cavity (J).

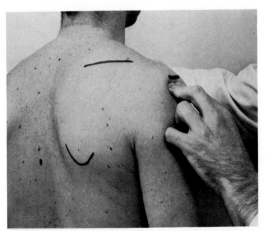

Fig 4–4.—Superficial landmarks of the shoulder. The spine of the scapula lies at the level of the third dorsal vertebra. The inferior angle lies at the level of the seventh rib and eighth dorsal vertebra. The rotator cuff is palpated just distal to the acromion process.

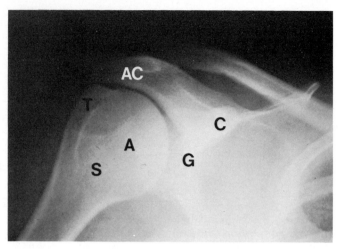

Fig 4–5. –Roentgenographic anatomy of the shoulder: *S* = surgical neck of the humerus; *A* = anatomical neck of the humerus; *T* = greater tuberosity; *C* = coracoid process; *AC* = acromion process; *G* = glenoid fossa.

ward behind the shoulder blades. Involvement of the acromioclavicular joint is tested by directing the patient to adduct the arm across the front of the chest and touch the opposite shoulder. Pain with this test suggests acromioclavicular or sternoclavicular disease. The strength of the shoulder, especially at 90° of abduction, is tested and compared to the opposite arm.

ROENTGENOGRAPHIC ANATOMY

The shoulder is routinely examined by anteroposterior views with the arm rotated externally and internally (Fig 4–5). A lateral view may be obtained by utilizing a transaxillary or transthoracic exposure.

DISORDERS OF THE ROTATOR CUFF

The tendons of the rotator cuff muscles fuse together near their insertions into the tuberosities of the humerus to form a musculotendinous cuff. With advancing age and repeated trauma, these tendons, especially the supraspinatus, undergo degeneration. This is most severe near the tendon insertion. Secondary changes, in the form of thickening and chronic inflammation, frequently develop in the overlying bursa.

A great deal of difficulty is encountered in diagnosing nonarticular soft tissue lesions of the shoulder. Tendinitis, bursitis, complete and incomplete rotator cuff ruptures, calcific deposits, and other lesions are all capable of producing similar signs and symptoms. A variety of terms have developed to describe these diseases: supraspinatus syndrome, chronic impingement syndrome, painful arc syndrome, and internal derangement of the subacromial joint. The treatment for all of these lesions tends to be similar except for complete rupture of the capsular rotator muscles, which causes loss of motor function. Surgical repair is frequently necessary for this lesion.

Chronic Strains and Tendinitis

At any age, a chronic strain of the musculotendinous unit may develop. Small tears of the rotator cuff may even be produced in the young athlete or laborer from repetitive use. Scarring and thickening of the involved area of tendon occurs with secondary irritation of the overlying bursa. Thickening of all of these tissues decreases the distance between the cuff and the overlying coracoacromial arch. Pain and crepitus may be noted when motions of the arm squeeze and pinch these tissues between the humerus and the overlying arch.

CLINICAL FEATURES

The major clinical manifestations are pain, tenderness, muscle spasm, and, occasionally, atrophy. The patient is frequently unable to lie on the affected shoulder and may feel a locking sensation with certain motions, especially abduction. The pain is often referred to the deltoid region.

Maximum tenderness is usually noted over the supraspinatus insertion as this is the most common area of involvement (Fig 4–6). The acromioclavicular joint may also be tender due to degenerative changes. There is usually little loss of muscle power. The pain and crepitus are most severe in the arc of motion between 60° and 120° of abduction. This is where the traumatized soft tissues are maximally compressed between the tuberosity and the overlying arch. The roentgenogram is usually normal, but some sclerosis may be present in the tuberosity secondary to long-standing local inflammation.

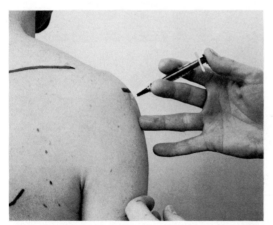

Fig 4–6.—Injection at the rotator cuff. The needle is placed at the point of maximum tenderness in the sulcus between the acromion and the humeral head.

TREATMENT

Relief of pain and restoration of function are the therapeutic goals. The most important part of the treatment program is rest. This allows the inflammatory process to subside, relieves pain, and restores function. Rest should not be complete, however, because stiffness is prone to develop in the shoulder joint, especially in the elderly patient.

Local steroid injections often relieve pain and swelling but should be used with caution, especially in the young patient; 1 to 2 ml of steroid mixed with equal amounts of lidocaine is injected, under sterile conditions, into the area of maximal tenderness, which is usually the supraspinatus tendon and acromioclavicular joint. The injection may be repeated every seven to ten days for one month. Aspirin and other anti-inflammatory drugs are often beneficial. Physical therapy in the form of diathermy or ultrasound is also helpful.

Function is restored by an exercise program directed at preserving muscle tone and preventing stiffness (Fig 4–7). Pendulum exercises are begun early but are performed only within the limits of pain. As pain subsides, the exercises are increased and further range-of-motion exercises are added. Swimming is an excellent means of restoring shoulder strength and motion. Work habits and other activities that cause compression and pinching of the inflamed tissue should be avoided. A sling may be worn initially between the exercises in order to rest the shoulder, but it is gradually discontinued as the exercises are increased.

Improvement is usually seen within three to five weeks. If it is not, a more serious cuff lesion such as a rupture should be suspected. Surgery is reserved for those cases that fail to respond to conservative treatment, and it consists of partial

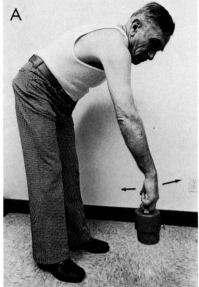

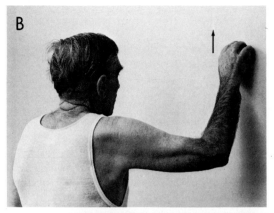

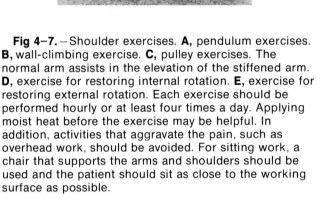

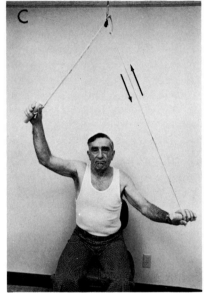

Fig 4–7.—Shoulder exercises. **A,** pendulum exercises. **B,** wall-climbing exercise. **C,** pulley exercises. The normal arm assists in the elevation of the stiffened arm. **D,** exercise for restoring internal rotation. **E,** exercise for restoring external rotation. Each exercise should be performed hourly or at least four times a day. Applying moist heat before the exercise may be helpful. In addition, activities that aggravate the pain, such as overhead work, should be avoided. For sitting work, a chair that supports the arms and shoulders should be used and the patient should sit as close to the working surface as possible.

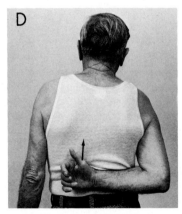

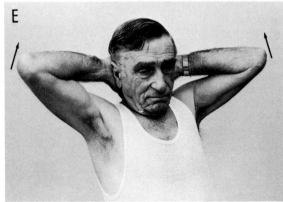

excision of the acromion, release of obstructing soft tissue, and repair of any rotator cuff tears.

Ruptures of the Rotator Cuff

Ruptures of the rotator cuff result from continued deterioration and degeneration (Fig 4–8). The tear may be partial or complete. Ruptures are uncommon before the age of 40, but may occur in the young athlete secondary to a sudden forceful motion of the shoulder.

CLINICAL FEATURES

A history is frequently obtained of a fall on the outstretched hand or an attempt at lifting a heavy object. A snap may be felt in the shoulder, and acute pain begins immediately after the injury. The pain may become progressively worse for the next few hours and the patient will note an inability to abduct or flex the shoulder, depending on the area of the tear. The pain is often referred down the deltoid muscle.

If the rupture is partial, the clinical findings are similar to those seen in chronic tendinitis. Even with complete rupture, the shoulder may have a full range of motion because of continued function of the other rotator muscles. Usually, however, with both partial and complete ruptures, there is significant weakness in abduction or flexion. The weakness is usually most severe in abduction because the muscle most commonly torn is the supraspinatus. If the tear is more anterior into the subscapularis, forward flexion will be weak. It may be impossible to actively abduct the arm more than 45° to 50°, after which further abduction is obtained by scapulothoracic motion. A painful "catch" may be noted on passive motion between 50° and 100° where compression of the swollen tissues between the tuberosity and the overlying arch occurs. Tenderness at the site of the tear is a common finding, and with complete ruptures a defect in the cuff may be palpated through the deltoid muscle. Passive range of motion is frequently normal in the pain-free shoulder.

Atrophy of the cuff muscles is frequently present and the "drop-arm" test may be positive. In this test, the arm is passively abducted to 90° and then released. If abduction is able to be maintained, slight downward pressure is applied to the forearm, and the strength of the affected shoulder is compared to the nor-

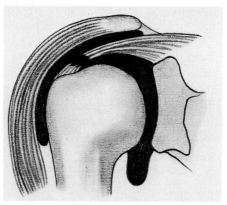

Fig 4–8.—Rupture of the rotator cuff.

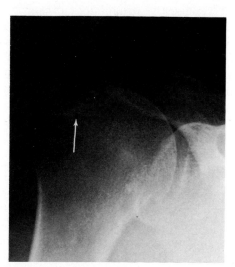

Fig 4–9.—Cystic changes and sclerosis frequently occur in the humeral head in chronic rotator cuff disorders.

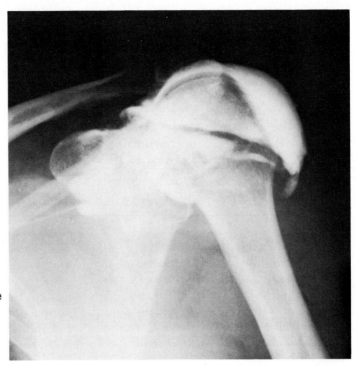

Fig 4–10. — Arthrogram of the shoulder revealing dye leakage through the rotator cuff into the subacromial bursa, indicating a complete rupture.

mal shoulder. If pain is severe during the examination, it can be relieved by lidocaine infiltration of the tender area and the strength measured again. Inability to maintain shoulder abduction with this test is suggestive of a rotator cuff tear.

Roentgenographic examination may reveal chronic changes in the tuberosity of the humerus (Fig 4–9). Degenerative changes may also be present in the acromioclavicular joint. Arthrography of the shoulder will help distinguish between complete and incomplete tears (Fig 4–10).

TREATMENT

Partial tears usually respond well to the conservative treatment program outlined for chronic tendinitis. Occasionally, it is necessary to surgically repair the rupture and remove any impinging structures beneath the coracoacromial arch.

Complete tears should also be repaired if they are sufficiently disabling. If retraction of the muscle is not severe, the re-sults are usually good. Frequently, however, there is very little loss of function and minimal pain. In these patients, especially if they are relatively inactive, operative intervention is probably not justified.

Calcific Deposits in the Rotator Cuff

Calcium deposits in the rotator cuff tendon are frequent causes of pain and stiffness in the shoulder. These deposits result from degenerative changes in the same area where ruptures take place and are most frequently found in the supraspinatus tendon. Many of them remain small and deep in the tendon and, consequently, do not irritate the overlying bursa. Others slowly increase in size until they contact the bursa and produce an inflammatory reaction and swelling of the bursa. Impingement of these swollen tissues on the overlying coracoacromial arch may increase the inflammation and pain. Intermittent mechanical locking of the shoulder may even occur.

CLINICAL FEATURES

The onset of symptoms may be gradual or acute. The pain is characteristically severe and accentuated by the slightest motion. Night pain and an inability to sleep on the shoulder are common complaints. The pain may radiate to the deltoid and even down the arm and forearm. It may subside suddenly when the milky deposit ruptures into the overlying bursa.

Examination in the acute stage reveals markedly limited motion and exquisite tenderness over the bursa and calcific deposit. There may be pronounced spasm of the rotator cuff muscles.

The symptoms and signs in chronic cases are less pronounced. Shoulder motion is frequently normal and muscle spasm is absent. Symptoms of intermittent impingement and tenderness of the rotator cuff are usually present, however.

Roentgenographic examination in internal and external rotation will usually reveal the deposit (Fig 4–11). If the deposit is anterior in the subscapularis muscle or posterior, a transaxillary view may be necessary to demonstrate it.

TREATMENT

The treatment is directed at relief of the inflammation and tension under the bursa from the swollen calcific mass. An injection of 2 ml of steroid mixed with equal amounts of lidocaine will often give dramatic relief. If the deposit appears soft, fluffy, and irregular on roentgenographic examination, aspiration and needling of the deposit may also be indicated. If the deposit is dense, round, and well circumscribed, however, this procedure is less helpful.

Aspiration and needling are performed with the patient under local anesthesia. An 18-gauge needle is partially filled with lidocaine or saline and inserted directly into the deposit. Multiple areas are then injected and aspirated. A fine, flaky

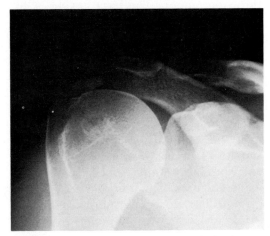

Fig 4–11. – Large calcific deposit in the rotator cuff.

material may be withdrawn. The aspiration and needling are repeated over several areas until all accessible material is withdrawn. A second large needle placed in the calcific mass can be used for aspiration while the first needle is used for injection. At the end of the procedure, 2 ml of steroid is left in the bursa.

Analgesics and sedatives are given as necessary. Continuous warm, moist packs are applied to the shoulder. Diathermy and ultrasound may also be beneficial. The arm is allowed to hang in a sling until the acute pain subsides, and pendulum exercises are then initiated within the limits of pain. Motion progresses as tolerated.

Surgical excision of the calcific deposit is reserved for cases that fail to respond to conservative treatment. The results are usually excellent.

DISORDERS OF THE BICEPS TENDON

Tenosynovitis

Tenosynovitis of the long head of the biceps is a common cause of shoulder pain in adults over 40. It may also occur in the young athlete from repeated strains, such as those caused by the throwing motion. The basic lesion is an inflammation in the tendon and its sheath in the bicipital groove. The disorder may be primary or secondary to disease of the overlying rotator cuff.

CLINICAL FEATURES

The most common symptom is pain over the anterolateral aspect of the shoulder that may be referred down the anterior aspect of the arm. Muscle spasm and limitation of motion are frequently present. The most constant physical finding is tenderness to palpation over the bicipital groove. Active and passive shoulder motions are often restricted because of pain. Maneuvers that stretch the biceps tendon or cause it to glide in the groove may reproduce the pain. Forceful external rotation with abduction or backward flexion of the extremity is often painful. Supination against resistance with the elbow flexed is also frequently uncomfortable (Fig 4–12). The roentgenograms are usually normal.

TREATMENT

In the acute stage, the treatment consists of rest, moist heat, and gentle range-of-motion exercises. All motions that stretch the biceps tendon should be

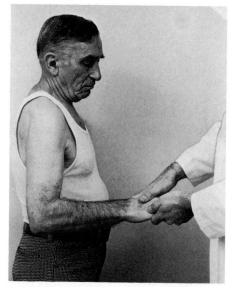

Fig 4–12.—Yergason's test. The forearm is supinated against resistance. Pain in the region of the bicipital groove is suggestive of bicipital tenosynovitis.

avoided. A sling may be used temporarily. Local steroid injections into the tendon sheath are frequently beneficial, and anti-inflammatory drugs are given as necessary.

The majority of cases respond well to conservative treatment. Surgery is recommended for those cases that fail to improve. Anchoring the tendon in the

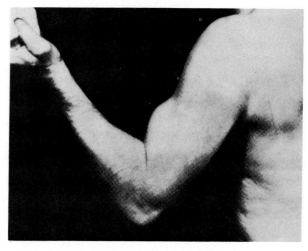

Fig 4–13.—Rupture of the long head of the biceps. A localized bulge is present in the arm. (From DePalma, A. F.: *Surgery of the Shoulder* [2nd ed.; Philadelphia: J. B. Lippincott Co., 1973].)

bicipital groove to prevent its motion will relieve the pain. The results are usually excellent.

Rupture of the Biceps Tendon

The biceps tendon may rupture as a result of advanced degeneration from chronic tendinitis. The rupture is usually complete and may follow a forceful contraction of the biceps muscle.

CLINICAL FEATURES

The onset is usually sudden. A sharp snap may be felt by the patient, followed by pain and weakness of the arm. The diagnosis is easily made by the observation of an abnormally large mass in the arm that represents the retracted muscle belly of the long head of the biceps (Fig 4–13). There may be some loss of elbow flexion power.

TREATMENT

No treatment is necessary in many cases. There is only minimal loss of function and usually little pain associated with this condition. In the young patient, however, surgical repair of the rupture is often indicated.

Subluxing Biceps Tendon

The biceps tendon may occasionally dislocate from the bicipital groove. The usual cause is a tear in the overlying subscapularis tendon as the result of degenerative changes, but the condition may result from a congenitally shallow groove. The disorder may also occur in the young patient on forceful external rotation and abduction of the shoulder. Recurrences are frequent and may be reproducible by the patient (Fig 4–14). Tenosynovitis frequently develops, which leads to pain and stiffness.

The only cure for this lesion is anchor-

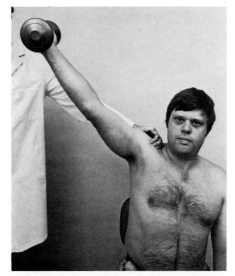

Fig 4–14. — Test for subluxing biceps tendon. With a weight in the hand, the arm is elevated and externally rotated. As the arm is slowly abducted from this position, a snap may be heard or felt in the bicipital groove.

ing the tendon in the bicipital groove surgically. The results are uniformly good.

FROZEN SHOULDER (ADHESIVE CAPSULITIS)

Frozen shoulder is a disorder characterized by the insidious onset of pain and restriction of motion. The disease tends to be chronic, and full recovery may take several months. The cause is unknown but bicipital tenosynovitis, rotator cuff tendinitis, and reflex sympathetic dystrophy have all been blamed.

CLINICAL FEATURES

The onset is usually gradual and begins in the fifth decade. The disorder frequently develops during a period of inactivity in the use of the extremity or following a relatively minor injury to the shoulder. Pain is a constant symptom but frequently does not occur until much of the shoulder motion has already been lost. It is usually well localized in the region of the rotator cuff and may radiate down the deltoid and anterior arm. It frequently interferes with sleep, especially when the patient attempts to lie on the affected shoulder.

Examination reveals an apprehensive patient who holds the arm protectively at the side. Spasm of the scapular muscles and trapezius is often present and varying degrees of deltoid and spinati atrophy may be noted. Generalized tenderness is present around the rotator cuff and biceps tendon. Shoulder motion is usually restricted to varying degrees, depending on the stage of the disease. The signs of reflex sympathetic dystrophy are often present in the involved extremity (edema of the hand, coolness, and discoloration).

The course of the disease is variable. Some patients recover relatively early in the disorder, but in many cases the condition is progressive over several months. In these patients, shoulder motion gradually decreases and the pain subsides. As soon as the pain diminishes, the shoulder begins to regain its motion. Recovery is slow, and complete recovery in less than six months is rare. Most patients will eventually regain full motion of their shoulder, however.

TREATMENT

The most important facet of treatment is prevention. Every attempt should be made to maintain motion in the shoulder during those periods of time when the patient may be inactive due to disease or injury. Once the disease process has begun, treatment is directed at the relief of pain. Bed rest, moist heat, sedation, and analgesics are prescribed as necessary. A local injection of a steroid/lidocaine mixture into the rotator cuff may also prove beneficial. Pendulum and overhead pulley exercises are begun as soon as possible.

Most patients will eventually respond to a well-supervised program of physical therapy. Those patients who fail to respond may benefit from careful manipulation of the shoulder under general anesthesia followed by aggressive range-of-motion exercises. Repeated cervical sympathetic blocks may also be indicated in those patients who have a significant sympathetic component to their symptoms. Surgical intervention is rarely necessary.

SNAPPING SCAPULA

Snapping scapula is an uncommon disorder in which an audible grating sound occurs with motion of the scapulothoracic joint. Normally, the serratus anterior and subscapularis muscles cushion the scapula from the underlying rib cage. The scapula is poorly protected at its medial border and at its superior and inferior angles, however. Abnormal angulations at these locations may cause pain and snapping sensations. Tumors of the scapula or ribs, bursae between these bones, and poor posture with sagging of the shoulder joint are other causes of crepitus in this area.

CLINICAL FEATURES

The onset is usually gradual, but the process is frequently precipitated by a traumatic event. The snapping is often palpable and painful. The origin of these noises can frequently be well localized by the patient to a specific area in the scapulothoracic articulation.

Roentgenograms of the scapula, including oblique views, are obtained to discover such lesions as exostoses and tumors when they are present.

TREATMENT

If the roentgenograms are normal, physical therapy, rest, and local steroid injections will often relieve the pain.

Correction of poor posture is also frequently beneficial. If the snapping is secondary to tumor or exostosis, and the pain and disability are sufficient to justify surgery, the involved area of the scapula is removed surgically.

GLENOHUMERAL DISLOCATION

Dislocations of the shoulder are most commonly anterior in location and usually result from a fall on the externally rotated, abducted arm (Fig 4–15). This force levers the humerus out of the glenoid cavity into its anterior position.

CLINICAL FEATURES

The diagnosis is usually not difficult. Clinically, the acromion is much more prominent than normal and there is absence of the normal fullness of the humeral head beneath the deltoid and acromion process. The humeral head may be palpated anteriorly deep to the pectoral muscles. Little motion of the shoulder is possible without severe pain. The integrity of the neurovascular structures of the arm should always be assessed.

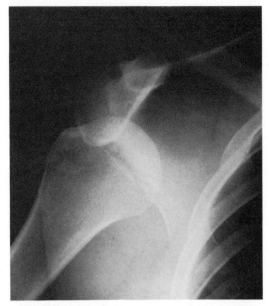

Fig 4–15.—Anterior dislocation of the shoulder.

TREATMENT AND PROGNOSIS

Shoulder dislocations are frequently reducible without general anesthesia if good muscular relaxation can be obtained. Gentle, straight traction on the arm is usually sufficient (Fig 4–16). If

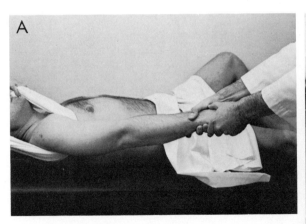
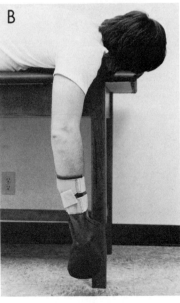

Fig 4–16.—Reduction of shoulder dislocation. **A,** straight traction is applied to the wrist with countertraction to the axilla. **B,** Stimson's method.

straight traction does not reduce the dislocation, Stimson's method may be used. The patient is placed in a prone position with the affected arm hanging over the side of the table. A 4.5- to 6.75-kg weight is tied to the wrist for traction. As the shoulder muscles relax, spontaneous reduction frequently occurs. If the shoulder remains dislocated, reduction with the patient under a general anesthetic is usually necessary. Open reduction is rarely required.

Primary dislocations in patients under the age of 30 have a high rate of recurrence. These recurrences frequently take place with little or no trauma and often can be reduced by the patient. In order to prevent recurrences and allow for proper healing of the anterior shoulder joint capsule after the initial injury, strict immobilization for four weeks is necessary in the acute dislocation. A shoulder immobilizer is satisfactory treatment, but the patient must not be allowed to externally rotate the arm (Fig 4–17). Recurrent dis-

locations usually require corrective surgery. The most common procedures used are those that restrict external rotation or reinforce the anterior shoulder joint capsule.

Primary dislocations in patients over the age of 40 are not complicated by recurrence but frequently result in shoulder joint stiffness. In this age group, light immobilization in a sling for one to two weeks is all the treatment that is necessary, and active motion is then encouraged in order to prevent stiffness.

ACROMIOCLAVICULAR DISLOCATION

Acromioclavicular dislocations and separations occur as the result of a fall on the shoulder or from a direct blow to the top of the shoulder. They are classified as complete or incomplete. A complete dislocation is present when both the acromioclavicular and coracoclavicular liga-

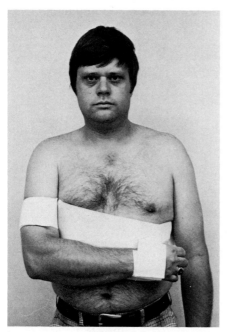

Fig 4–17.—Shoulder immobilizer.

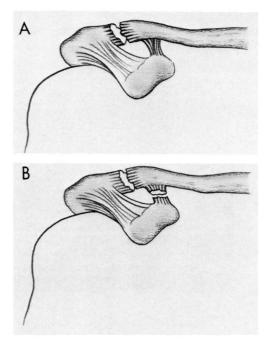

Fig 4–18.—**A,** incomplete dislocation of the acromioclavicular joint. The coracoclavicular ligaments are intact. **B,** complete dislocation.

ments are disrupted (Fig 4–18). Incomplete separations are those in which only the acromioclavicular joint ligaments are disrupted.

CLINICAL FEATURES

These injuries are characterized by tenderness and swelling over the acromioclavicular joint. The outer clavicle is usually elevated in both complete and incomplete dislocations (Fig 4–19). Downward traction on the arm may increase the deformity.

Complete dislocations may be differentiated from incomplete dislocations by an anteroposterior roentgenogram with a 9-kg weight hanging from both arms. If complete rupture of the coracoclavicular ligaments has occurred, widening between the coracoid process and the clavicle will be present on the affected side (Fig 4–20).

TREATMENT

Reduction of the incomplete separation by manual pressure is usually easy but maintenance of the reduction is frequently difficult. Strapping between the elbow and clavicle may maintain the reduction, but usually no treatment is necessary for these injuries. A sling is used for a few days to minimize the pain, and active shoulder motion is begun as tolerated. The outer end of the clavicle may remain prominent, but this is usually painless and does not interfere with function. If it does, the tip of the clavicle may be surgically removed at a later date. Complete acromioclavicular dislocations usually require surgical intervention with reduction of the dislocation and repair of the ruptured ligaments.

STERNOCLAVICULAR DISLOCATION

Sternoclavicular dislocations are uncommon injuries that occur as the result of a fall on the shoulder. The anterior dislocation is more common. The rare posterior dislocation may cause pressure on the anterior structures of the neck, leading to dyspnea and vascular compression that may require immediate reduction.

The injury usually produces a tender, visible prominence at the sternoclavicular joint. Some discomfort with shoulder motion is usually present.

Anterior dislocations are reduced by traction and manipulation, but the reduction is frequently difficult to maintain. Recurrence after the reduction is common, but, except for minor cosmetic deformity, no function is lost. Surgical intervention, therefore, is rarely justified in the acute case. If posttraumatic arthritis occurs, surgical excision of the medial 1 to 2 cm of clavicle will usually relieve the symptoms.

SHOULDER PAIN

In previous portions of this chapter, the musculoskeletal causes of shoulder pain have been described. Since shoulder pain is not only frequent but also is often due to diverse mechanisms and to referral pain, this subject deserves special attention. Numerous authors have stated in the past that shoulder pain may be referred to the shoulder via the phrenic

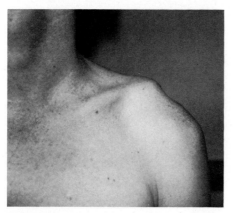

Fig 4–19.—Clinical deformity with acromioclavicular dislocation.

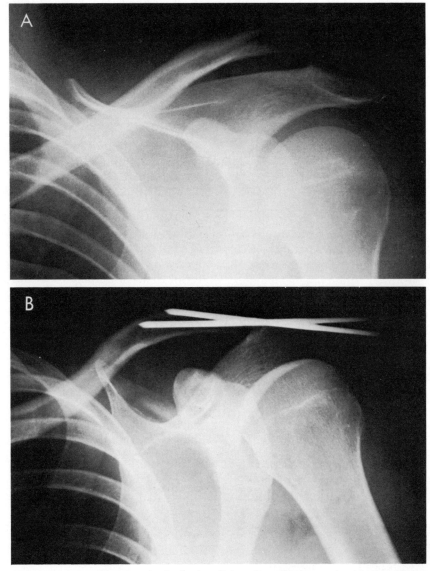

Fig 4–20. — **A,** complete acromioclavicular dislocation. **B,** the postoperative appearance. The pins are removed in seven to eight weeks.

nerve, and it is well documented in anatomical texts that the phrenic nerve contains afferent as well as efferent nerve fibers. The physician must be constantly aware of the importance of recognizing that shoulder pain may be referred from areas of disease that have their origin in cervical, intrathoracic, or diaphragmatic areas. The primary concern of this portion of the chapter is with a group of disorders that represent referral pain to the shoulder and that the physician must be able to extract from the history of his patient.

The diagnosis may be obvious insofar as the patient may have a history of carcinoma and now is seen with bone pain localized in the shoulder area. The diagnostic workup should be limited in this case, as metastatic disease with a probable lytic bone lesion would be the most likely diagnosis. However, pain on top of the shoulder may be the only signal with a liver abscess, which is threatening to perforate the diaphragm. Referral pain may be to any particular area of the shoulder, but it is most commonly pain on top of the shoulder, in the supraspinous fossa, over the acromion, or over the clavicle, that is in the region of distribution of the cutaneous branches of the fourth cervical nerve.

When a gastric ulcer perforates, the escaping fluid may indeed impinge on the lower surface of the diaphragm. This in turn irritates the terminations of the phrenic nerve on one or both sides, and can be the cause of pain on top of one or both shoulders. Pain, therefore, can be referred to the shoulder in cases of subphrenic abscess, diaphragmatic pleurisy, acute pancreatitis, gallstones, ruptured spleen, and in some cases of appendicitis with peritonitis and of pelvic inflammatory disease with perihepatic inflammation, so-called Fitz-Hugh-Curtis syndrome. As was previously mentioned, the pain is felt either in the supraspinous fossa, over the acromion or clavicle, or in the subclavicular fossa. There is good anatomical evidence to support the nerve distribution over the diaphragm and over the acromioclavicular region, so that lesions affecting a certain portion of the diaphragm may cause pain over the corresponding part of the shoulder area on the same side of the body. In general, pain on top of both shoulders indicates a median diaphragmatic irritation. The physician must be extremely careful not to be trapped by the patient's description of the shoulder pain as "arthritis." Cope (1963) well describes in his text that when the diaphragm is irritated by a neighboring lesion, as blood from a ruptured spleen, tenderness may be elicited by pressure on the corresponding phrenic nerve in the neck.

As was previously mentioned, perforation of the gastric duodenal or intestinal ulcer may indeed refer pain to the top of the right shoulder. However, if the pain is felt on both shoulders at the onset of the attack, it suggests that the perforation has occurred in the anterior portion of the stomach, causing irritation on the median portion of the diaphragm. In the cases of pyloric duodenal ulcer, the shoulder pain is usually felt in the right supraspinous fossa, or on the corresponding side.

It is extremely important in the initial evaluation of a patient who has had serious abdominal injury for the physician to ask about shoulder pain. Injury to solid viscera, such as the liver, spleen, pancreas, or kidney, usually causes some type of hemorrhage. Since the hemorrhagic material may cause irritation of the diaphragm, the significance of pain on top of the shoulder is paramount.

There may, of course, be intrathoracic causes of shoulder pain, which must be sought out by the physician if the history is consistent. A 45-year-old man with a history of heavy smoking who is admitted with shoulder pain must indeed be thought of as having either Pancoast's syndrome or bronchogenic carcinoma with metastasis to the bony shoulder. Neoplasms at the extreme apex of the lung may invade contiguous structures, producing Pancoast's syndrome. In this condition, pain is the most common initial complaint by the patient. The pain is usually felt in the shoulder on the involved side, and may also be present in the scapular or infrascapular area, upper anterior part of the chest, arm, neck, and axilla. Other components of this well-known syndrome include Horner's syndrome, muscle weakness of the upper extremities on the involved side, and sensory disturbances also in the upper extremities. The pain is explained by the neoplastic involvement of the pleura, ribs, spinal column, and brachial plexus.

One may also see shoulder pain as the result of disease present in areas distant from the shoulder that are not intrathoracic or diaphragmatic. The woman who is admitted with a history of carcinoma of the breast and previous therapy, which may have included a mastectomy, and who has shoulder pain, surely must be thought to have a lytic lesion in the shoulder area until proved otherwise. The patient who has had a previous history of cervical or degenerative osteoarthritis, or who has sustained a significant injury causing an acute cervical disc syndrome, can indeed have shoulder pain referral. The physical findings may also include muscle spasm, some subjective and/or objective muscle weakness, and straightening or loss of the cervical curve.

Of course, distant metastasis from other areas is also not uncommon, although bone pain resulting from osseous metastasis is especially common to the ribs, spinal column, and pelvis. Those carcinomas or neoplasms that have a propensity to produce osseous metastasis include lung, breast, medullary thyroid carcinoma, prostatic carcinoma, and Hodgkin's disease. The physician must be extremely suspicious of any middle-aged or elderly person who is seen with a fracture involving the area of the shoulder with a history of minimal or no trauma. One must also mention Paget's disease as a cause of localized bone pain. Lesions in the upper extremities in Paget's disease may appear as nerve palsy syndromes. However, since osteogenic sarcoma in adults most often arises in pagetic lesions, the patient may indeed be seen with persistent pain because of the sarcomatous elevation of the periosteum. Since many patients with Paget's disease are totally asymptomatic during the course of their disease, the onset of localized pain by these patients in the extrem-

ities, including the shoulder, would suggest the sarcomatous change that may have taken place.

Reflex neurovascular dystrophy, or so-called shoulder-hand syndrome, is a very poorly understood disorder in terms of cause. The patient has pain and stiffness in the shoulder and, together with the pain, swelling and vasomotor phenomena may occur within the hand on the involved side. This syndrome can only be presumed to be caused by reflex sympathetic stimulation analogous to that proposed for so-called causalgia. These patients in general are usually above the age of 50, and often have had an associated acute illness prior to the onset of this particular syndrome. Some of the more common preceding events include acute myocardial infarction, trauma to the distal upper extremity, cerebrovascular accident, or pulmonary disease. These patients all show a marked variability in the intensity of the pain, duration of the acute symptoms, and the extent, if any, of dystrophic change. A variant or frequent complication is a frozen shoulder, and this is probably due to the dystrophic changes that may occur.

There is no specific therapy for this syndrome. Aggressive physical therapy, including an active exercise program, which is facilitated by analgesic medication, should be instituted at the onset of the syndrome. If the pain becomes refractory and impedes the patient's ability to perform the physical therapy, a trial of corticosteroids is indicated. Generally, prednisone or one of its equivalents is used in relatively small doses of 10 to 20 mg/day. If the patient continues to have pain in spite of the physical therapy, analgesics, and the use of corticosteroid therapy, one might employ the stellate ganglion block.

Although most causes of shoulder pain are musculoskeletal in origin, it behooves the physician to obtain again a thorough history from his patient in order to be able to fully evaluate the other possible causes of referral shoulder pain. The physician must constantly be aware of the possibility of complications of even infectious disease as being a cause of referral shoulder pain. A good example of this is the young patient who has a one- to two-week history of severe sore throat, chills, fevers, myalgias, and who has been previously unsuccessfully treated with penicillin. The onset in this patient of abdominal pain, and also left-sided shoulder pain, surely must suggest to the physician the diagnosis of infectious mononucleosis with spontaneous splenic rupture. The physician must indeed maintain a high index of suspicion for all causes of shoulder pain in order to accurately diagnose and treat his patient's condition.

BIBLIOGRAPHY

Bateman, J. E.: The diagnosis and treatment of ruptures of the rotator cuff, Surg. Clin. North Am. 43:1523, 1963.

Bush, L. H.: The torn shoulder capsule, J. Bone Joint Surg. 57A:256, 1975.

Cope, Z.: *The Early Diagnosis of the Acute Abdomen* (12th ed.; Oxford, England: Oxford University Press, 1963).

DeDeuxchaisnes, C. N., and Krone, S. M.: Paget's disease of bone: Clinical and metabolic observation, Medicine 43:233, 1964.

DePalma, A. F.: *Surgery of the Shoulder* (2d ed.; Philadelphia: J. B. Lippincott Co., 1973).

Grant, J. C. B.: *A Method of Anatomy* (6th ed.; Baltimore: Williams & Wilkins Co., 1958).

Hammond, G.: Complete acromionectomy in the treatment of chronic tendinitis of the shoulder, J. Bone Joint Surg. 53A:173, 1971.

Kessel, L., and Watson, M.: The painful arc syndrome: Clinical classification as a guide to management, J. Bone Joint Surg. 59B: 166, 1977.

Kozin, F., et al.: The reflex sympathetic dystrophy syndrome: I. Clinical and histologic studies: Evidence for bilaterality, response to corticosteroids, and articular involvement, Am. J. Med. 60:321, 1976.

McLaughlin, H. L.: The "frozen" shoulder, Clin. Orthop. 20:126, 1961.

Moseley, H. F.: *Ruptures of the Rotator Cuff* (Springfield, Ill.: Charles C Thomas, Publisher, 1952).

Neer, C. S.: Anterior acromioplasty for the chronic impingement syndrome in the shoulder, J. Bone Joint Surg. 54A:41, 1972.

Parsons, T. A.: The snapping scapula and subscapular exostosis, J. Bone Joint Surg. 55B: 345, 1973.

Quigley, T. B.: The nonoperative treatment of symptomatic calcareous deposits in the shoulder, Surg. Clin. North Am. 43:1495, 1963.

Steinbrocher, O.: The Painful Shoulder, in Hollander, J. L., and McCarty, D. J., Jr. (eds.): *Arthritis and Allied Conditions* (8th ed.; Philadelphia: Lea & Febiger, 1972).

5 / The Elbow

THE ELBOW is a strong, hinge joint that allows flexion and rotation of the forearm. It also provides the bony origin for most of the extrinsic muscles of the wrist and hand. It is frequently affected by inflammatory and traumatic conditions that seriously alter its function.

ANATOMY

The elbow joint is formed by the articulation between the humerus and the radius and ulna (Fig 5–1). The humerus widens distally to form the lateral and medial condyles. The capitellum of the lateral condyle articulates with the radial head and the trochlea articulates with the ulna. The head of the radius also articulates with the lateral ulna and is held in position by the orbicular ligament. Medi-

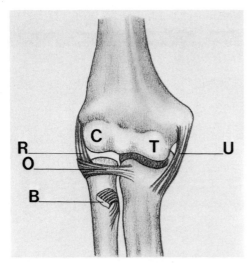

Fig 5–1.—Bony and ligamentous anatomy of the elbow: *R* = radial collateral ligament; *O* = orbicular ligament; *B* = biceps insertion; *U* = ulnar collateral ligament; *C* = capitellum; *T* = trochlea.

al and lateral collateral ligaments provide additional stability.

Adjacent to each condyle are the epicondyles, which are the bony attachments for many forearm muscles. The flexor-pronator muscle group takes its origin from a common tendon that attaches to the medial epicondyle, and the extensor-supinator group arises in a similar manner from the lateral epicondyle. Posteriorly, the triceps attaches to the olecranon; anteriorly, the biceps and brachialis attach to the radius and ulna, respectively.

Three major nerves cross the elbow joint on their way into the forearm. The median nerve passes deep in the antecubital fossa medial to the biceps and brachialis, and the radial nerve passes lateral to them. The ulnar nerve reaches the forearm by coursing posteriorly in a groove between the medial epicondyle and the olecranon process, where it is easily palpated. It is also vulnerable to injury in this superficial location.

EXAMINATION

The tip of the olecranon process and the epicondyles form useful bony landmarks (Fig 5–2). When the elbow is fully extended and viewed from behind, these points form a straight, transverse line. With the elbow flexed, they form an isosceles triangle. Just distal to the lateral epicondyle lies the radial head. These two points, along with the olecranon process, form another triangle on the posterolateral aspect of the joint. This triangle is occupied by the anconeus muscle. This area usually bulges when the joint is

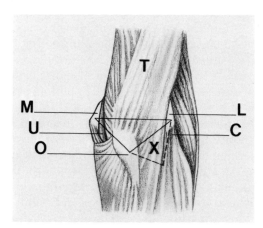

Fig 5–2.—The flexed elbow from behind: *T* = triceps; *M* = medial epicondyle; *U* = ulnar nerve; *L* = lateral epicondyle; *C* = common extensor tendon; *X* = the posterolateral triangle. The isoceles triangle between the epicondyles and the olecranon *(O)* is altered in most fractures and dislocations of the elbow except the supracondylar fracture, where all three points move together.

distended by fluid and is an excellent site for joint aspiration.

With the forearm in the supinated position, an angle is formed with the arm at the elbow joint. This is referred to as the "carrying angle" and normally measures 15° to 20° (Fig 5–3). Alterations in this angle may occur following injury or infection, especially in the young, and may lead to cubitus valgus or varus.

ROENTGENOGRAPHIC ANATOMY

The roentgenographic features of the elbow are well visualized by standard anteroposterior and 90° flexion lateral views (Fig 5–4). Comparison views of the opposite elbow should be obtained whenever necessary.

TENNIS ELBOW

Tennis elbow, or epicondylitis, is one of a large group of musculoskeletal disorders commonly termed "overuse syndromes." It is an inflammatory condition

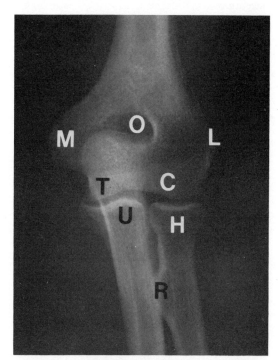

Fig 5–4.—Roentgenographic anatomy of the elbow: *M* = medial epicondyle; *O* = olecranon fossa; *L* = lateral epicondyle; *T* = trochlea; *C* = capitellum; *U* = coronoid process of the ulna; *H* = radial head; *R* = radial tuberosity. Regardless of the position of the elbow, the long axis of the radius always passes through the capitellum.

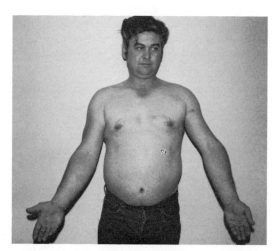

Fig 5–3.—Gunstock deformity (cubitus varus) of the left elbow with reversal of the carrying angle due to an old fracture with malunion.

characterized by pain at the origin of the flexor muscles at the medial epicondyle or the extensor muscles at the lateral epicondyle. The cause is unknown, but minor tears in the tendinous attachments of these muscles are often present. The disorder is common in those individuals whose activities require repeated use of the extensor or flexor mechanism of the forearm. The lateral side is more commonly involved.

CLINICAL FEATURES

The onset is usually gradual. A dull ache appears over the affected epicondyle that is worsened with use of the involved muscles. Activities that require rotation and grasping, such as opening a jar, increase the pain. The pain often radiates into the forearm. Extension or flexion of the hand against resistance will reproduce the pain at the affected epicondyle. The point of maximum tenderness can usually be well localized by digital pressure applied to the epicondyle. The roentgenograms are usually normal.

TREATMENT

The treatment is similar to that for other "musculotendinous overuse syndromes."

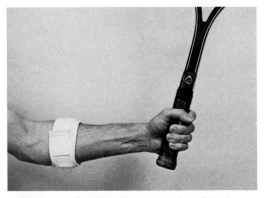

Fig 5–5. — Tennis-elbow dressing. The dressing should be applied approximately 2.5 cm below the epicondyle and fit snug enough to partially relieve the strain on the affected muscles.

The most important aspect of treatment is rest, and this can frequently be obtained merely by avoiding the offending activity. The inflammation may be further decreased by the application of moist heat or ultrasound. Aspirin, 8 to 10 tablets per day, is given as necessary. Local infiltration of the affected area with 1 to 2 ml of a steroid/lidocaine mixture will often give permanent relief. The injection is placed in the area of maximum local tenderness and may be repeated at weekly intervals for two to three weeks. A special tennis-elbow dressing may also be effective (Fig 5–5). If these modalities are not effective, the elbow and wrist should be immobilized in a long arm cast. The cast is applied so that the wrist is immobilized in a position that maintains relaxation of the affected muscles. For the more common lateral epicondylitis, the cast is applied with the elbow flexed 90°, the forearm supinated, and the wrist slightly dorsiflexed.

Tennis players can prevent recurrences by proper technique. The handle of the tennis racket should be large enough to prevent undue torque from being applied to the racket during the act of striking the ball. The ball should also be struck in the center of the racket face, and the body, rather than the arm, should be used for power.

The disease is usually self-limited, but symptoms may persist for several weeks before full recovery occurs. Conservative treatment is effective in most cases. Surgery is reserved for resistant cases and usually consists of resection of the injured portion of the tendon and repair.

OSTEOCHONDRITIS DISSECANS

Osteochondritis dissecans is a condition in which a portion of subchondral bone undergoes avascular necrosis. This segment of bone, with its overlying articular cartilage, may partially or completely separate from the adjacent bone and

6 / The Wrist and Hand

THE IMPORTANCE OF the wrist and hand is evidenced by the fact that the rest of the upper extremity functions primarily to place the hand in a position where it can operate most effectively. Treatment of the wide variety of disorders that occur in the hand requires an understanding of the complicated anatomy and functional physiology.

ANATOMY

Skin, Fascia, and Nail

The skin on the dorsum of the hand is loose and overlies a subcutaneous space through which pass many veins and most of the lymph vessels of the hand. This abundance of lymph vessels accounts for the dorsal lymphedema that commonly occurs secondary to infection in the palm or fingers.

The palmar skin, however, is firmly attached to the underlying palmar aponeurosis, which is continuous with the palmaris longus tendon (Fig 6–1). This thick fascia sends extensions into the fingers and serves to protect the important deeper structures of the hand. It may become nodular and shortened in Dupuytren's contracture.

The nail of each finger originates close to the distal interphalangeal joint and is surrounded on the sides and at the base by thick folds of tissue, the paronychium and the eponychium, respectively. It covers a rich capillary bed that may be tested to determine the circulation of the extremity. The nail should be retained, whenever possible, in fingertip injuries.

Blood Supply

Most of the blood supply to the hand enters on the palmar aspect through the radial and ulnar arteries. Each of these arteries terminates in a superficial and a deep branch. The superficial branches join to form the superficial palmar arch, which is located at the level of the base of the first web space. The deep palmar arch, which is located 1 cm proximal to the superficial arch, is formed by the junction of the deep branches. The arches are so named because of their position relative to the flexor tendons. Many branches and anastomoses from these arches provide the blood supply to the fingers and hand. In the fingers, digital vessels lie just ventral to the flexor skin crease of the interphalangeal joints (Fig 6–2).

Muscles of the Hand

Motions of the wrist and fingers are controlled by groups of muscles that are classified as either intrinsic or extrinsic. Intrinsic muscles arise within the hand and are responsible for the delicate movements of the fingers. Extrinsic muscles are those that take origin within the forearm.

EXTRINSIC MUSCLES

Motion at the wrist is accomplished by the various wrist flexors and extensors. In addition to providing wrist motion, these muscles stabilize the wrist in slight dorsiflexion, a position that allows maximum function of the extrinsic flexors.

Nine finger flexors and the median

53

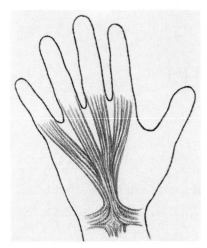

Fig 6–1.—The palmar aponeurosis.

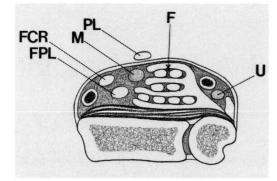

Fig 6–3.—Structures proximal to the wrist joint. The ulnar nerve *(U)* and artery continue distally through the ulnar tunnel of Guyon. The nine finger flexors *(F, FPL)* and median nerve *(M)* pass through the carpal tunnel beneath the transverse carpal ligament. Note the superficial location of the median nerve and the sublimi to the long and ring fingers. FCR = Flexor carpi radialis; PL = Palmaris longus.

nerve pass into the hand through the carpal tunnel beneath the transverse carpal ligament (Fig 6–3). Five deep flexors pass to the distal phalanx of each finger and thumb and four superficial flexors pass to the middle phalanx of each finger. Each of these finger flexors can be tested individually (Fig 6–4).

The finger flexors pass beneath a series of ligaments between the distal palmar crease and the distal interphalangeal joint. These annular ligaments or "pulleys" prevent the tendon from bowstringing. Tendon repair in this area called "no-

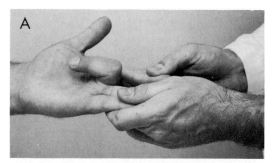

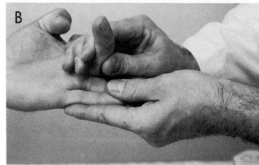

Fig 6–4.—**A,** the sublimis is functioning if the proximal interphalangeal joint can be flexed while the adjacent fingers are held extended. **B,** the profundus is functioning if the distal interphalangeal joint can be flexed while the rest of the finger is stabilized.

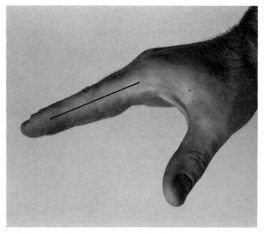

Fig 6–2.—The neurovascular bundle is situated just ventral to the flexor skin crease.

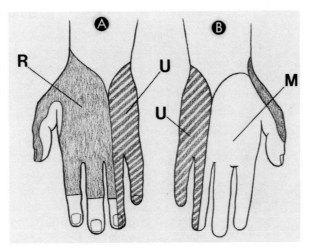

Fig 6–5. – Dorsal **(A)** and palmar **(B)** sensation of the hand:
R = radial nerve; *U* = ulnar nerve; and *M* = median nerve.

man's-land" is often unrewarding because of adhesions that form between the lacerated tendon ends and these ligaments.

The extensor tendons pass dorsally over each finger and thumb and insert into the phalanges. They extend the proximal phalanges and assist the intrinsic muscles in interphalangeal joint extension. The thumb extensors are easily palpated at the anatomical "snuffbox."

INTRINSIC MUSCLES

The thenar (median nerve) and hypothenar (ulnar) muscles act primarily to position the thumb and small finger for the purpose of pinch. The rest of the intrinsic muscles (interossei and lumbricals) insert into the proximal phalanges and extensor hoods and assist in flexion of the metacarpophalangeal joints and extension of the interphalangeal joints.

Nerve Supply

The ulnar nerve provides the motor supply to all of the intrinsic muscles of the hand except the two radial lumbricals and the thenar muscles. It also provides sensation to the entire ulnar 1½ fingers (Fig 6–5). Its function is easily evaluated by testing finger abduction and palpating the belly of the first dorsal interosseous muscle (Fig 6–6).

The thenar muscles and the two radial lumbricals are supplied by the median nerve, which also supplies sensation to the palmar aspect of the radial 3½ fingers as well as the tips of these fingers on their dorsal aspect. Its function is evaluated by testing opposition of the thumb to each finger and observing the thenar muscles for contractions.

The radial nerve has no intrinsic muscle supply but does provide sensation to the dorsum of the hand over the radial 3½ fingers. It supplies motor function to the extrinsic wrist and finger extensors.

Bones and Ligaments

The carpal bones contribute to the mobility of the hand by allowing flexion, extension, and radial and ulnar deviation to occur. The carpal bones are eight in number and are arranged into a distal and proximal row. Strong ligaments bind them together anteriorly, one of the strongest being the transverse carpal ligament. At the metacarpophalangeal and interphalangeal joints, strong collateral ligaments provide mediolateral stability.

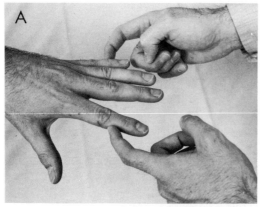

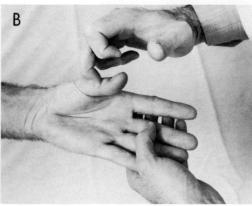

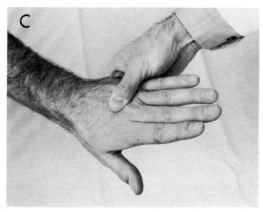

Fig 6–6. – **A,** testing for ulnar motor function. **B,** testing for median nerve function by determining thenar muscle strength. **C,** testing for radial nerve function by examining wrist extension against resistance.

ROENTGENOGRAPHIC ANATOMY

The 27 bones of the hand are visualized by anteroposterior, lateral, and oblique roentgenograms when appropriate (Fig 6–7).

CARPAL TUNNEL SYNDROME

Carpal tunnel syndrome, or compression of the median nerve at the wrist, is a common entity. It occurs as the result of compression of the nerve between the flexor tendons and the transverse carpal ligament. Usually, no cause is found, but the disorder is seen in association with hypothyroidism, synovitis of the wrist, rheumatoid and gouty arthritis, and aberrant or anomalous muscles in the wrist. It is sometimes seen following fractures of the wrist and is not uncommon in the third trimester of pregnancy. When it does occur late in pregnancy, the symptoms tend to subside after delivery. The syndrome is bilateral in up to 50% of cases.

CLINICAL FEATURES

The onset is usually spontaneous, with gradually increasing night pain being common. The night pain is frequently the reason the patient seeks medical attention and occurs because of a slight increase in swelling at the wrist with inactivity. The pain may radiate into the forearm, arm, and even the shoulder. Numbness and tingling occur along the median nerve distribution, but the sensory impairment rarely involves all 3½ fingers supplied by the median nerve. A sense of weakness and clumsiness in the use of the hand is common. All of these symptoms may be precipitated by various manual activities such as typing or painting. They frequently subside after shaking and moving the hand or allowing it to hang downward.

Physical examination usually reveals some sensory disturbance along the

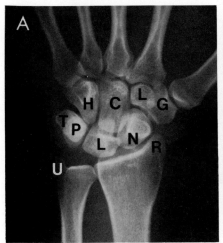
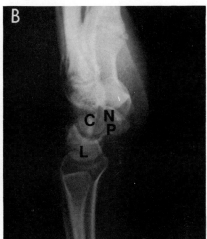

Fig 6–7.—Roentgenographic anatomy of the wrist: H = hamate with its prominent hook; C = capitate; L = lesser multangular (trapezoid); G = greater multangular (trapezium); T = triquetrum; P = pisiform; L = lunate; N = navicular (scaphoid); U = ulnar styloid; and R = radial styloid. On the lateral view, note that the capitate, lunate, and distal radius are in a direct line.

median nerve. Tinel's sign and Phalen's test are often positive (Fig 6–8). Atrophy of the thenar muscles is seen in long-standing cases.

Roentgenograms of the wrist are helpful in ruling out local bony abnormality. Electromyography and nerve conduction studies may be of benefit but are frequently unnecessary to establish the diagnosis in classical cases. The nerve conduction studies will reveal delayed conduction across the wrist.

TREATMENT

If repetitive trauma is a factor in the onset of symptoms, cessation of that trauma may serve to alleviate the symptoms in some cases. Injection of the carpal canal (avoiding the median nerve!) will occasionally give some relief as well. Intermittent splinting and anti-inflammatory medication may also be beneficial.

If symptoms persist, surgical release of the transverse carpal ligament is indicated. This is usually followed by prompt and permanent relief of pain. Improve-ment of sensory and motor function may take several weeks or months. No disability results from sectioning the ligament and the results are uniformly good.

ULNAR TUNNEL SYNDROME

Pain along the ulnar border of the hand secondary to compression of the ulnar nerve in its "tunnel" is much less common than median nerve compression. It may result from pressure on the nerve by soft tissue tumors, ganglia, constricting bands or muscles, or thrombosis of the ulnar artery. The symptoms and signs are similar to those found with carpal tunnel syndrome except that they are ulnar nerve in distribution. Sensation to the dorsum of the hand and fingers to the second phalanges is usually intact, however, because the dorsal sensory branch of the ulnar nerve passes to the back of the hand proximal to the ulnar tunnel.

The treatment is the same as that for carpal tunnel syndrome, and surgical release of the ulnar tunnel is usually necessary.

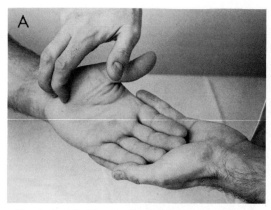 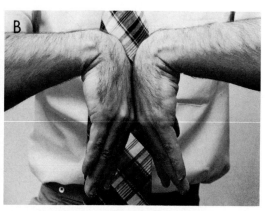

Fig 6–8.—A, Tinel's sign. Percussion of the median nerve at the carpal tunnel may reproduce the pain and tingling along the median nerve distribution. **B,** Phalen's test. The symptoms may also be reproduced after one minute of acute wrist flexion against resistance.

HYPOTHENAR HAMMER SYNDROME

Occlusion of the ulnar artery at the wrist may produce symptoms similar to those seen with ulnar tunnel syndrome. This disorder is usually secondary to some repetitive trauma to the ulnar aspect of the hand such as that which occurs when the hand is used as a mallet. This produces a thrombosis of the ulnar artery and results in ischemic manifestations such as pain, pallor, paresthesias, and decreased temperature of the affected digits. Local tenderness may be present and Allen's test is frequently positive (Fig 6–9).

Treatment is directed at avoiding the offending practice. The symptoms may resolve in many cases without any further treatment. Surgical resection of the thrombosed segment may be necessary if symptoms fail to respond to conservative treatment.

GANGLION

The ganglion is the most common soft tissue mass in the hand. It is always found adjacent to a joint or tendon sheath and may occur in any area of the body. The cause is unknown, but the cyst contains a mucinous material and usually has a stalk that can be traced to a tendon sheath or joint. Ganglion cysts are occasionally seen in children but frequently subside spontaneously in this age group.

CLINICAL FEATURES

A history of trauma is often elicited. Local pain and a feeling of weakness may be experienced by the patient. The mass may change in size, and this change is usually related to the level of activity of

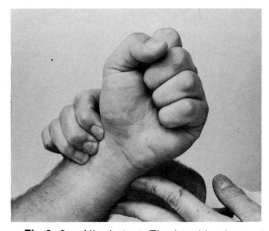

Fig 6–9.—Allen's test. The hand is elevated. The radial and ulnar arteries are occluded and the patient clenches the fist for 20 seconds. The arteries are released one at a time. Release of either artery will usually allow rapid restoration of the circulation to the hand. If one artery is occluded, however, revascularization of the hand will be delayed or absent.

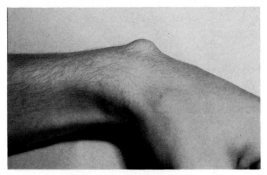

Fig 6–10. — Ganglion cyst.

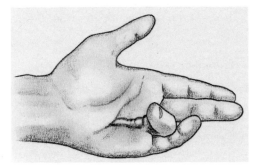

Fig 6–11. — Dupuytren's contracture. A flexion deformity of the finger is present, with nodular thickening of the fascia to the ring finger.

the patient. Ganglia are most common on the dorsum of the wrist. They are more prominent with the wrist flexed and are usually freely movable (Fig 6–10).

TREATMENT

A cure may be effected by aspirating or puncturing the cyst in multiple areas and injecting it with a steroid compound. A compression dressing is then applied for 48 to 72 hours.

If symptoms persist, excision of the cyst is indicated. The surgical procedure involves total removal of the cyst, its stalk, and a small portion of the adjacent joint capsule or tendon sheath. Methylene blue injected into the cyst may help to localize the stalk. Recurrences are not uncommon, but the rate should be low if the cyst is adequately removed.

DUPUYTREN'S CONTRACTURE

Dupuytren's contracture is a disease of the palmar fascia in which progressive contractures of the fascia occur, leading to a flexion deformity of the distal palm and fingers. The cause is unknown, but it is often hereditary and bilateral. It is more common in males and may be associated with fibrous contractures elsewhere in the body, especially in the plantar fascia of the foot. Pathologically, the contracture consists of proliferating vascular fibrous tissue that later develops into mature collagen.

CLINICAL FEATURES

The disorder is asymptomatic. Deformity and interference with the use of the hand by the flexed, contracted fingers are the most common complaints. The process usually begins on the ulnar side of the hand, often starting at the ring finger. An isolated nodule may appear in this area that eventually hardens and disappears. The overlying skin becomes adherent to the fascia and a strong fibrous cord develops that extends into the finger (Fig 6–11). In the later stages of the disorder, the cord begins to contract, pulling the finger into flexion. Multiple fingers may be affected.

TREATMENT

The treatment is surgical. Fasciectomy is indicated as soon as joint contracture occurs. If performed early, complete restoration of extension can be anticipated.

STENOSING TENOSYNOVITIS

Tenosynovitis is a common condition that results from repetitive overuse or direct trauma. The resultant inflammation and irritation hinders the normal gliding motion of the tendon. Several distinct syndromes can be described depending on the site of the involvement.

Many of them occur in the hand and some are associated with rheumatoid arthritis.

de Quervain's Disease

Tenosynovitis frequently occurs in the first dorsal extensor compartment of the wrist (Fig 6–12). The extensor pollicis brevis and abductor pollicis longus occupy this compartment and are involved where they cross over the radial styloid.

CLINICAL FEATURES

Pain and tenderness are usually present at the first dorsal compartment and crepitus with motion of the tendon may be noted. The pain may radiate up the forearm and down into the thumb. Active and passive motion of the thumb aggravate the pain, and local thickening of the tendon sheath is frequently present. Characteristically, pain is reproduced by passive stretching of the affected thumb tendons (Fig 6–13).

TREATMENT

The treatment in mild cases includes salicylates, immobilization, avoidance of the offending activity, and steroid injections into the tendon sheath. Moist heat is applied as necessary.

The symptoms usually subside with conservative treatment, but if they persist, surgical release of the tendon sheath is indicated.

Trigger Finger

If swelling of the flexor tendon and sheath occur, passage of the tendon through the constricted sheath may be difficult (Fig 6–14). This may result in snapping or "triggering" of the affected finger at the metacarpophalangeal joint as the swollen, nodular tendon passes through the constricted sheath. The symptoms are frequently worse after rest and improve with active use of the finger. The triggering effect itself is seen distal to the affected area and the finger may even lock completely. A congenital form is occasionally seen in the thumb of children. The examination usually reveals tenderness, swelling, and a firm mass at the proximal flexor pulley.

The treatment is the same as that for de Quervain's disease. Surgical release is frequently necessary but many cases, especially those that occur in children, recover spontaneously.

Extensor Carpi Radialis Tenosynovitis

Pain and tenderness affecting the radial wrist extensors is occasionally seen in heavy laborers. The symptoms, signs, and treatment are similar to those in de Quervain's disease.

ULNAR NERVE PARALYSIS

Paralysis of the ulnar nerve may occur from several causes, but the most common is chronic trauma to the nerve where it passes behind the elbow. The nerve is most superficial at this location and is easily subjected to external pressure. A cubitus valgus deformity at the elbow secondary to a growth plate fracture or infection may also cause paralysis by progressive stretching of the nerve in its

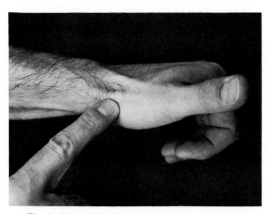

Fig 6–12. — The first dorsal compartment.

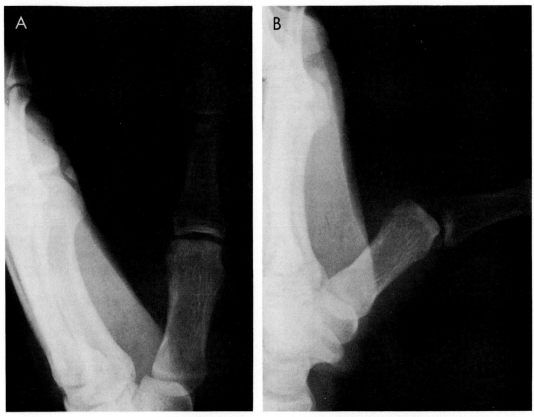

Fig 6–20.—Normal **(A)** and stress **(B)** roentgenograms of the thumb with complete rupture of the ulnar collateral ligament.

The treatment of all fingertip injuries is directed toward the coverage of the deeper tissue. This may be accomplished by simple closure, free grafts, or flaps. Wounds should not be allowed to heal by the "open" treatment without closure or coverage. Epithelialization of the wound will eventually occur but may take up to 12 weeks, and the resultant skin coverage is usually thin and tender and breaks down easily.

SIMPLE CLOSURE

Simple closure is effective when skin loss is minimal and sufficient looseness of the surrounding skin and soft tissue is present to permit suturing of the wound without undue tension. A small portion of the distal phalanx may be removed with a rongeur. The scar line should be kept on the dorsal aspect if possible in order to prevent a tender scar from being present on the volar aspect of the finger. Never trim "dog-ears." They will usually disappear with time, and trimming them may compromise healing.

FREE GRAFTS

Free grafts are usually split thickness or full thickness in nature. The thinner grafts tend to "take" better than thicker grafts but do not afford the protection of a full-thickness graft. Although they may heal over bone or tendon, secondary revisions are often necessary. Their use should be limited to dorsal wounds or those without exposure of bone or tendon. These thin grafts may be obtained

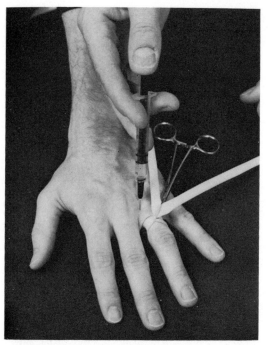

Fig 6–21. — Metacarpal block. The anesthesia should be instilled into the web space.

tip is not necessary. As healing progresses, full-thickness grafts may become dark after a few days. This should not be a cause for alarm, because the deeper portion is usually viable in spite of the appearance of the more superficial layers.

FLAP GRAFTS

Extensive wounds may require local flaps. A variety of flap grafts are available for use depending on the need. These grafts provide more bulk and protection and are used when subcutaneous tissue is needed, for example, over bone and tendon. They are occasionally used by the experienced surgeon.

Crush Injuries

These injuries are the result of direct violence to the tip of the finger. A painful subungual hematoma or fracture of the distal phalanx may occur (Fig 6–22). The treatment of these injuries is directed at the soft tissues. Isolated painful hematomas may be drained by gently drilling a hole into the nail with a No. 11 blade. A

from a number of areas. The donor area often ends up being unsightly after healing, however, and should be chosen carefully. The thigh or lateral aspect of the buttock are satisfactory donor sites.

Full-thickness grafts provide better protection for the volar aspect of the finger but have the same limitations as split-thickness skin grafts when used over bone and tendon. They are less sensitive and may be used on volar injuries. The flexor creases of the wrist and elbow are excellent donor sites. The donor wound is easily closed without undue tension in these areas. The graft should include no subcutaneous tissue. As with all grafting procedures, it is wise to plan backward and be certain that the graft will completely cover the area of the wound. If the patient brings in the amputated fingertip, it may be used as a full-thickness graft if it is in good condition. All fat must be removed prior to application. In children under 5 years of age, defatting the

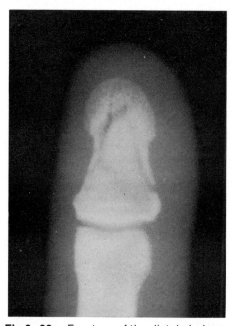

Fig 6–22. — Fracture of the distal phalanx.

heated paper clip may also be used. The hematoma should not be drained, however, when a fracture of the phalanx is present.

Fracture fragments are stabilized by the adjacent soft tissue and can usually be ignored. A compression dressing and ice are applied, and the hand is elevated to combat swelling. Warm soaks are started in 48 to 72 hours and gentle motion is encouraged. Recovery is usually rapid.

Extensor Tendon Injuries

The extensor mechanism of each finger is a complex system, only a part of which is the extrinsic tendon itself. Restoration of normal function requires accurate diagnosis and repair. All skin lacerations over the hand should be thoroughly inspected for tendon injury, but special attention should be paid to lacerations over the metacarpophalangeal joint. Extensor tendon lacerations in this area are particularly difficult to diagnose because the injury frequently occurs with the metacarpophalangeal joint in flexion, and the examination is usually carried out with the finger in extension. The tendon laceration will then lie at a different level than the skin laceration and often goes undetected. With any extensor tendon injury, there is variable loss of active extension of the finger.

Lacerations in the extensor complex must be repaired accurately, and there should be no hesitation to extend the wound proximally or distally in order to properly visualize the ends of the tendon. Direct end-to-end repair using nonabsorbable suture such as wire or nylon is desirable. The finger and wrist are splinted in extension in order to remove tension from the suture line. Immobilization is maintained for approximately four weeks.

Flexor Tendon Injuries

Flexor tendon injuries are diagnosed by history and examination. Partial or

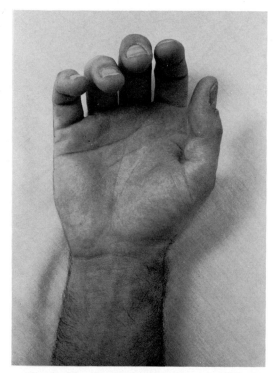

Fig 6–23.—The position of rest. With the hand lying on a flat surface, the fingers will maintain a position of slight flexion. When the flexor tendons are lacerated, the affected finger will rest in extension.

complete loss of finger flexion will be accompanied by a typical posture of the finger (Fig 6–23). There are often associated digital nerve injuries.

Repair of flexor tendon injuries is a complex problem that should be undertaken only in the operating room by an experienced surgeon. Primary repair of these injuries is indicated when the laceration occurs distal to the sublimis insertion or proximal to the distal palmar crease. Primary tendon repair between these two points, in so-called no-man's-land, is frequently unrewarding because adhesions are likely to form between the lacerated tendon ends and the flexor sheath and pulleys (Fig 6–24). In selected cases of sharp wounds, primary tendon repair may be undertaken in this area. Otherwise, simple closure of the

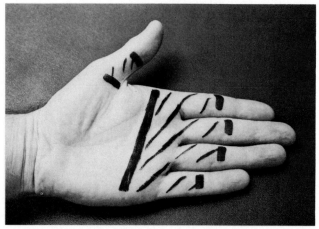

Fig 6–24.—No-man's-land,
the critical area of the annular ligaments.

skin laceration followed by secondary tendon grafting in six to eight weeks is often preferable.

HAND INFECTIONS

Felon

A felon is an infection of the closed space of the pulp of the distal phalanx (Fig 6–25). It occurs secondary to a local puncture wound and is characterized by rapidly increasing pressure and pain. Osteomyelitis of the distal phalanx and extension of the infection into the flexor sheath or adjacent joint may result. Early incision and drainage is indicated. A short 24-hour trial of conservative treatment with antibiotics and hot packs may be attempted, but if symptoms do not rapidly diminish early drainage is advisable.

A metacarpal block is adequate anesthesia. A tourniquet is applied to the base of the finger and a direct incision is made into the point of maximum tenderness and swelling. The incision does not have to be any longer than 5 to 10 mm. If no specific "point" can be detected, a straight lateral incision, which may be extended around the tip of the finger, is made (Fig 6–26). The "fish-mouth" incision should not be used. Routine care of the wound after drainage includes dressing changes every two to three days and

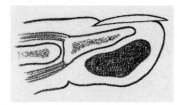

Fig 6–25.—Felon. The pus accumulates in the pulp of the distal phalanx.

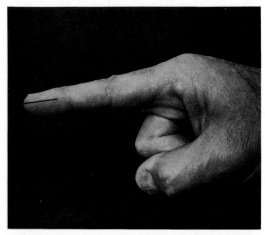

Fig 6–26.—Drainage of felon. The incision is placed posterior to the neurovascular bundle.

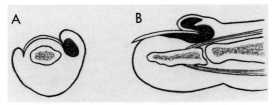

Fig 6–27.–Paronychia. **A,** the abcess is present beneath the eponychium. **B,** the infection has penetrated under the nail and extended proximally.

maintenance of antibiotic therapy. The wound will usually be healed in two weeks.

Paronychia

Paronychia is an infection of the distal phalanx that occurs along the edge of the nail. The organism, usually *Staphylococcus,* is introduced by biting the nail or by a rough manicure. Local signs of infection such as redness, swelling, and tenderness are invariably present (Fig 6–27).

Acute paronychia will usually require drainage although antibiotics and local care will occasionally result in a cure. Once the pus has localized, incision and drainage are indicated. This is easily accomplished by passing a scalpel between the nail and the adjacent eponychium with the patient under local anesthesia. If the infection has penetrated under the

nail, a small portion of it may have to be excised. Incision and drainage through the eponychium should be avoided.

Once the infection spreads under the nail, a subungual abscess results. In this case, drainage is only effective if the proximal part of the nail is excised (Fig 6–28). The nail will usually regrow. Chronic paronychia is treated in a similar manner.

Tendon Sheath Infections

Infection may occur inside a flexor tendon sheath from extension of a felon or directly from a puncture wound. The rapid increase in pressure due to the accumulation of pus may obliterate the blood supply to the tendon, resulting in necrosis and complete loss of function of the tendon. The infection may also spread through the rest of the hand. Early diagnosis and treatment are therefore important.

CLINICAL FEATURES

The patient with suppurative tenosynovitis is febrile and often in a toxic condition. The disorder can usually be diagnosed by the presence of the four cardinal signs of Kanavel: (1) the finger is uniformly swollen, (2) the finger is held in slight flexion for comfort, (3) intense pain is present on passive extension of the

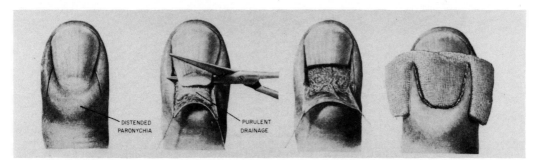

Fig 6–28.–Drainage of paronychium when a subungual abscess is present. Lateral incisions are made through the eponychium and the base of the nail is removed. (From Milford, L.: The Hand, in Crenshaw, A. H. [ed.]: *Campbell's Operative Orthopaedics* [5th ed.; St. Louis, C. V. Mosby Co., 1971].)

finger, and (4) marked tenderness is present along the course of the inflamed sheath.

TREATMENT

Early treatment with high doses of antibiotics, elevation, and splinting may result in a cure. In addition, wide incision and drainage are usually necessary to prevent sloughing of the tendon and further spread of the infection.

BIBLIOGRAPHY

Bowers, W. H., and Hurst, L. C.: Gamekeeper's thumb, J. Bone Joint Surg. 59A:519, 1977.

Boyes, J. H.: *Bunnell's Surgery of the Hand* (5th ed.; Philadelphia: J. B. Lippincott Co., 1970).

Conklin, J. E., and White, W. L.: Stenosing tenosynovitis and its possible relation to the carpal tunnel syndrome, Surg. Clin. North Am. 40:531, 1960.

Dinham, J. M., and Meggitt, B. F.: Trigger thumbs in children, J. Bone Joint Surg. 56B:153, 1974.

Entin, M. A.: Repair of extensor mechanism of the hand, Surg. Clin. North Am. 40:275, 1960.

Flatt, A. E.: *The Care of Minor Hand Injuries* (3d ed.; St. Louis: C. V. Mosby Co., 1972).

Herndon, W. A., Hershey, S. L., and Lambdin, C. S.: Thrombosis of the ulnar artery in the hand, J. Bone Joint Surg. 57A:994, 1975.

Kaplan, E. B.: *Functional and Surgical Anatomy of the Hand* (2d ed.; Philadelphia: J. B. Lippincott Co., 1965).

Milford, L.: The Hand, in Crenshaw, A. H. (ed.): *Campbell's Operative Orthopaedics* (5th ed.; St. Louis: C. V. Mosby Co., 1971).

Nelson, C. L., Sawmiller, S., and Phalen, G. S.: Ganglions of the wrist and hand, J. Bone Joint Surg. 54A:1459, 1972.

Nevasier, R. J., Wilson, J. N., and Lievano, A.: Rupture of the ulnar collateral ligament of the thumb (gamekeeper's thumb), J. Bone Joint Surg. 53A:1357, 1971.

Rodrigo, J. J., Kiebauer, J. J., and Doyle, J. R.: Treatment of Dupuytren's contracture, J. Bone Joint Surg. 58A:380, 1976.

Sakellarides, H. T., and DeWeese, J. W.: Instability of the metacarpophalangeal joint of the thumb, J. Bone Joint Surg. 58A:106, 1976.

Smith, R. J.: Post-traumatic instability of the metacarpophalangeal joint of the thumb, J. Bone Joint Surg. 59A:14, 1977.

7 / The Back

BACK PAIN is one of the most frequent conditions requiring medical treatment. It is also the most expensive ailment between the ages of 30 and 60 years and one of the most difficult to treat. Back pain may be due to a variety of disorders, including gynecologic, genitourinary, and gastrointestinal diseases, but the most common causes are lumbar strain and disorders of the lumbar disc.

ANATOMY

The vertebrae, discs, and ligaments of the dorsal and lumbar spine are similar in most respects to their counterparts in the cervical spine. The lumbar vertebrae are larger and thicker, however, due to their weight-bearing function (Fig 7–1). Anterior and posterior longitudinal ligaments are applied to the respective surfaces of the vertebral bodies, and posterior stability is aided by supraspinous and interspinous ligaments and the ligamentum flavum. The discs account for over one third of the total height of the lumbar spine and account for most of the normal lordosis.

Spinal nerves exit the canal by passing through intervertebral foramina, each foramen consisting of the inferior aspect of the pedicle above and the superior aspect of the pedicle below the level of exit. In the lumbar spine, disc disease usually affects the nerve root exiting one level below, because that is the nerve that actually passes over the disc (Fig 7–2). Thus, a herniated disc between the fourth and fifth lumbar vertebrae commonly affects the fifth nerve root and not the fourth.

EXAMINATION

Examination of the back is performed with the patient standing, sitting on the examining table, and in the supine position. The patient is first observed in the standing position. Any list or excessive kyphosis or lordosis is noted. Next, the chest is measured in full inspiration and expiration. Normal expansion is greater than 5 cm but may be less than 2.5 cm in ankylosing spondylitis. The iliac crests are then palpated to determine if they are level. If they are not, footboards of varying thicknesses may be placed under the shorter extremity to assess the amount of shoe lift necessary to level the pelvis. The shoulders are also observed for evenness, although the dominant shoulder is frequently lower in the normal population. The spine and sacroiliac joints are palpated and percussed for spasm and tenderness. Any varicosities in the lower extremities are also noted. The range of motion is then slowly tested. With the patient bending forward as far as possible, flexion is measured as the distance between the fingertips and the floor. This calculation represents a combination of lumbar spine mobility and hamstring flexibility. While the patient is flexed forward, the back is viewed from behind to detect any scoliosis, and from the side to detect any persistence of the normal lumbar lordosis that might be present secondary to protective muscle spasm. Extension and right and left bending are then measured. Pain on bending toward the affected side frequently signifies disc disease, whereas pain on bending away from the affected side frequently denotes

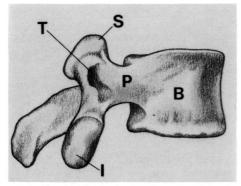

Fig 7–1.—A typical lumbar vertebra: *S* = superior articular facet; *I* = inferior articular facet; *P* = pedicle; *T* = transverse process; and *B* = body.

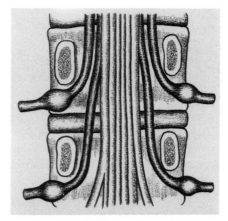

Fig 7–2.—Relationship of nerve roots to discs in the lumbar spine.

muscle strain. The gait pattern is then observed and the ability to walk on the heels (L5 root) and balls of the feet (S1 root) is tested.

In the sitting position, a complete neurologic examination of the lower extremities is performed. Reflexes, motor strength, and sensation are tested. The thighs and calves are measured to detect any muscular atrophy. Discrepancies of one-half in. in the thigh and one-fourth in. in the calf are significant. Straight leg raising in the sitting position is also tested and compared to straight-leg-raising tests that will be performed in the supine position. The peripheral pulses are palpated and any abnormalities in the vascular status of the extremity are noted.

In the supine position, the hip is placed through a full range of motion and thoroughly tested to rule out primary hip abnormality. The straight-leg-raising tests are then performed and the leg lengths are measured (Fig 7–3). Next, with the patient on the side, manual pressure is applied to the iliac crest (pelvic compression test). Reproduction of pain in the sacroiliac joints or symphysis pubis with this maneuver may suggest disorders of these areas.

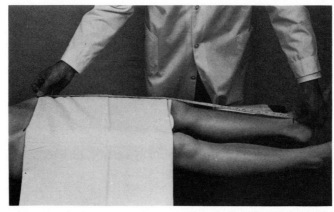

Fig 7–3.—The lower extremities are measured between the anterior superior iliac spines and the medial malleoli with the leg in neutral alignment. Discrepancies under 1 cm are probably not significant.

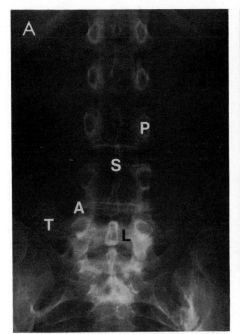

Fig 7–4.—Anteroposterior **(A)** and lateral **(B)** view of the lumbar spine: S = spinous process; P = pedicle; T = transverse process; L = lamina; A = articular facet joint; B = body; and I = intervertebral foramen.

ROENTGENOGRAPHIC ANATOMY

The evaluation of disorders of the lumbar spine should include a standard roentgenographic examination. The roentgenographic features are well visualized by the following: (1) anteroposterior view (Fig 7–4), (2) lateral view (see Fig 7–4), and (3) oblique views in both directions (Fig 7–5). In addition, a spot lateral view of the lumbosacral space may be necessary.

LUMBAR DISC SYNDROMES

The pattern of disc deterioration in the lumbar spine is similar to that which occurs in the cervical spine. In the lumbar spine, however, acute soft disc herniation is the most common cause of pain, whereas in the cervical spine, symptoms are usually secondary to spondylosis. Ninety-five percent of disc lesions in the lumbar spine occur at the fourth and fifth spaces, with most of the remainder occurring at the third space. With repetitive trauma, progressive degeneration of the nucleus pulposus occurs, which may lead to protrusion or complete extrusion of a portion of the disc contents into the neural canal. This usually occurs in the area of greatest weakness at the posterolateral aspect of the disc (Fig 7–6). Chronic disc deterioration may also occur, resulting in spur formation, disc space narrowing, and degenerative changes in the facet joints and between adjacent vertebral bodies.

A rare but serious complication of lumbar disc disease is the cauda equina syndrome. This results from a massive central disc protrusion and may produce variable degrees of permanent paralysis in the lower extremities. Bladder and bowel function may also be severely impaired. This condition is a true emergency and usually demands immediate surgery.

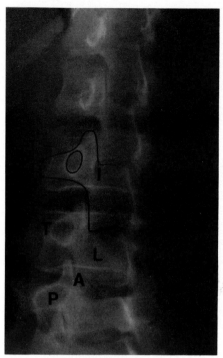

Fig 7–5. — Oblique view: *A* = articular facet joint; *I* = isthmus or pars interarticularis; *T* = transverse process; *L* = lamina; and *P* = pedicle. The oblique view visualizes the so-called Scottie dog. Spondylolysis occurs through the isthmus.

CLINICAL FEATURES

The onset of symptoms is variable. One specific traumatic episode may produce symptoms, but because of the progressive nature of the disease process in the disc, the symptoms usually occur gradually. The most common complaint is low back pain, which is often deep and aching in nature. The pain is aggravated by activity and relieved by rest. Coughing, sneezing, or other actions that increase the stress on the disc tend to intensify the pain. The back pain is often localized near the disc and may be referred to the iliac crest or buttock.

Low back pain may occur in combination with radiating pain or the two pain patterns may occur separately. Radicular pain characteristically spreads over the

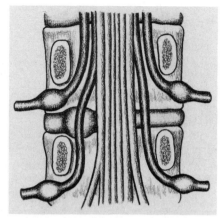

Fig 7–6. — Lumbar disc protrusion. Note that herniation affects the root that exits one level below.

buttock and passes down the posterior or posterolateral aspect of the thigh and calf and may even spread onto the foot. Both types of pain usually improve with bed rest. If little or no relief of pain occurs with rest, inorganic causes should be considered. Relentless pain that is not relieved or may even be aggravated by

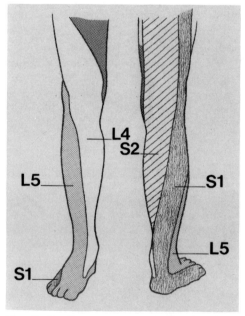

Fig 7–7. — Dermatomes of the lower extremity.

recumbency should lead one to suspect a spinal cord tumor.

Paresthesias, in the form of numbness and tingling, are common and are usually more marked in the distal portion of the extremity. They may follow a specific dermatome pattern (Fig 7–7).

Examination often reveals restriction of low back motion. Bending toward the affected side frequently exacerbates the pain. Variable degrees of local tenderness and muscle guarding are present. In an attempt to relieve tension on the nerve root, the patient may list or bend away from the painful side and stand with the affected hip and knee slightly flexed. A characteristic clinical picture may be present, depending on the level of nerve root involvement (Table 7–1). The sensory examination may reveal diminished sensation along the affected dermatome. The various tests measuring sciatic nerve root tension are frequently positive (Fig 7–8).

The diagnosis usually becomes appar-

ent on the basis of the history and examination. Plain roentgenograms of the lumbar spine are usually normal. The diagnosis may be confirmed by electromyography, discography, ascending lumbar phlebography, and myelography (Fig 7–9). The myelogram is not a procedure without some morbidity, however, and is usually indicated only if surgical intervention is contemplated or if other serious spinal abnormality is suspected. Spinal fluid analysis may show a slight increase in protein content.

TREATMENT

The initial treatment is always conservative. The objective is to "unload" the disc, and this is accomplished only by strict, complete bed rest. Rest for 23 hours a day on a firm mattress is begun and continued for a minimum of ten to 14 days. While the patient is in bed, the hips and knees are kept moderately flexed. Lying on the abdomen, which increases the lumbar lordosis, is avoided. Hip flex-

TABLE 7–1.—CLINICAL FEATURES OF COMMON LUMBAR DISC SYNDROMES

DISC	PAIN	SENSORY CHANGE	MOTOR WEAKNESS, ATROPHY	REFLEX CHANGE
L3–L4 (L4 root)	Low back, posterolateral aspect of thigh, across patella, anteromedial aspect of leg	Anterior aspect of knee, anteromedial aspect of leg	Quadriceps (knee extension)	Knee jerk
L4–L5 (L5 root)	Lateral, posterolateral aspect of thigh, leg	Lateral aspect of leg, dorsum of foot, first web space, great toe	Great toe extension, ankle dorsiflexion, heel walking difficult, (footdrop may occur)	Minor (posterior tibial jerk depressed)
L5–S1 (S1 root)	Posterolateral aspect of thigh, leg, heel	Posterior aspect of calf, heel, lateral aspect of foot (3 toes)	Calf, plantarflexion of foot, great toe; toe walking weak	Ankle jerk
Cauda equina syndrome (massive midline protrusion)	Low back, thigh, legs; often bilateral	Thighs, legs, feet, perineum; often bilateral	Variable; may be bowel, bladder incontinence	Ankle jerk (may be bilateral)

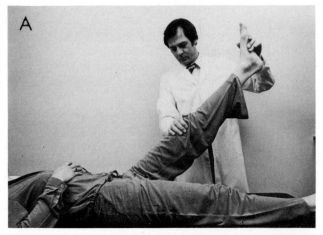

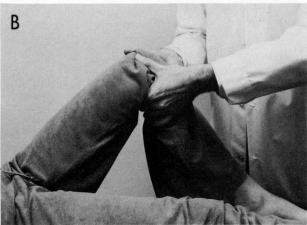

Fig 7–8.—Tests of nerve root tension, the most important examination in herniation of the lumbar intervertebral disc. **A,** the foot is slowly raised, keeping the knee straight, until sciatic pain is produced. A positive test includes the following: (1) pain produced before 70° is reached, (2) aggravation of the pain by dorsiflexion of the ankle, and (3) relief of the pain by flexion of the knee. **B,** the popliteal compression test is then performed by flexing the knee and applying pressure to the popliteal nerve in the fossa. Reproduction of leg pain by this maneuver is further evidence of nerve root irritation. If the patient can extend the leg to 90° while sitting but the same test is impossible in the supine position, malingering should be suspected. If raising the leg on the contralateral side reproduces pain in the affected leg, disc herniation should be strongly suspected.

ion and pelvic tilt exercises are begun within the limits of pain (Fig 7–10). Salicylates, analgesics, and moist heat are used as necessary. If physical therapy is necessary or if the patient cannot follow the strict regimen of bed rest at home, hospitalization should be considered. Pelvic traction (6.75 to 13 kg), diathermy, and massage are then prescribed. If im-

provement occurs, which it does in the majority of cases, the exercise program is expanded and gradual resumption of ambulation is allowed. A lumbosacral corset may be temporarily used, but it is always best to encourage patients to develop their own musculature and range of motion. The brace is discontinued as soon as possible. Recurrences are pre-

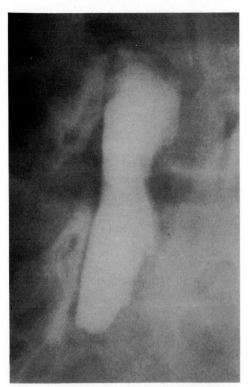

Fig 7–9.—Abnormal lumbar myelogram revealing a large extradural defect in the dye column consistent with disc herniation.

CHEMONUCLEOLYSIS

In 1964, enzymatic dissolution of the nucleus pulposus was introduced for the treatment of the herniated lumbar disc. This procedure involves injecting the affected disc with chymopapain, a derivative of the papaya plant, which digests the nucleus pulposus. Preliminary reports of its use in selected cases appeared encouraging, but a recent double-blind study has left its use in doubt. It continues to be used in several centers and may still offer an alternative to laminectomy in the future.

Chronic Lumbar Disc Disease

A high percentage of adults over the age of 40 have degenerative disc disease at one or more levels on roentgenographic examination (Fig 7 – 12). Significant thinning of the disc is often present, accompanied by osteophyte formation. These roentgenographic changes are common in the general population and are present in many asymptomatic individuals. Degenerative changes in the adjacent facet joints and surrounding soft tissues may, however, lead to intermittent low back pain and even nerve root irritation.

Chronic low back pain of this nature will usually respond to conservative management. Salicylates, rest, moist heat, and the use of a lumbosacral corset may be the only treatment necessary. Flexion exercises will correct associated muscular and postural problems. When signs of nerve root irritation with radicular pain are present, compression of the root by a small, acute, soft disc herniation or degenerative spur should be suspected. Surgical intervention is occasionally indicated to relieve nerve pressure under these circumstances. Arthrodesis of the adjacent vertebrae may also be indicated to relieve chronic low back pain by stabilizing the degenerated painful disc

vented by a proper exercise program and the avoidance of stress to the lower part of the back (Fig 7 – 11).

The condition of the majority of patients will improve with conservative treatment. Surgery is reserved for those patients who have major or progressing neurologic deficits or those with intractable pain who fail to respond to conservative management. The disc is removed through a small laminotomy approach and the nerve root is explored. With a positive history, physical findings, myelogram, and electromyogram, a 90% to 95% success rate can be assured. In the absence of one or more of these, the cure rate for surgery declines. Patients must also be cautioned that although their leg pain will disappear postoperatively, some mild, intermittent low back pain may persist.

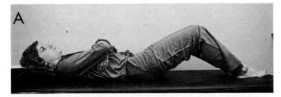

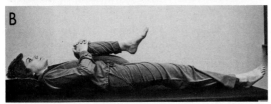

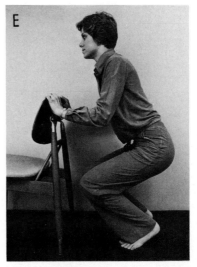

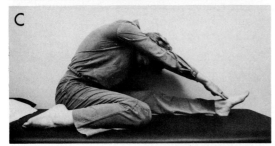

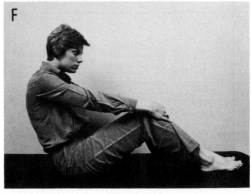

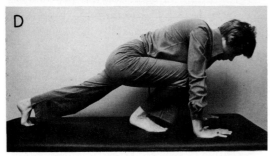

Fig 7–10. — Low back exercises. **A,** pelvic tilt, performed to decrease the lumbar lordosis and raise the anterior aspect of the pelvis. The small of the back is pressed to the floor and the abdominal and buttock muscles are tightened. **B,** hip flexion, performed to stretch the tight posterior spinal musculature and unload the posterior disc. Each knee is drawn up and pulled firmly to the chest several times and held for 10 to 20 seconds. The exercise is then repeated using both knees. After the acute pain has subsided, the remainder of the exercises are performed: **C,** hamstring stretching exercises; **D,** hip flexor stretching exercises; **E,** quadriceps strengthening and heel cord stretching exercise; and **F,** abdominal strengthening exercise. All exercises are performed on a carpeted floor and should be repeated in sets of five to ten at least three times daily.

segment. Conservative treatment is usually successful in most cases, however.

LUMBAR STRAIN

Muscular or ligamentous injury is the most common cause of low back pain. It may follow single or multiple traumatic episodes. Incomplete muscular tears or ligament sprains occur, leading to pain and tenderness over the affected area. These injuries respond well to rest and symptomatic treatment over a one- to two-week period. When the injury is superimposed on a chronic pattern of low back pain or lumbar disc disease, the treatment is often more lengthy, however.

A variety of factors predispose to chronic repetitive low back strains. Obesity, poor muscular tone, faulty work habits, the wearing of high-heeled shoes, and the lack of a daily exercise program are among the contributing factors. Most of these cause the center of gravity of the body to be shifted forward, which leads to an increase in the lumbar lordosis. This places an added strain on the discs, ligaments, and muscles in order to maintain an upright posture.

Obesity contributes to chronic low back pain in other ways. First, it is known that intra-abdominal pressure aids the erector spinae muscles in keeping the lumbar spine erect and decreases intradiscal pressure. Obese patients have poor

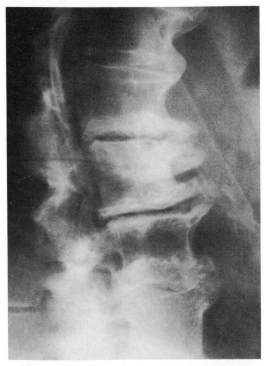

Fig 7–12.—Chronic degenerative disc disease in an adult with only minimal symptoms.

abdominal muscular tone and thus do not benefit from this action. Obese patients also typically have an increase in their lumbar lordosis, which further adds stress to the lower part of the back.

With a daily program of proper postural exercises, weight loss, and a general exercise program, most patients with chronic back pain will be able to rehabilitate the lower part of the back. Full cooperation is necessary.

SPONDYLOLISTHESIS

Spondylolisthesis is a term applied to a disorder, usually in the lumbar spine, in which a gradual slipping of one vertebra on another occurs. Several types have been described (congenital, degenerative, pathologic, traumatic, and spondylolytic). Most spondylolisthesis, however, is secondary to spondylolysis, which represents a defect in the pars interartic-

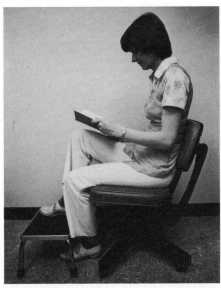

Fig 7–11.—Correct sitting posture. At least one knee should be kept higher than the hips. In addition to proper sitting posture, the following guidelines are helpful to decrease the lumbar lordosis and prevent strain: (1) maintain the proper weight, (2) avoid high-heeled shoes, (3) avoid sleeping on the abdomen, (4) place one foot on a stool when standing at work, (5) lift with the knees and not with the back, and (6) avoid lifting objects above the waist or away from the body.

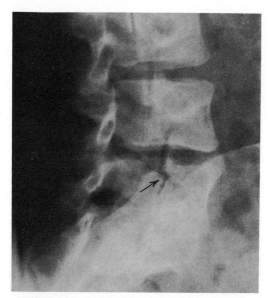

Fig 7–13. — Bony defect *(arrow)* in the isthmus or neck of the "Scottie dog" present in spondylolysis.

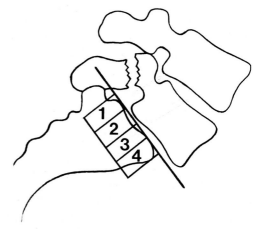

Fig 7–14. — Meyerding's classification of spondylolisthesis. The amount of slippage is graded 1 to 4. Grade 1 represents 25% forward displacement; grade 2, 25% to 50%; grade 3, 50% to 75%; and grade 4, greater than 75%.

ularis or isthmus of the vertebra (Fig 7–13). This defect has a definite hereditary predisposition and usually becomes manifest as the result of repetitive stresses to the lower part of the back. Spondylolisthesis is classified according to the amount of forward slippage of the affected vertebra (Fig 7–14).

CLINICAL FEATURES

Spondylolysis may be symptomatic even without spondylolisthesis and both conditions may be associated with lumbar disc herniation. The disorder is often asymptomatic, however, frequently being discovered incidentally on roentgenograms taken for other purposes. The symptoms usually begin gradually in the second or third decade. Low back pain, sometimes radiating into the buttocks, occurs with activity and is relieved by rest. Symptoms of nerve root irritation may also be present with radiation of the pain into the extremities. These symptoms often progress in severity, especially in the teenager.

Examination reveals guarding of the lower part of the back and spasm of the paraspinal muscles. With moderate forward slippage, the lumbar lordosis appears increased and the buttocks may appear more prominent. A palpable

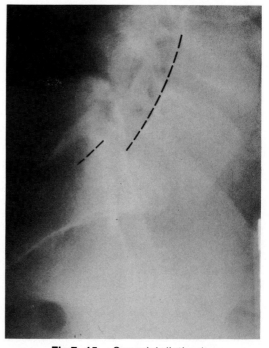

Fig 7–15. — Spondylolisthesis.

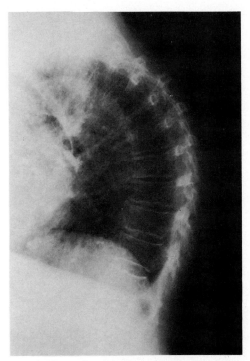

Fig 7–21. — Roentgenogram of an elderly patient with senile kyphosis.

eases of the discs and vertebral bodies are the most common causes. Congenital kyphosis is rare and is usually secondary to a localized malformation of the spine.

Senile Kyphosis

Senile kyphosis results from multiple areas of disc degeneration at the thoracic level. It is relatively common in the elderly patient and may be symptomatic. Roentgenograms will often reveal thinning of the disc and osteoporosis with mild wedging deformities (Fig 7–21).

Treatment is directed toward maintaining good posture. Exercises that strengthen the back and abdominal muscles are often helpful. The use of a light spinal brace will frequently relieve the symptoms.

Postural Round Back

Faulty posture is common in adolescents and young children. It probably occurs as a result of minor muscular imbalances and weakness. The typical picture is one in which the patient, often a teenager, shows an increase in the normal dorsal kyphosis, lumbar lordosis, and an increased pelvic inclination. The shoulders are often rounded and drooped, and the abdomen may be protuberant. The scapulae are frequently prominent. The kyphosis is typically supple in contrast to the nonflexible, fixed kyphosis in Scheuermann's disease.

Roentgenograms of the dorsal spine are usually unremarkable. No wedging or end-plate irregularities tend to be present.

After ruling out other causes of kyphosis, the patient is started on an exercise program to overcome contractures and decrease the lumbar lordosis (Fig 7–22). The disorder usually responds well to the exercises.

Scheuermann's Disease

Scheuermann's kyphosis is a fixed kyphosis that develops near the time of puberty. The cause is unknown, but the deformity is caused by typical wedging abnormalities in the dorsal spine that result in a decrease in the anterior height of the vertebrae.

CLINICAL FEATURES

Poor posture is a common complaint, and fatigue and pain usually accompany the deformity. The family history is often positive.

Examination reveals an increase in the normal kyphosis of the dorsal spine usually associated with local tenderness. There may be tightness of the hamstring, pectoral, and iliopsoas muscles. In contrast to postural round back, this kyphosis is fixed. The abdomen may be protuberant, and there is usually an increase in the lumbar lordosis. The results of the neurologic examination are usually normal.

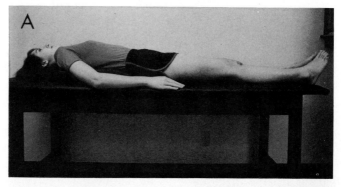

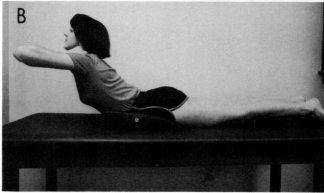

Fig 7–22.—Exercises for postural round back. **A,** the resting position with a pillow under the dorsal spine. **B,** scapular adduction and thoracic hyperextension exercise that stretches the pectoral muscles and contracted anterior soft tissues. In addition, the low back exercises previously described are performed to correct excessive lumbar lordosis.

A positive diagnosis is possible only with a roentgenographic examination. Wedging of the vertebrae, irregularity of the end-plates and typical Schmorl's nodules are seen on the lateral view, usually between T2 and T12 (Fig 7–23). Synostoses and osteophyte formation are not uncommon in the adult patient.

TREATMENT

Conservative treatment consisting of a Milwaukee brace and postural exercises will usually result in a cure. The brace is worn for approximately one year full time and is used at night for an additional year. Hamstring stretching and pelvic tilt exercises are initiated. Severe deformity with pain or neurologic symptoms are indications for surgery at any age. The surgery is similar to that performed for scoliosis.

Long-term results of conservative treatment are generally favorable when the disease is confined to the dorsal spine. There is an increased incidence of back pain with curves that are low in the dorsal spine or upper lumbar spine. The working capacity for the patient is usually not affected, however.

DISCITIS

Discitis is an infectious or inflammatory disease of unknown cause. An infectious basis is strongly suggested. The process most commonly occurs in the midlumbar spine of children about the age of 6. A history of trauma or infection elsewhere may be present.

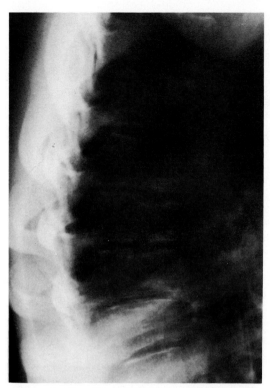

Fig 7–23. — Roentgenogram of Scheuermann's disease. End-plate irregularities and mild wedging deformities are present.

CLINICAL FEATURES

The symptoms consist of low back pain that often radiates into the abdomen or lower extremities. The child has difficulty walking and standing and may even refuse to walk or sit at all. A slight limp may be present.

Examination reveals restriction of motion in the lumbar spine associated with hamstring spasm and a flattening of the normal lumbar lordosis. Local tenderness in the midlumbar region is usually present. The child is often irritable and may run a low-grade fever. Nausea and vomiting occasionally occur.

There is a positive blood culture in approximately 50% of patients, and the organism is usually *Staphylococcus*. Needle aspiration of the affected disc will sometimes reveal the same organism.

There is usually an increase in the sedimentation rate and WBC count. The bone scan is usually abnormal, and plain roentgenograms frequently reveal single disc space narrowing with irregularity of the adjacent end-plates. Eventually, fusion may even occur between the involved vertebrae.

TREATMENT

Treatment consists of antibiotics, bed rest, and the application of a body cast. Treatment is continued until the systemic signs of infection, such as the sedimentation rate, temperature, and WBC count, are normal. The prognosis is usually good.

LUMBOSACRAL ANOMALIES

A variety of minor congenital abnormalities may exist in the lumbar spine and at the lumbosacral junction. The majority of these occur at the lumbosacral region and most are asymptomatic. Facet joint asymmetry, variations in the number of lumbar vertebrae, spina bifida occulta, and transitional lumbosacral vertebrae are among the more common anomalies seen on routine roentgenograms. Only the transitional vertebra appears to be related to low back pain.

The transitional vertebra (lumbarized S1 or sacralized L5) may produce pain at the false joint that forms at the articulation between its elongated transverse process and the sacrum (Fig 7–24). The disc between this vertebra and the sacrum is usually markedly thinned but is rarely the cause of symptoms. The treatment is usually conservative. A lumbosacral corset may be beneficial by restricting motion at this area.

MEDICAL CAUSES OF LOW BACK PAIN

One of the most common maladies to present itself to the family physician is the complaint of low back pain. In other

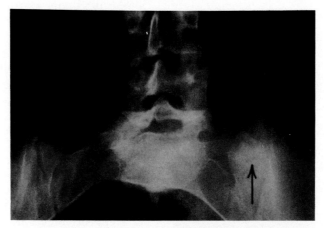

Fig 7–24. – Transitional lumbosacral vertebra.
A false joint is present *(arrow).*

areas of this text we have approached the musculoskeletal causes of low back pain and have presented the conservative and surgical methods of treatment. It is the purpose of this section to deal with those causes of low back pain that are other than musculoskeletal in origin and that may have a relationship to systemic disease. Statistical analyses have shown in general that 18% to 20% of the population have had back pain at one time or another during their lives. Statistics also show that approximately 10% to 11% of this group had roentgenograms taken and approximately 5% had already worn a brace, while approximately 0.7% had already undergone an operation for low back pain.

By definition, low back pain refers to any pain in the lumbosacral area of the spine or the areas of the paraspinous muscles, and it may or may not radiate into the hip or the leg. This section will stress those medical causes that may have similar presentations to the musculoskeletal causes of low back pain but that may have much greater import insofar as the primary underlying diagnosis and ultimate prognosis. Although musculoskeletal causes of low back pain are far more common than the medical causes we will discuss, it behooves the physician to

keep these other causes in mind for early recognition and management on the patient's behalf.

HISTORY

As with all chief complaints in medicine, an accurate recorded history must be obtained and is of particular importance for those patients presenting with low back pain. A particularly thorough history is needed from the person with chronic low back pain who has consulted many physicians in the past. It is extremely important that the history is complete and goes into those areas of systemic symptoms that may be related to the patient's chief complaint. There are many history forms available, developed to save the physician time in dealing with this painstaking problem. The forms, of course, do not supplant the physician and his one-on-one taking of the history from his patient. The forms do encourage the patient to think about his disease, and it would save some office time if the forms had been previously reviewed. The history must contain social and socioeconomic status, ethnic group, past medical history, medications, past medical illnesses, allergies, any recent illnesses prior to the onset of the chief complaint, and, if the patient is female, a gynecologic and obstetric history. It is critically important not to forget the family history, which should include questions regarding skin disorders such as psoriasis, colitis, arthritis disorders, or eye disorders present in other members of the family. The history should designate the time of onset of the problem and any associated circumstances, as well as any previous history of back pain, and if the present pain is similar or dissimilar to that experienced previously. Previous hospitalizations and/or procedures such as myelography should be noted. The onset of the pain should be coordinated with the type of pain and its relationship to activity, rest, and medications that may have been tried by the patient. The description of the pain, as well as its point of maximum intensity and any points of radiation, should be well documented. The change in the patient's particular ability to work, perform daily duties, participate in sports, or inability to relax because of the pain are critical data for the overall analysis of the severity of pain in this particular patient. If the patient is a woman, the relationship of the onset of the pain to the key portions of the menstrual cycle, to her age, and to her obstetric history is often helpful. The relationship of the back pain to any previous trauma, including obstetric trauma, such as in forceps or breech deliveries, or multiple gestations, should be reported. Systemic symptoms should be sought for such things as weight loss, malaise, tiredness, fever, and associated symptoms, particularly in the gastrointestinal system, such as diarrhea, or in the genitourinary system, such as dysuria or urethral discharge. Any history obtained of weight loss, skin or eye disorders, and symptoms of other joint involvement should call to the physician's attention the possibility of an underlying systemic collagen vascular disease. There is no doubt that low back pain has a strong psychological component and therefore any emotional stress or strain and its treatment should be sought in the history. A careful history can often elicit crucial information requiring immediate management. As an example, the diagnosis of spinal cord compression should always be considered even before any neurologic signs occur in any patient with a known carcinoma in whom back pain and tenderness develops, or in any patient with acute back pain who is found to have a lytic lesion of a vertebral body.

PHYSICAL EXAMINATION

Because a physician is looking for other than musculoskeletal causes of low back pain, a physical examination must be complete, with the patient undressed. Some critical information can be obtained by a physician's observation of the patient prior to the physical examination. The patient's age, appearance, coordination, and symmetry should be observed. The patient's complexion can be easily assessed as to pallor, ruddiness, or cyanosis. Disturbances of gait or disfigurements of joints should be noted. As an example, hypertrophic osteoarthropathy could suggest the underlying problem of chronic lung disease, cyanotic heart disease, or carcinoma of the lung. A careful examination of the skin can reveal diagnostic rashes such as psoriasis or the pathognomonic rash of ulcerative colitis, pyoderma gangrenosum. The old saying that "the eyes have it" may indeed be true if the patient is a young man with a red, painful, tearing eye, arthritis, and a urethral discharge as complaints.

Examination of the heart should include auscultation for murmurs of associated disease; a good example is the aortic insufficiency that may be seen in a patient with ankylosing spondylitis. Examination of the lungs should include auscultation for wheezes, diaphragmatic excursion for possible air trapping or decreased excursion secondary to ankylosing spondylitis, and auscultation for a localized wheeze to suggest the possibility of an obstruction secondary to a metastatic or primary carcinoma of the lung. Examination of the abdomen should include palpation for hepatomegaly and/or splenomegaly, and for any other masses that might suggest the possibility of primary or metastatic disease. Examination of the man is not complete without performing a rectal examination for a full evaluation of the prostate gland. Examination of the woman should include breast, pelvic, and rectal examinations with a Papanicolaou smear, Thayer-Martin culture if indicated, and bimanual examination for full evaluation of both tubes and ovaries and rectal shelf area. The neurologic examination can be critical, but neurologic findings may appear late and in many instances the physician should not wait until the appearance of these findings before definitive diagnosis is made and treatment instituted. Examination of the external genitalia of the man and woman, and rectal examination to include guaiac of the stool is necessary, and again, depending on the age of the patient, may be critical in the overall evaluation and diagnosis. As an example, a young man with bone pain, possibly pelvic symptoms, and a testicular mass has a testicular carcinoma with metastasis until proved otherwise.

No one part of the physical examination is virtually diagnostic. Only the entire physical examination as performed by the physician and evaluated by him in a reasonable period of time can ultimately give indications as to the underlying medical problem and its diagnosis and management. But, assuming that the rest of the physical examination has been duly covered by physicians in the past, let us now focus briefly on the physical examination as it relates to the lower part of the back. Height, weight, and chest expansion should be measured and recorded. Decrease in chest expansion is seen as one of the earliest physical findings of ankylosing spondylitis (an expansion of less than 2.5 cm should indicate this condition). As mentioned previously, often just watching the patient walk across the room in his or her underwear will give more information than a lengthy examination with the patient on the examining table fully clothed. The physician should look for the presence of asynchronous arm swing. With low back pain causing paravertebral muscular spasm, one sees rotation of the pelvis and an abnormality of gait. Physical examination of the back should include functional leg tests and Trendelenburg's tests to distinguish back pain and hip pain. Both in children and adults, one should always examine the back for the presence of scoliosis. If one examines a patient in the upright position and asks the patient to flex forward, one will note that the lordotic curve disappears in a normal person; however, people with conversion hysteria and malingerers, unlike those with a real muscle spasm, exhibit reverse lordosis on forward bending. Asynchronous motion of the bony skeleton generally points to underlying abnormality. With the patient standing bent forward in a flexed position, the physician can easily press or reach the interspinal space and localize tenderness and pain. Moderate or severe spasm will cause an involuntary motion. Areas of tenderness are also sought over the greater trochanter or the ischial tuberosity, the iliac crest, and the sacroiliac joints. Point tenderness over the sacroiliac joint in a patient with a history of drug abuse should serve to alert the physician to a diagnosis of osteomyelitis.

Examination of the lower back is not complete without a neurologic examination to record the tendon reflexes, particularly the patellar and Achilles tendons. As was previously mentioned, these tendon reflex changes may indeed be late in the course of the illness and the presence of the reflexes may not necessarily relate to the seriousness of the cause of the underlying back pain. In general, the patellar reflex is decreased or absent with a L3 or L4 spinal nerve compression. The Achilles tendon reflex is usually absent in L5–S1 nerve abnormality. Weakness of the extensor hallux longus muscle is usually a problem of the fifth lumbar spinal nerve, which would indicate a lesion of the L4–L5 interspace. Since the majority of lumbosacral disc disease takes place at the L5 or S1 level, the examination of the Achilles tendon reflex and extensor hallucis longus muscle function are critical in low back examination and in determining the cause of pain in the patient. Examination of the reflexes to show hyperactivity may well indicate an intraspinous lesion, such as a metastatic lesion in the cord area. Sensory deficits should be tested but these are sometimes difficult to evaluate because of the patient's subjective assessment of this particular examination. However, the particular findings of lower extremity numbness, evidence for neurologic deficit in testing the pinprick, and the light touch in the perianal area and the patient's history of incontinence should surely suggest the possibility of spinal cord compression, whether it is by primary or metastatic tumor.

PROBLEMS COMMON TO THE PEDIATRIC PATIENT

Since the family physician's practice includes pediatrics, certain common orthopedic problems particular to the pediatric patient should be mentioned first. In most pediatric patients who present to the physician with low back pain, the back pain is secondary to musculoskeletal causes. Pain in the lumbosacral spine is a much more common complaint than pain in the thoracic or cervical spine. The physical examination and history should again be complete, and bilateral comparison is often the simplest, most efficient way to determine the present location and extent of any abnormality. Causes of low back pain in children will be discussed in their order of frequency and importance.

Sprained Back or Low Back Derangement

A sprained back or low back derangement is characterized by the absence of neurologic findings, intact motor power, reflexes, sensation, and normal straight-leg-raising test results. Tenderness may be elicited by palpation and is usually localized within the paraspinal muscles. The condition usually subsides within seven to ten days and is best treated conservatively with application of heat, utilization of analgesics, and rest. Bracing of the spine often is not necessary, and perhaps careful neglect is the best treatment. Low back derangement or sprained back can be the result of a severe automobile accident, and one must be on the lookout then for nerve compression or acute disc herniation, or more serious injuries involving transection and/or contusion of the spinal cord.

Spondylolisthesis and Spondylolysis

Spondylolisthesis and spondylolysis occur much more frequently in teenagers, and the pain is usually complained of by the patient after strenuous activity, such as in sports. The two entities have been discussed earlier.

Scoliosis

Lateral curvature of the spine, or scoliosis, occurs not uncommonly in the pediatric patient but is usually not a cause of low back pain. Even when the curves are unusually excessive, back pain may appear, but it is relatively uncommon in the pediatric patient.

Scheuermann's Disease

Scheuermann's disease, or round back syndrome, is not uncommon in the pediatric patient, and does tend to produce pain in the thoracic spine area. If the condition is not excessive, it is best left alone. An excessive curve is probably best treated with a Milwaukee brace.

Tumors

Two tumors that may occur in the pediatric age group are osteoid osteomas and osteoblastomas, both of which are benign tumors of the bone. They usually involve the posterior elements of the vertebrae, and only rarely the vertebral bodies themselves. They can be a cause of back pain, and may cause mild scoliosis. Diagnosis is best performed by roentgenograms, and if pain is not removed by salicylate analgesics, surgery is usually recommended. Surgical removal usually produces instant and lasting relief of the pain.

Congenital Anomalies of the Spine

In general, congenital anomalies of the spine in the pediatric age group are seldom causes for the chief complaint of back pain by the patient. Spina bifida occulta is seldom, if ever, a cause of back pain in this age group. Of course, inspection of the back is extremely important to at least identify other congenital anomalies that may have significant neurologic deficits associated with them, such as Faun's beard, which is a doughy, fatty mass in the midline of the back, sometimes covered by excessive hair. This is good evidence for a lipoma that may extend to the spinal cord and produce neurologic symptoms.

Disc Space Infection

With the increase in drug abuse in our teenage population, disc space infection is not an uncommon cause of back pain as an initial complaint. The chief complaint of the patient is usually localized to the area of the underlying infection, and there is a definite tenderness on palpation of the spine over the infected disc space. Roentgenograms are usually not tremendously beneficial, although occasionally one may notice disc space narrowing. There is usually mild leukocytosis and an elevated sedimentation rate. Management is through identification of the inciting bacterial agent and institution of appropriate antibiotic therapy. This particular disease process will be covered more thoroughly in the section on osteomyelitis.

Lumbar Disc Syndrome

Although lumbar disc syndrome is a common cause of back pain in adults, it is usually rare in children. The physician should consider this as a cause of low back pain in the pediatric age group, but the diagnosis may be difficult since neurologic signs are usually less evident than on the adult examination. Here it is extremely important that the physician utilize comparison of both sides, since this is the only way small discrepancies in the neurologic examination will be noticed. In general, the treatment is the same, being conservative, with bed rest, analgesics, muscle relaxants, and appropriate consultation obtained if conservative therapy does not cause resolution of the symptoms.

Others

Other potential causes of low back pain in the pediatric age group include leg length discrepancy of greater than 2.5 cm, spinal tumors, and kidney stones. Renal stones are rare in children, and underlying metabolic disorders, such as cystinuria, should be looked for by the physician. The pain of renal stone is usually characteristic, being severe and acute in onset, unilateral, with well-documented radiation into the inguinal area. The finding of microscopic hematuria and positive Murphy's kidney punch are diagnostic.

MEDICAL CAUSES OF BACK PAIN IN THE ADULT

In the adult, other medical causes of low back pain must include ankylosing spondylitis, multiple myeloma, carcinoma with metastasis, or primary spinal lesions, postmenopausal osteoporosis, with or without compression fractures, Paget's disease, renal stone, renal vein thrombosis, acute pyelonephritis, pelvic inflammatory disease, pelvic congestion syndrome, and osteomyelitis. The physician must also consider that the back pain may be referral pain from other areas. Examples of this would be the back pain of acute pancreatitis or of a dissecting aortic aneurysm.

Ankylosing Spondylitis

Ankylosing spondylitis is frequently familial, much more common in men than in women, and represents a chronic inflammation of the joints of the axial skeleton that is usually manifested by the onset of morning stiffness and progressive stiffening of the spine. Probably one of the most important developments to change our concept of ankylosing spondylitis has been the discovery recently of a nearly 100% association between ankylosing spondylitis and the HLA-B27 antigen. This new laboratory test provides a very useful method for the physician to screen those patients with either a familial history of the disease or those young men who present with low back pain suggestive of ankylosing spondylitis. The test is still relatively expensive, and for that reason cannot be used yet for mass screening.

As was mentioned earlier, this disease is usually seen in relatively young males between the ages of 15 and 30 at the time of onset. The difficulty in making the initial diagnosis is due to the insidious onset of the disease. The patient may have been to many physicians prior to the time that he sees his present physician, and often many types of therapy have been prescribed without success. The medical history again becomes paramount, and it is important to attempt to extract a history, particularly of early morning stiffness and of episodes of aching low back pain. Although this disease is more common in men, any woman who has ulcerative colitis has an extremely high chance of developing ankylosing spondylitis at some point during her lifetime. It is also important to extract from the history that the pain is usually located in the low buttocks and thigh region, but rarely radiates into the hip, calf, or foot. Often, the disease is mild and there may be few systemic symptoms, but in a severe form, fatigue, weight loss, anorexia, fever, and any other systemic complaints may accompany the onset. Even though peripheral joint involvement may be present before the development of pain in the sacroiliac joint, the definitive diagnosis can only be presumptive until the sacroiliac joint is involved to such a degree to be demonstrated roentgenographically.

CLINICAL SIGNS

Clinical signs include sacroiliac tenderness and some limited motion of the lumbar spine in all planes of movement. An important physical finding is the loss of chest expansion because of rib cage involvement, and this can be easily checked by the physician by measuring chest expansion at the nipple line before and after deep inspiration. Observation of the patient at the time of the initial examination may allude to the possible diagnosis, since many of these patients have changed their posture and developed a thoracic kyphosis in order to ease the lower back pain.

Virtually any of the other joints of the axial skeleton may be involved, but most commonly the hips, shoulders, knees, wrists, metacarpophalangeal, and metatarsophalangeal joints are the secondary joints usually seen. When there is involvement of the hips and shoulders one may see permanent damage, but in the other joints the process often resolves without any residual disability or deformity, and this is similar to the arthritis that may be seen with inflammatory bowel disease.

It is important to note that usually no skin lesions occur with ankylosing spondylitis but that an anterior uveitis occurs in approximately 25% of the patients. There is usually no urethritis to help distinguish it from Reiter's syndrome. Other extraskeletal involvement in ankylosing spondylitis may include the development of aortic insufficiency or apical pulmonary fibrosis.

ROENTGENOGRAPHIC FINDINGS

Just as one of the early physical findings of ankylosing spondylitis is a decrease in chest expansion, so sclerosing of the sacroiliac joint is the roentgenographic finding. These joints will lose their clear-cut margin on roentgenograms, and as healing takes place following the inflammation there may be a complete fusion represented on the roentgenograms of the sacroiliac joint. One usually sees, as a manifestation of early changes in the spine, only demineralization of the vertebral bodies. However, as the disease progresses, one may see calcifications of the anulus fibrosus and the paravertebral ligaments, which gives rise to the so-called bamboo-spine appearance characteristic of ankylosing spondylitis.

HLA-B27 ANTIGEN

The current availability of the HLA-B27 antigen is critical in the diagnosis of ankylosing spondylitis. This antigen oc-curs in nearly 100% of white patients with ankylosing spondylitis, regardless of sex. It is critical to note, in spite of this strong association, that the presence of a positive HLA-B27 antigen does not reflect disease, and therefore is not a diagnostic criterion of ankylosing spondylitis. Other laboratory findings suggestive of the disease include an elevated sedimentation rate, mild hypochromic anemia, elevation of CSF protein, the presence of IgG antiglobulins, and an elevated creatinine phosphokinase level in the serum.

EXTRASKELETAL MANIFESTATIONS

In general, the extraskeletal manifestations are those of uveitis, aortic insufficiency, and apical pulmonary fibrosis. Because this is a chronic or long-standing disease, the development of secondary amyloidosis is not uncommon and should be particularly considered in those patients in whom chronic renal disease develops. Another late but uncommon manifestation of ankylosing spondylitis occurs with the involvement of the cauda equina; the patient may present with incontinence of urine, pain, and sensory loss in the sacral nerve distribution.

In summary, the diagnosis of ankylosing spondylitis should be based on the history as obtained from the patient, limitation of motion of the lumbar spine, point tenderness of the sacroiliac joints, limitation of chest expansion to 2.5 cm or less, roentgenographic changes of early sclerosis or late changes of fusion of the sacroiliac joints, and the presence, although this is not a diagnostic criterion, of the HLA-B27 antigen.

DIFFERENTIAL DIAGNOSIS

Differential diagnosis of ankylosing spondylitis must include Reiter's syndrome, psoriatic arthropathy, arthritis associated with chronic inflammatory bowel disease, and rheumatoid arthritis. The history again seems to be the most important differential point in screening patients for ankylosing spondylitis. The young man with insidious back pain of at least three months' duration, who complains of morning stiffness and who may give a history of improvement of the back pain with exercise, is surely at high risk of suspicion for having ankylosing spondylitis. Psoriatic arthropathy, although similar, usually has late involvement of the sacroiliac joints and involves both the small and the large joints, particularly of the upper extremity, and has very specific skin lesions associated with it. Although aortitis may occur in psoriatic arthropathy, urethritis is absent, as is pulmonary fibrosis. Reiter's syndrome is similar to psoriatic arthropathy in that sacroiliac joint involvement usually occurs late. In Reiter's syndrome, the small and large joints, particularly of the lower extremity, are affected, and skin lesions are usually specific. Uveitis may occur, and urethritis is present at least at some point in the illness. Aortitis may occur, but pulmonary fibrosis has not been reported. The arthritis associated with inflammatory bowel disease usually involves the large joints, particularly hips and shoulders, and sacroiliitis may be present early in the illness. Skin manifestations may be nonspecific or pathognomonic. In the patient with chronic ulcerative colitis, the skin lesion of pyodermic gangrenosum is at least very suggestive of the chronic underlying illness. It should be mentioned again that in those women with chronic ulcerative colitis the incidence of development of ankylosing spondylitis at some point during their lifetime is a significant possibility. In chronic inflammatory bowel disease, uveitis may occur but is uncommon. Urethritis is usually not present, and aortitis is rare.

TREATMENT

From both the physician's and the patient's perspective, diagnosis of ankylos-

ing spondylitis is at least partially gratifying insofar as specific therapy is available and the patient's relief of symptoms is often dramatic. In general, the drugs utilized in the treatment of ankylosing spondylitis are all anti-inflammatory agents. The salicylates should be utilized first, since these are least expensive and may offer dramatic relief to the patient. However, if the pain is severe, usually indomethacin is the drug of choice, and is particularly effective in alleviating the joint symptoms. The initial dose of indomethacin should be 25 mg twice daily, and this should be increased weekly to the lowest effective dose. The suggested maximum dose should not exceed 25 mg four times daily. One should be particularly cognizant of the side effects of indomethacin, which include headache, fatigue, nausea, vomiting, peptic ulcer disease, and depression. Phenylbutazone is extremely effective but, because of the complications of agranulocytosis and other hematologic abnormalities, it should be used with caution.

There are a number of nonsteroidal anti-inflammatory agents currently on the market. These agents, because of their anti-inflammatory effect, could be of benefit, but good studies are not yet available to show their effectiveness.

Probably the most important mode of therapy for the patient, in addition to the drug therapy, is exercise. The patient must be kept active and supported in his previous exercise activities. Swimming, sports, maintenance of ideal weight, and postural training must all be stressed. Just as in other illnesses, despite optimal management the patient may progress with irreversible deformities, and surgical techniques now are available to help correct the flexion deformities of the spine and to relieve chronic hip pain by replacement of the hip with a prosthesis. The decision to perform a hip replacement must be reviewed with the patient very carefully since ankylosis about the prosthesis does occur and has been reported in as many as 50% of the patients.

Early diagnosis, good long-term management, frequent follow-ups (including helping the patient to understand his disease), use of exercise, and the appropriate anti-inflammatory drugs usually will provide the patient with a normal life span. Death may occur as a complication of this long-standing disease, either by the development of aortic insufficiency or by the development of secondary amyloidosis and chronic renal disease. Since the valvular disease is a specific pathologic entity, it behooves the physician to examine for this frequently; if it is discovered, the patient should be educated as to the use of prophylaxis to prevent subacute bacterial endocarditis. It is important to stress to the patient that the usual course of the disease is not life-threatening, and that he should be able to maintain his current life-style and work load. This is extremely important in the way of supportive therapy.

Multiple Myeloma

Another disease that must be considered in the differential diagnosis of low back pain is multiple myeloma. This disease has been well described in numerous medical texts, and will only be reviewed here. Multiple myeloma is found in increasing incidence in patients over the age of 40. Men are affected twice as commonly as women. The early manifestations of the disease include systemic symptoms of weakness, anorexia, and weight loss. As the disease advances, other organ systems become involved resulting in bone pain, anemia, renal insufficiency, neurologic deficits, and/or bacterial infections. Usually, multiple lesions are found in bone, but in about 10% of the cases a single skeletal defect may be found. Although the classic lesion of multiple myeloma affecting the bone is

the so-called punched-out lesion with sharply demarcated edges on radiologic examination, the physician should be extremely suspicious of any middle-aged man who presents with back pain and diffuse osteoporosis not compatible with his age (Fig 7–25). Lesions of multiple myeloma may be found in any part of the bony skeleton, but in general they are more common in the skull, spine, ribs, and pelvis. As mentioned earlier, in about 25% of the cases there is generalized demineralization of the bones without focal punched-out lesions, and the physician should definitely be aware of this. Because of this demineralization or because of the punched-out lesions, pathologic fractures occur frequently, and there may be entire collapses of vertebral bodies resulting in nerve root or spinal cord compression. Hypercalcemia is not an uncommon laboratory finding.

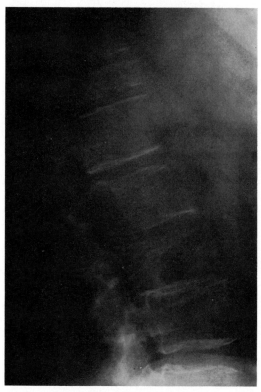

Fig 7–25. – Multiple myeloma.

In approximately half of the cases of patients with plasma cell disease the urine contains the Bence Jones protein, which has the unique property of precipitating in an acid pH when the temperature is between 4.4 and 15.6 C and redissolving when the temperature is raised to 32.2 C. The clinical diagnosis of multiple myeloma is based principally on the presence of the typical bone lesions, the characteristic dysproteinemia on serum protein electrophoresis, Bence Jones proteinuria, and the plasma cell infiltration of the marrow, peripheral blood, or other tissues. Because of the dysproteinemia, the patient may present with repeated episodes of pneumonia, meningitis, or urinary tract infection. The infections are often pneumococcal in origin and are apparently related to the patient's inability to synthesize normal amounts of specific antibody in response to the bacterial challenge.

One usually also sees a normochromic anemia, with systemic symptoms of anemia being among the initial complaints. Characteristically, the patient has a rapid sedimentation rate secondary to rouleau formation of the RBCs, and bloodgrouping procedures are difficult to carry out on these persons. Because of plasma cell proliferation in the marrow, one may also see leukopenia or thrombocytopenia. Plasmacytosis may be seen, but other causes, such as connective tissue disorders, neoplasm, cirrhosis of the liver, and some hypersensitivity states, must be excluded. It is well known that amyloidosis is often associated with multiple myeloma. This is so-called secondary amyloidosis. In men, particularly over the age of 40, who present with otherwise unexplained cardiac enlargement, congestive heart failure, or nephrotic syndrome, amyloidosis should be considered. In those patients with a previous history of multiple myeloma who may present with renal failure or nephrotic syndrome, the diagnosis of amyloidosis should be obvious. The ultimate diagnosis, of course, depends on obtaining a biopsy specimen and histologic staining for amyloid.

Simple, routine screening procedures for multiple myeloma consist of measuring the ESR and the serum concentrations of alkaline phosphatase and calcium. It should be mentioned that in this disease the alkaline phosphatase concentration is usually normal. The calcium concentration is elevated in only 25% to 40% of the patients, and the ESR can be normal in up to 20% to 30% of patients. Whenever there is low back pain, particularly in men over the age of 40, even in the absence of osteolytic lesions a serum electrophoresis for detection of M components and urine electrophoresis for detection of Bence Jones protein are indicated in order to rule out multiple myeloma.

Since patients with multiple myeloma may have hypercalcemia, hypercalciuria, and hyperuricemia, the importance of ambulation and adequate hydration in their treatment cannot be overstressed. Every effort should be made not to immobilize the patient and allow him to become bedridden with pain when first seen. Since plasma cell tumors are characteristically radiosensitive, x-ray therapy has been shown in the past to be of extreme help in the control of localized symptomatic lesions. Of the therapeutic drugs presently available in the treatment of multiple myeloma, melphalan (Alkeran), cyclophosphamide (Cytoxan), and prednisone are the drugs most useful for long-term treatment. An oncologist should be consulted since the treatment of these patients is long term and requires the expertise of more than one physician. Recently it has been shown that in a few patients who become refractory to continuous melphalan or cyclophosphamide therapy, some remissions have been achieved with a combination of cyclophosphamide and adriamycin. One can measure response to chemotherapy by objective signs of improvement, including decrease in concentration of abnormal M-type serum globulins, decreased Bence Jones proteinuria, hematologic improvement of the anemia, and cessation of further skeletal destruction as seen on roentgenograms.

Paget's Disease

Paget's disease is a nonmetabolic bone disease of unknown origin that causes excessive bone destruction and repair with associated deformities. Up to 3% of patients over the age of 50 may show localized lesions, but clinically important disease is much less common. Bone pain is usually the first symptom that the patient presents with; however, kyphosis, bowed tibias, large head, waddling gait, frequent fractures, and neuropathies may also be seen. Serum calcium and phosphate levels are normal and the alkaline phosphatase level is elevated. Roentgenograms usually show dense expanded bones. One must differentiate this disease from primary bone lesions, such as osteogenic sarcoma or multiple myeloma, and secondary bone lesions, such as metastatic carcinoma and osteitis fibrosis cystica. Overall, the prognosis of the mild form of this disease is good, and the most frequent complications are sarcomatous changes or renal complications secondary to hypercalciuria. The treatment generally consists of a high-protein diet with adequate vitamin C intake; a high calcium intake is generally desirable, and the use of antimetabolic hormones for osteoporosis should be considered. Salicylate analgesics usually are helpful in controlling the bone pain, and sodium fluoride has been tried in refractory cases. For progressive disease with symptomatology, thyrocalcitonin and mithramycin have recently been investigated and used.

Others

It should be mentioned briefly that the physician must not forget the well-documented back pain that occurs with acute pyelonephritis, renal vein thrombosis, and renal stone. The patient who presents with sudden onset of chills, fever, urinary frequency and urgency, and pain and tenderness in the costovertebral angle must be considered to have acute pyelonephritis. The elderly patient, often bedridden or in a nursing home, who contracts an illness that has the complication of dehydration and who then presents with acute onset of flank pain and back pain, an enlarging flank mass, and associated massive proteinuria should indeed be considered to have renal vein thrombosis. Of course, renal vein thrombosis can also be caused by renal carcinoma with renal vein metastasis and obstruction. It should be stressed that any elderly patient who presents with a nephrotic syndrome should be suspected of having multiple myeloma or renal vein thrombosis.

Low Back Pain in Women

Just as low back pain is one of the more frequent complaints heard by the family physician, it is also a common complaint in any gynecologic practice, though even the most common causes are musculoskeletal in origin. As regards pelvic causes of backache, retrodisplacement of the uterus may be associated with backache, especially when there is marked retroflexion of the uterus. Endometriosis and pelvic inflammatory disease frequently are associated with significant low backache and this pain may cause the patient to seek medical aid. Large posterior tumors in the pelvis may be painful by virtue of pressure or impingement on the sacral plexus. A very dangerous backache, of course, may occur with malignancies of the pelvis, especially carcinoma of the cervix. This usually indicates

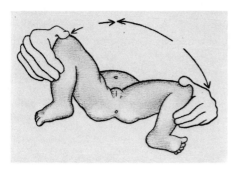

Fig 9–5.—Restricted abduction of the right hip.

eral and, although the cause is unknown, heredity appears to play a role. Females are affected nine times more often than males, and firstborns or children born by breech deliveries also have a higher incidence of the disorder. It is occasionally present in association with clubfoot and congenital muscular torticollis deformities.

Pathologically, abnormalities are seen in both the acetabulum and femoral head. The acetabulum may be more shallow in contour and more vertically inclined than normal, resulting in insufficient coverage and inadequate containment of the femoral head. The femur is often excessively anteverted, and the hip joint capsule may also be lax.

CLINICAL FEATURES

The clinical picture ranges from mild dysplasia, with minimal clinical findings, to subluxation and even to frank disloca-

tion. Complete dislocation is rarely present at birth, however, but may develop with weight bearing. The physical findings vary according to the amount of instability and the age of the patient.

In the newborn child, dysplasia is much more common than dislocation. The most important physical finding in this age group is limitation of abduction of the flexed hip (Fig 9–5). Any limitation of abduction to less than 50° or 60° is considered abnormal. The newborn child normally has a slight flexion contracture of the hip and knee, but the hips should be able to be fully abducted to lie flat on the examining table. If this is not possible, congenital hip dysplasia should be suspected. Asymmetry of the gluteal skin folds may also be noted. The various tests denoting hip instability are frequently positive (Fig 9–6). When positive, these tests suggest that the dysplasia may progress to dislocation if the condition is not treated.

When complete dislocation is present, there is frequently loss of the normal flexion contracture of the hip, and the affected extremity appears shorter (Fig 9–7). If weight bearing has begun, a painless limp is often the initial symptom. Hip motion, especially abduction, is limited, and abnormal piston mobility or "telescoping" may be present. The Trendelenburg test is usually positive. This test takes advantage of the fact that normally, when standing on one leg, contraction of

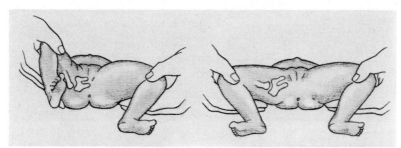

Fig 9–6.—Ortolani's test for congenital dislocation of the hip. A "click" is palpable or audible as the hip is reduced by abduction. If the test is negative, the examination should always be repeated in two to four months.

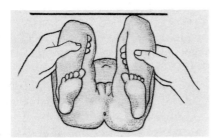

Fig 9–7.—Galeazzi's or Allis' sign. The child is placed on a firm surface with the hips and knees flexed. The knee will appear lower on the dislocated side.

the abductor muscles on the side bearing weight will cause the opposite side of the pelvis to be elevated. If the hip is dislocated, these muscles no longer work effectively, and when the child stands on the affected leg, the opposite side of the pelvis drops downward instead.

The roentgenographic examination is usually not very helpful when the patient is under 3 months of age unless a complete dislocation is present. After this

age, a delay in the ossification of the femoral head is frequently noted (Fig 9–8). The acetabulum may be more inclined vertically, and the acetabular index is often increased. If subluxation or dislocation has occurred, upward and outward displacement of the femoral head will be seen.

TREATMENT

Any suggestion of instability or stiffness in the hip of the newborn warrants treatment. The treatment is initiated as soon as possible and varies with the age of the patient and the degree of dysplasia. Early detection is of utmost importance as conservative treatment is more likely to succeed in the infant. The older the child is over the weight-bearing age, the more likely surgery will be necessary and the less likely a normal functional result will ensue. Whenever any doubt exists, treatment and follow-up are indicated.

The objective of treatment is to reduce

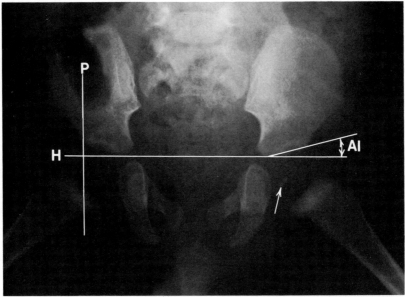

Fig 9–8.—Roentgenogram of the pelvis: P = Perkin's vertical line; H = Hilgenreiner's horizontal line, and the acetabular index *(AI)*. The ossification center of the capital femoral epiphysis should lie in the inferior medial quadrant formed by Perkin's and Hilgenreiner's line. The *AI* normally measures less than 30°. Here, ossification of the capital epiphysis on the dysplastic hip has been delayed compared to the left *(arrow)*.

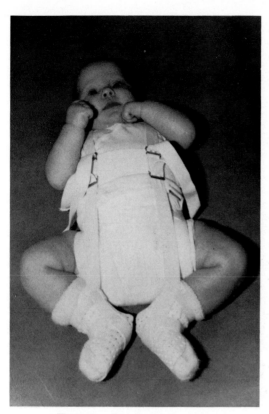

Fig 9–9. — The Pavlik harness.

much pressure on the femoral head, which may lead to avascular necrosis.

Failure to obtain or maintain a stable reduction necessitates surgical intervention. The objective is to reduce the hip by either closed or open methods and maintain the reduction by casting or osteotomy.

LEGG-CALVE-PERTHES DISEASE

Perthes disease or coxa plana is a self-limited disorder of the hip in which a portion of the ossific nucleus of the femoral head undergoes avascular necrosis. Eventually, the infarcted, necrotic bone is absorbed and replaced by normal bone. The cause of this condition is unknown but some cases follow transient synovitis of the hip. The disorder usually occurs between the ages of 4 and 10, and males are more commonly affected. Fifteen percent of cases are bilateral, and the condition is rare in blacks.

The disease is frequently divided into three stages. The early stage of the disease is characterized by inflammation and synovitis of the hip joint and early ischemic changes in the ossific nucleus of the femoral head. Roentgenograms taken at this stage reveal soft tissue swelling that may result in lateral displacement of the femoral head. An increase in the opacity of the ossific nucleus is usually present (Fig 9–10).

In the second, regenerative or fragmentation stage, the necrotic area begins to be replaced by viable bone. This phase lasts from one to two years. The roentgenographic appearance during this stage is one of fragmentation and compression of the femoral head with secondary widening of the femoral neck.

Reossification and healing occur in the third stage, which varies in duration beyond one year. The roentgenogram in this stage shows disappearance of the rarefaction while normal bone continues to reform. The final roentgenographic

the femoral head into the acetabulum and maintain that reduction. By maintaining the hip in the reduced position, normal development of the hip joint structures and acetabulum is encouraged. A variety of external devices are available for the treatment of the hip with moderate instability and stiffness. The most functional is the Pavlik harness, which maintains the hip in a more natural "human" position, allows active motion, and prevents full extension in the adducted position (Fig 9–9). The harness is usually worn for six weeks plus one week for each week in which the diagnosis has been delayed. This device does not force the hip into the excessive abduction that can occur when using triple diapers or many of the other abduction splints. This position of extreme abduction may actually be harmful to the hip by exerting too

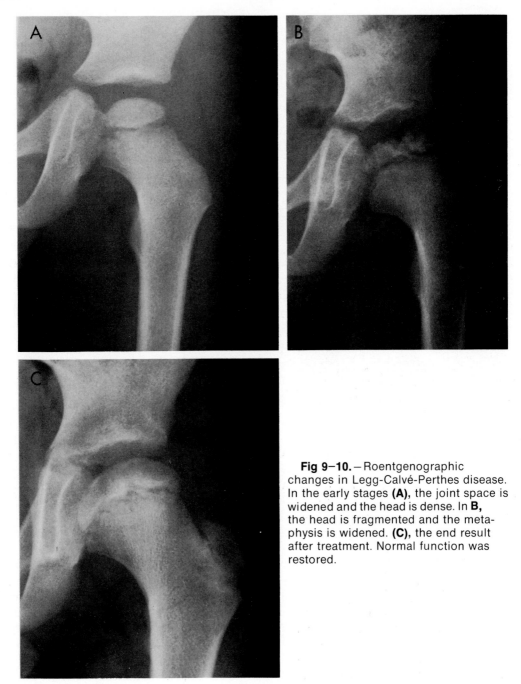

Fig 9–10. — Roentgenographic changes in Legg-Calvé-Perthes disease. In the early stages **(A),** the joint space is widened and the head is dense. In **B,** the head is fragmented and the meta-physis is widened. **(C),** the end result after treatment. Normal function was restored.

appearance depends on several factors, including the age of the patient, the degree of involvement, and the adequacy of treatment. The femoral head may be normal in shape or irregular and flat (coxa plana).

CLINICAL FEATURES

The onset is gradual and the initial complaint is usually a painful limp. The pain is often referred down the inner aspect of the thigh to the knee. The discomfort is frequently relieved by rest and aggravated by weight bearing.

Examination reveals moderate restriction of motion secondary to the synovitis. Abduction and internal rotation are especially limited. Pain is present at the extremes of motion, and tenderness is usually noted over the anterior hip joint.

TREATMENT

The ultimate goal of treatment is to prevent deformity of the femoral head from occurring while healing is progressing. If deformity can be prevented, the chances of degenerative joint disease developing at a later date are lessened. The immediate goals of treatment are the relief of pain, maintenance of joint motion, and containment of the femoral head in the acetabulum. If the head is contained in the acetabulum while it is reforming, the acetabulum will "mold" the head and prevent significant deformity from occurring. These goals of treatment are usually accomplished by the use of a brace that allows motion but contains the head in the acetabulum (Fig 9–11). The brace must be worn continuously for two to three years.

Surgery may be necessary in certain selected cases, but is usually reserved for those patients who fail to respond to conservative treatment. An osteotomy of the femur or innominate bone is performed in an attempt to provide "coverage" of the femoral head.

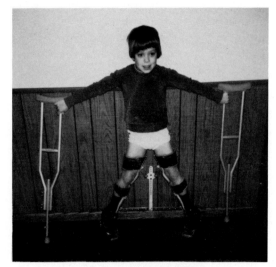

Fig 9–11.—Abduction brace.

The prognosis is dependent on the age of the patient, the degree of involvement, and the adequacy of treatment. Young patients with minimal involvement who are treated early do very well with few sequelae. Older patients, over the age of 8, frequently have some permanent restriction of motion, a slight limp, and a more irregular or flattened femoral head. A few patients will later develop degenerative arthritis.

SLIPPED CAPITAL FEMORAL EPIPHYSIS

Slipped capital femoral epiphysis is a disorder of unknown cause in which weakening of the epiphyseal plate of the upper femur occurs, resulting in upward and anterior displacement of the femoral neck. The actual amount of displacement will vary. In most cases, the slippage is gradual and some elements of healing are usually present.

The condition is seen most commonly in boys between the ages of 11 and 16 during their rapid growth spurt. The disorder is bilateral in 25% of cases and frequently occurs in two distinct body types. The first is the slender, tall, rapidly growing boy and the second is the large, obese boy with underdeveloped sexual characteristics. The presence of the disorder in these two body types suggests a hormonal cause, but none has ever been proved.

CLINICAL FEATURES

The onset is generally gradual, and symptoms usually occur even when little displacement is present. Discomfort in the hip and knee and a painful limp with activity are the most common initial complaints.

Examination reveals tenderness over the hip joint capsule. An external rotation deformity of the lower extremity may be present, and internal rotation, abduction, and flexion are usually restricted. Pain is

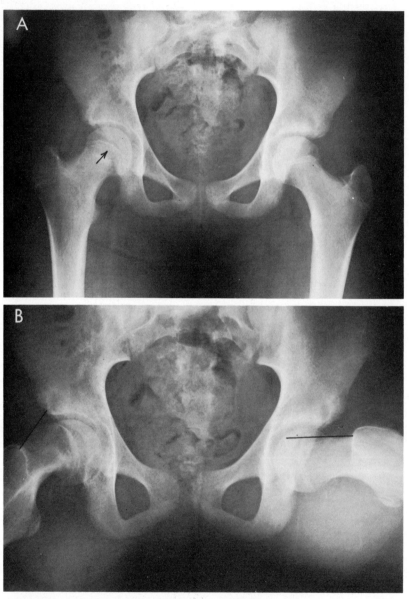

Fig 9–12.—Slipped capital femoral epiphysis. Widening of the epiphyseal plate *(arrow)* and displacement of the femoral head are present.

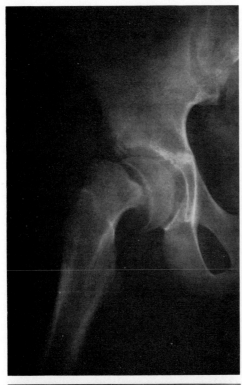
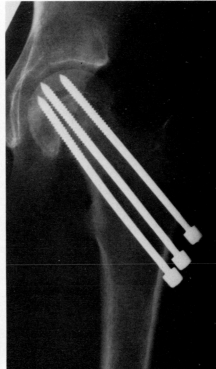
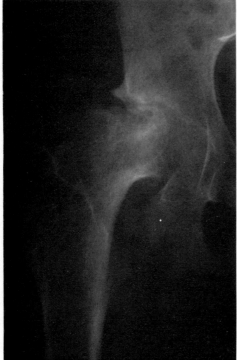

Fig 9–13 (above left). — Acute traumatic separation of the upper femoral epiphysis.

Fig 9–14 (above). — Postoperative roentgenogram following pinning for slipped capital femoral epiphysis.

Fig 9–15 (left). — Avascular necrosis following acute traumatic slipped capital femoral epiphysis. Reconstructive surgery was eventually required.

present at the extremes of motion, and the hip tends to rotate externally and abduct as it is flexed (Whitman's sign).

In the early "preslipping" stage, the roentgenogram characteristically reveals irregular widening of the epiphyseal plate and joint swelling (Fig 9–12). As displacement occurs, a line drawn along the superior or anterior neck of the femur will transect less of the femoral head than normal. This may be more readily seen on the lateral view. More severe degrees of slippage are usually easily diagnosed.

A condition similar to slipped capital femoral epiphysis is termed acute traumatic separation of the upper femoral epiphysis (Fig 9–13). This is actually an epiphyseal fracture and has a much poorer prognosis than the gradual slippage that occurs in slipped capital femoral epiphysis.

TREATMENT

As soon as the diagnosis is made, surgery is indicated. The patient is immediately placed on crutches and weight bearing is prohibited. Traction in the hospital may be necessary to reduce the acute component of the slippage. In order to prevent further slippage from occurring, the femoral head is fixed to the neck using small pins (Fig 9–14). Weight bearing is prohibited for several months until the epiphyseal plate closes. Severe deformities may also require osteotomy of the femur.

The prognosis is usually good, except in those cases with acute traumatic separation. Slight shortening of less than 1.25 cm may result along with a mild external rotation deformity. The internal fixation devices are usually removed after the epiphyseal plate closes in one to two years. In cases with acute traumatic separation, avascular necrosis of the femoral head is a common complication, and this usually results in severe traumatic arthritis of the hip (Fig 9–15).

ACUTE CARTILAGE NECROSIS

An occasional complication of slipped capital femoral epiphysis is acute necrosis or lysis of the articular cartilage of the hip joint. The articular surfaces of both the acetabulum and femoral head may be involved up to one year after the slippage. This condition appears to be directly related to the severity of the slippage. The cause of this process is unknown, but destruction and degeneration of the hyaline cartilage occurs. A painful fibrous ankylosis of the hip joint is frequently the end result.

TRANSIENT SYNOVITIS

Transient or "toxic" synovitis is a self-limited, nonspecific inflammation of the synovium of the hip joint that occurs in children. It is a common cause of pain in the hip in children under 10 years of age. The cause is unknown, but a viral infection is suspected. Its importance lies in its similarity to other hip joint disorders, especially septic arthritis.

CLINICAL FEATURES

The onset is frequently acute and may follow a traumatic event or a recent upper respiratory infection. A painful limp is characteristic, and the pain is frequently referred to the inner aspect of the thigh and knee joint. A few patients will have night pain.

The hip is typically held in a position of slight flexion, abduction, and external rotation so that the hip joint capsule is under the least amount of tension. Pressure and discomfort are thereby reduced. Passive motions, especially internal rotation and abduction, are restricted. Temperatures of 37.3 to 38.3 C may be present.

The roentgenogram may reveal swelling of the capsule and adjacent soft tissue. Slight widening of the joint space

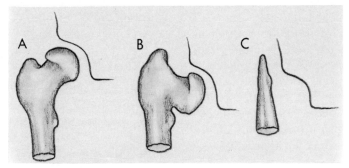

Fig 9–16. – **A,** the normal neck-shaft angle.
B, coxa vara. **C,** proximal focal femoral deficiency.

may also be present, but there are no changes in bone texture.

Laboratory findings are usually minimal, although there may be a slight increase in the WBC count. Aspiration and culture of the hip joint fluid are negative.

TREATMENT

Bed rest, gentle skin traction, and the elimination of weight bearing are indicated. The relief of pain and discomfort is usually rapid, and motion is restored in two to four days. Crutches are used for two to four weeks, and the patient is observed closely for up to two years because Perthes' disease will develop in a significant percentage (5% to 10%). Antibiotics are used only when the disorder is associated with an infection elsewhere.

COXA VARA

Coxa vara is an abnormality of the upper femur consisting of a decrease in the normal angle of inclination below 110° to 125° (Fig 9–16). This may result from a wide variety of acquired and congenital conditions and usually results in a shortened extremity.

Acquired Forms

These are the most common types of coxa vara. Included in this category are Perthes' disease, slipped capital femoral epiphysis, rickets, osteomalacia, and various injuries to the upper femur. Each disease has its own clinical and roentgenographic features.

Congenital Forms

Congenital local disturbances in the growth of the proximal femur may also lead to shortening and a significant coxa vara deformity. These disorders usually fall into three distinct classifications.

CONGENITAL COXA VARA (INFANTILE, CERVICAL, DEVELOPMENTAL)

This disorder is the result of faulty development of the femoral neck, which leads to the varus deformity. The cause is unknown. The disorder is frequently bilateral and becomes manifest after weight bearing has begun.

The child usually presents with a painless limp. If the disorder is bilateral, a "duck-waddle" gait may be present. In this gait pattern, the body sways from side to side. Abduction and internal rotation of the affected extremity are usually restricted, and the leg may be from 2.5 to 5 cm shorter than normal. The lumbar lordosis is usually exaggerated, and with continued weight bearing the varus deformity may progress.

The roentgenographic examination usually reveals a decrease in the neck-shaft angle. In addition, a triangular defect in the inferior aspect of the femoral neck may be present.

The treatment of mild deformities in which the neck-shaft angle is greater than 100° consists of a shoe lift, exercises to release contractures, and periodic reexamination. A brace that prohibits weight bearing may be necessary. More severe deformities require an osteotomy of the upper femur to correct the angulation.

CONGENITAL BOWED FEMUR WITH COXA VARA

This type of coxa vara is characterized by lateral bowing of the femur. The coxa vara is usually not as severe as that found with congenital coxa vara but the shortening of the extremity may reach 10 to 15 cm. The treatment consists of equalizing the extremities by shoe lifts.

CONGENITAL SHORT FEMUR WITH COXA VARA

This uncommon disorder is also known as proximal focal femoral deficiency. Portions of the proximal femur are either completely absent or severely underdeveloped and shortening of the limb may reach 25 to 37.5 cm by adulthood. Bracing is necessary in the young child, and amputation of the lower part of the leg, followed by prosthetic fitting to equalize the leg lengths, is usually the definitive treatment.

DEGENERATIVE ARTHRITIS

Degenerative arthritis confined to the hip joint is a common affliction in the middle and later years of adult life. The cause is not completely understood, but obesity, trauma, congenital hip dysplasia, avascular necrosis of the femoral head, and slipped capital femoral epiphysis are all factors in its onset.

Pathologically, the articular cartilage becomes progressively thinned and worn away. New bone proliferation around the femoral head and acetabulum occurs, and the synovium becomes chronically thickened and congested.

CLINICAL FEATURES

The clinical course is gradual, and both hips may be affected. The onset of symptoms may be precipitated by a relatively minor injury. Pain after activity and stiffness after rest are characteristic. The stiffness frequently subsides with activity and the pain frequently subsides with rest. The pain is often referred to the knee joint region. With the passage of time, the pain increases, sometimes even occurring at rest. Crepitus and grating in the hip may develop, and a painful limp is common.

Examination reveals tenderness over the anterior and posterior hip joint and restriction of motion, especially internal rotation and abduction. Pain is usually present at the extremes of motion. A flexion contracture frequently develops. This can be measured by the Thomas test. In this test, the patient is placed in a supine position and the opposite thigh is flexed up to the chest to eliminate motion at the pelvis and lumbar spine. The angle

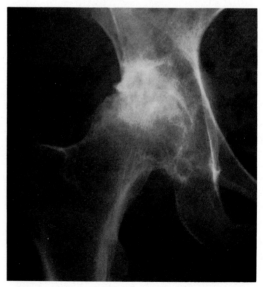

Fig 9–17. — Degenerative arthritis of the hip.

formed between the affected thigh and the examining table is the amount of flexion contracture of the hip.

The roentgenographic findings are characteristic (Fig 9–17). Irregular sclerosis, joint space narrowing, and osteophyte formation are prominent features.

TREATMENT

Conservative treatment will frequently eliminate symptoms and improve motion. The regimen requires a cooperative patient. Salicylates are prescribed in sufficient doses to relieve pain and reduce the inflammatory response. Ten to 12 tablets are usually required daily. Obesity must be corrected, and the joint placed at rest. Intermittent bed rest and the use of a cane when ambulatory are frequently sufficient. The cane is usually used in the hand opposite the affected extremity, and pressure is applied to the cane at the same time that weight is being borne on the painful hip. Buck's traction and moist heat are also helpful. Gentle range-of-motion exercise, such as swimming, will often overcome contractures and restore motion. The treatment plan may have to be repeated at intervals.

A variety of surgical procedures are available for those patients who fail to respond to conservative treatment. The most common procedures are arthrodesis, especially in the young patient, and total hip arthroplasty. The goal of each of these procedures is the elimination of pain. In addition, joint replacement will often improve hip joint motion. The indications for each procedure will vary according to the age and occupation of the patient.

AVASCULAR NECROSIS

Avascular or aseptic necrosis of the femoral head is an uncommon condition that occurs in the third to fifth decade. It is characterized by the development of an area of bone necrosis in the anterosuperior weight-bearing portion of the femoral head. The cause is unknown, but the condition is frequently bilateral and is more common in men. It is often seen in association with gouty arthritis, chronic alcoholism, and chronic renal disease, and in those patients who have undergone long-term steroid therapy. It probably occurs secondary to a circulatory disturbance to the femoral head. Following the initial infarction, collapse and fragmentation may occur, which lead to deformity of the femoral head and degenerative arthritis.

CLINICAL FEATURES

The onset is gradual, with pain and a slight limp being common. A history of trauma is usually absent. Joint motion becomes progressively restricted.

The roentgenogram reveals an increase in the density of the superior portion of

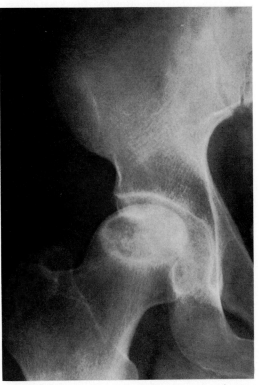

Fig 9–18. — Avascular necrosis of the femoral head.

the femur (Fig 9–18). A radiolucent zone is frequently present between the avascular segment and the surrounding bone. The joint space is usually well preserved until late in the disease, when degenerative arthritis intervenes.

TREATMENT

The goal of treatment is to prevent collapse of the femoral head and encourage repair of the necrotic area. With minimal involvement, prolonged abstinence from weight bearing by the use of crutches may allow replacement of the avascular segment, but bone grafting to hasten this reconstitution is frequently necessary. Later in the disease, when collapse has occurred, prosthetic replacement is indicated.

BURSITIS

Several bursae are present about the hip joint. The one most subjected to irritation and pain is the trochanteric bursa. This sac lies between the greater trochanter and the overlying tendinous portion of the gluteus maximus muscle. Inflammation of the sac is common in the elderly patient and is characterized by local pain over the trochanter that frequently radiates down the lateral aspect of the thigh to the knee. This pain pattern may cause confusion with lumbar disc disease. Local tenderness is usually present and hip motion, especially internal rotation and abduction, may be painful. It is difficult for the patient to lie on the affected side.

Treatment consists of moist heat, rest, and anti-inflammatory agents. Ultrasound to the affected area may be beneficial, and a local injection of a steroid/lidocaine mixture into the area of maximum tenderness is frequently curative.

MERALGIA PARESTHETICA

Meralgia paresthetica is an uncommon disorder characterized by pain and paresthesias occurring along the course of the lateral femoral cutaneous nerve of the thigh. This nerve enters the leg beneath the inguinal ligament and supplies sensation to the anterolateral aspect of the thigh. Painful involvement of the nerve may be confused with hip and low back disorders. The cause of this condition is unknown, but direct pressure or constriction of the nerve at its point of exit into the thigh is thought to play a role.

CLINICAL FEATURES

The disorder is sometimes seen in obese patients or those who wear tight corsets or undergarments. Hypersensitivity, burning, tingling, and pain that occurs with activity or direct pressure over the nerve are characteristic. The symptoms are often relieved by rest.

The pain may be aggravated by passive extension of the hip. A slight decrease in sensation over the anterolateral aspect of the thigh is sometimes noted and pain may be reproduced with pressure on the nerve medial to the anterior superior iliac spine.

TREATMENT

Symptoms usually subside over a variable length of time. Weight loss and the avoidance of constricting garments are advised. Injection of the nerve distal to the inguinal ligament 1.25 cm medial and 2.5 cm below the anterosuperior iliac spine with a local anesthetic may relieve symptoms. Surgical release or even removal of the nerve may occasionally be necessary for intractable cases, but the surgical results are only fair.

PROTRUSIO ACETABULI (OTTO PELVIS)

Abnormal intrapelvic protrusion of the acetabulum is a relatively uncommon disorder of unknown cause. It may be present on a congenital basis or develop secondary to trauma or arthritis. It is fre-

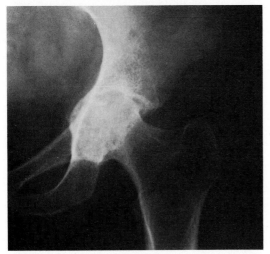

Fig 9–19.—Protrusio acetabuli. The medial acetabular wall protrudes and the femoral head has migrated medially.

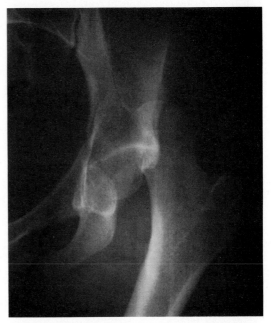

Fig 9–20.—Posterior dislocation of the hip.

quently bilateral and is characterized by abnormal deepening of the acetabulum, which allows the femoral head to be displaced further into the pelvis.

CLINICAL FEATURES

The onset is usually gradual, with progressive restriction of hip motion occurring over several years. Eventually, with the onset of degenerative arthritis, pain becomes a prominent symptom. Complete ankylosis of the joint frequently occurs.

The roentgenogram reveals abnormal protrusion of the medial wall of the acetabulum with thinning and degenerative changes (Fig 9–19).

TREATMENT

Traction and the avoidance of weight bearing are indicated in early cases. Arthrodesis in the unilateral case or total hip replacement may be necessary for disabling pain.

DISLOCATIONS OF THE HIP

Dislocations of the hip are the result of severe trauma and are usually posterior

in direction (Fig 9–20). They commonly result from the knee being struck while the hip and the knee are in a flexed position. This force drives the femoral head out of the joint posteriorly. These injuries are frequently associated with fractures of the posterior acetabular wall.

CLINICAL FEATURES

With posterior dislocation, the hip is characteristically held in a position of flexion and internal rotation. All motions are painful. There may be an associated injury of the ipsilateral knee.

TREATMENT

In the dislocated position, great tension is placed on the blood supply to the femoral head. Avascular necrosis may even result if the dislocation is not promptly reduced. In order to prevent this complication, early reduction within six to twelve hours is indicated. The reduction can usually be accomplished by traction on the flexed hip with countertraction on the pelvis. A general anesthetic is usually necessary. If closed reduction fails, or an acetabular fragment is present that is of sufficient size to produce instability, open reduction is indicated.

The reduction is frequently maintained by skeletal traction until sufficient soft tissue and bony healing have occurred to prevent redislocation. Weight bearing is prohibited for an additional two to three months.

BIBLIOGRAPHY

Aadalen, R. J., et al.: Acute slipped capital femoral epiphysis, J. Bone Joint Surg. 56A: 1473, 1974.

Aegerter, E., and Kirkpatrick, J. A.: *Orthopedic Diseases* (3d ed.; Philadelphia: W. B. Saunders Co., 1968).

Amstutz, H. C., and Wilson, P. D., Jr.: Dysgenesis of the proximal femur (coxa vara) and its surgical management, J. Bone Joint Surg. 44A:1, 1962.

Cattaral, A.: The natural history of Perthes' disease, J. Bone Joint Surg. 53B:37, 1971.

Coleman, S. S.: Treatment of congenital dislocation of the hip, J. Bone Joint Surg. 47A: 590, 1965.

Curtis, B. H., et al.: Treatment for Legg-Perthes' disease with the Newington ambulation-abduction brace, J. Bone Joint Surg. 56A:1135, 1974.

Epstein, H. C.: Posterior fracture-dislocations of the hip, J. Bone Joint Surg. 56A:1103, 1974.

Friedenberg, Z. B.: Protrusio acetabuli, Am. J. Surg. 85:764, 1953.

Gage, J. R., and Winter, R. B.: Avascular necrosis of the capital femoral epiphysis as a complication of closed reduction of congenital dislocation of the hip, J. Bone Joint Surg. 54A:373, 1972.

Gore, D. R.: Iatrogenic avascular necrosis of the hip in young children, J. Bone Joint Surg. 56A:493, 1974.

Grant, J. C. B.: *A Method of Anatomy* (6th ed.; Baltimore: Williams & Wilkins Co., 1958).

Hermel, M. B., and Albert, S. M.: Transient synovitis of the hip, Clin. Orthop. 22:21, 1962.

Ilfeld, F. W., and Makin, M.: Damage to the capital femoral epiphysis due to Frejka pillow treatment, J. Bone Joint Surg. 59A:654, 1977.

Marcus, N. D., Enneking, W. F., and Massan, R. A.: The silent hip in idiopathic aseptic necrosis (treatment by bone-grafting), J. Bone Joint Surg. 55A:1351, 1973.

Mitchell, G. P.: Problems in the early diagnosis and management of congenital dislocation of the hip, J. Bone Joint Surg. 54B:4, 1972.

Petrie, J. G., and Bitenc, I.: The abduction weight-bearing treatment in Legg-Perthes' disease, J. Bone Joint Surg. 53B:56, 1971.

Ramsey, P. L., Lasser, S., and MacEwen, G. D.: Congenital dislocation of the hip: Use of the Pavlik harness in the child during the first six months of life, J. Bone Joint Surg. 58A:1000, 1976.

Smith, K., Bonfiglio, M., and Dolan, K.: Roentgenographic search for avascular necrosis of the head of the femur in alcoholics and normal adults, J. Bone Joint Surg. 59A: 391, 1977.

Solomon, L.: Drug-induced arthropathy and necrosis of the femoral head, J. Bone Joint Surg. 55B:246, 1973.

Somerville, E. W.: Perthes' disease of the hip, J. Bone Joint Surg. 53B:639, 1971.

Stewart, M. J., and Milford, L. W.: Fracture-dislocation of the hip, J. Bone Joint Surg. 36A:315, 1954.

Tachdjian, M. O.: *Pediatric Orthopedics* (Philadelphia: W. B. Saunders Co., 1972).

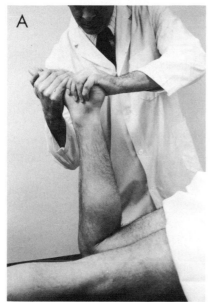
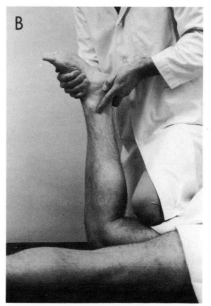

Fig 10–8.—Apley's test. The patient is prone and the knee is flexed 90°. **A,** to test for meniscus injury, the "grinding" test is performed. Downward pressure is applied to the foot as it is rotated. The joint is then flexed and extend-ed. A painful response may indicate meniscus damage. **B,** the foot is then lifted and the joint is distracted. Pain with rotation in this position may indicate ligamentous disease rather than meniscus injury.

will compress out the joint effusion and they should always be performed with the knee in the extended position in order to prevent patellofemoral pain from developing. Gentle range-of-motion exercises are started in two to three days. Swimming is an excellent exercise for increasing motion and decreasing muscle spasm and discomfort. As pain subsides and motion returns, weight-bearing activities are gradually resumed, but quadriceps exercises are continued for two to four weeks.

There are few indications for aspiration of the knee and even fewer indications for the injection of steroids in the treatment of the acute injury. The protective responses of the patient should be maintained, and it is better to reduce swelling by quadriceps contractions and to rehabilitate the knee through exercises.

Surgery is reserved for those cases of true irreducible locking, or cases with recurrent or persistent signs and symp-toms of meniscus injury. The meniscus is removed in order to prevent irreversible articular damage from occurring. The results are usually excellent, and most patients are able to resume normal activities six to eight weeks after surgery.

Discoid Meniscus

Because of a failure in normal development, a meniscus, usually the lateral, may be elliptical rather than semilunar. The most common clinical finding in this disorder is an audible click that occurs with motion of the knee joint. The click may be present in infancy, but the disorder is usually not otherwise symptomatic at this age. The meniscus frequently wears away so that the clicking disappears.

Occasionally, however, symptoms persist into adulthood, with clicking and aching pain at the lateral joint margin being common complaints. A palpable degenerative cyst may even form in the

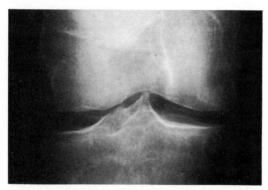

Fig 10–9.—Calcification of the meniscus.

meniscus. Local tenderness at the lateral joint space is usually present.

Meniscectomy may be necessary in the adult with persistent symptoms. Infants usually require no treatment.

Calcification of the Menisci

The meniscus can become calcified from a variety of causes (Fig 10–9), the most common being degeneration and trauma. However, calcification can also occur in several other conditions, including degenerative arthritis, ochronosis, and pseudogout. The calcification is usually not painful in itself. The symptoms are those that result from the primary disorder, and treatment is directed at that disorder.

CYSTS

Only two types of cystic lesions, the popliteal cyst and the cyst of the semilunar cartilage, occur with any frequency around the knee joint. The popliteal or Baker's cyst is an enlargement of the semimembranous bursa that is normally present in the medial aspect of the popliteal space. It may occur in any age group. In children, the cyst appears to be a primary lesion, in contrast to adults in whom most of these cysts are secondary to an intra-articular abnormality of the knee. This intra-articular abnormality, frequently a posterior tear of the medial meniscus or rheumatoid arthritis, causes an increase in the joint fluid. This chronic effusion opens the normal anatomical communication between the joint and cyst and allows fluid to escape into the semimembranous bursa.

CLINICAL FEATURES

In children, the symptoms are usually related to the effects of direct pressure of the cyst on the adjacent soft tissues. Local discomfort is common. In adults, the symptoms are related not only to the effects of the pressure of the cyst but also to the primary intra-articular abnormality. Many cysts are asymptomatic, however. The cyst commonly changes in size, depending on the activity of the patient and the amount of swelling in the knee.

Examination will reveal a cystic mass of variable size lateral to the medial hamstrings in the popliteal fossa. Local tenderness may be present. Other findings of primary joint disease may be present, especially in adults.

The roentgenogram is usually normal. Arthrographic studies, however, will usually reveal the cyst (Fig 10–10).

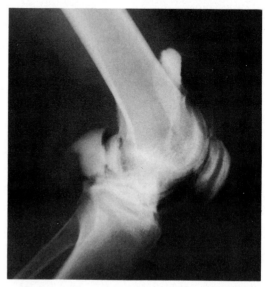

Fig 10–10.—Arthrogram revealing a large popliteal cyst.

TREATMENT

In children with primary cysts, the treatment should be conservative. There is a high rate of spontaneous disappearance of the cyst in this age group and an equally high rate of recurrence following surgical excision. Aspiration and injection of the cyst may be attempted but it is usually not necessary because the cyst frequently disappears in one to two years.

In adults, every attempt should be made to detect any underlying joint abnormality. Cyst excision without correction of the intra-articular abnormality is followed by a high rate of recurrence of the cyst. Correction of the intra-articular disease will also frequently make cyst excision unnecessary as the cyst becomes asymptomatic following elimination of the cause of the chronic effusion. Older patients are often treated successfully by aspiration alone.

Cysts may also develop in a meniscus, usually the lateral, as a result of degeneration or trauma. The patient is generally a young adult who has a history of pain and a gradually enlarging mass over the lateral joint line. A knee effusion may be present. Treatment consists of meniscectomy and cyst excision.

LESIONS OF THE LIGAMENTS

Ligamentous injuries to the knee are among the most serious of all knee disorders. Because of the importance of the ligaments in stabilizing the joint, early diagnosis of the injury is mandatory. Any delay in diagnosis and treatment may lead to a chronically unstable knee, which predisposes it to early traumatic arthritis.

The mechanism is usually one of forceful stress against the knee with the extremity bearing weight. A valgus stress against the knee may sprain or tear the medial collateral ligament, and a varus stress will injure the lateral collateral ligament. Tears of the cruciate ligaments, menisci, and capsule may also occur in conjunction with the collateral ligament injury.

CLINICAL FEATURES

The history of the injury is often difficult to reconstruct but will provide clues to the type of force applied to the knee. After the injury, the ability to bear weight on the extremity is often lost. Swelling from an acute ligament or capsular tear is usually immediate due to hemorrhage. A "pop" or tearing sensation may be heard or felt. Incomplete tears or sprains are often more painful than complete ligamentous ruptures.

Patients with chronically unstable knees due to old injuries often complain of the knee going out or giving way and of their not being able to depend on the extremity. These symptoms are always most noticeable during vigorous activities. A chronic effusion is often present.

The examination is of utmost importance in the acute injury. Any swelling or discoloration is noted. The lesion can frequently be localized by palpation alone. The palpation should begin away from the suspected area in order to promote cooperation. A point of maximum tenderness is often present along the course of the collateral ligament or capsule.

The knee should always be tested for stability with the patient relaxed in the supine position. If the examination cannot be adequately performed because of pain or hamstring spasm, it may have to be repeated with the patient under local or general anesthesia. The injured knee is always compared to the opposite, uninvolved knee. The tests are performed in the following sequence:

1. Abduction-adduction stress testing at 30° of knee flexion. With the knee

flexed 30°, the cruciate ligaments are relaxed. This prevents them from producing a false negative test. The medial and lateral ligaments can then be tested by applying valgus and varus stresses to the knee (Fig 10–11). If no laxity exists when the knee is tested in 30° of flexion, it can usually be assumed that no significant injury to the cruciate ligaments is present either, because injury to the cruciate ligament without injury to the collateral ligament is uncommon. If laxity exists in either direction with testing, however, the test reflects an injury to the collateral ligament.

2. Abduction-adduction stress testing at 0°. Valgus and varus stresses are applied in the same manner as when the knee was tested at 30° of flexion. If the knee was stable at 30°, it will also be stable at 0° because the collateral ligaments are intact. With the knee in extension, however, the cruciate ligaments tighten

and by themselves can prevent the joint from opening in spite of a collateral ligament tear. Therefore, if the knee is stable in extension, the cruciate ligaments are probably intact. If it is not, a very serious knee injury has occurred with a significant cruciate ligament tear being present in addition to the collateral ligament injury.

3. Drawer signs. Anteroposterior and rotatory instability are tested by determining how much abnormal excursion of the tibia is present when anterior and posterior stresses are applied to the tibia with the knee in a flexed position (Fig 10–12). Anterior drawer testing is performed with the foot in external rotation, neutral rotation, and internal rotation. Abnormal forward excursion of the tibia with the foot in either position is highly suggestive of a significant injury to the anterior cruciate ligament and joint capsule. The posterior drawer test is then performed by applying backward pressure against the tibia. Abnormal laxity with this test is present with posterior cruciate and posterior capsular injuries.

Roentgenographic examination may reveal avulsion fractures pulled off by the injured ligament (Fig 10–13). Stress films may also be helpful in determining whether complete or incomplete ligamentous disruption is present. Roentgenograms should always be obtained in the growing child below the age of 15 with open epiphyses to rule out a fracture of the distal femoral epiphysis that may simulate collateral ligament injury (Fig 10–14). Arthrography may reveal leakage of dye out of the capsule, but the test is usually not necessary if a good clinical examination is performed.

TREATMENT

Minor ligament sprains are treated in the same manner as meniscus injuries. Immobilization in a compression dress-

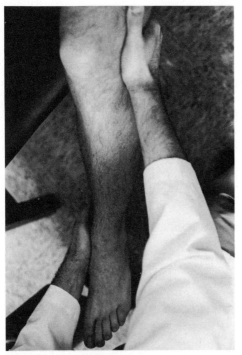

Fig 10–11.—Abduction stress test at 30°. To test the lateral collateral ligament, a varus stress is applied.

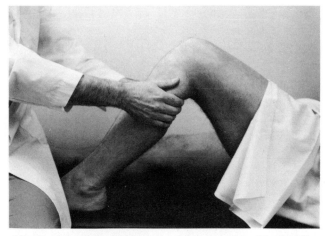

Fig 10–12. — The drawer test is performed with the hip flexed 45° and the knee flexed 90°

ing with ice and elevation for two to three days are followed by quadriceps exercises and heat to promote absorption of swelling and restoration of motion.

Minor sprains are easily differentiated from complete ruptures, but small partial ruptures are frequently difficult to diagnose. When there is certainty that a complete rupture does not exist, partial tears may be treated by plaster immobiliza-

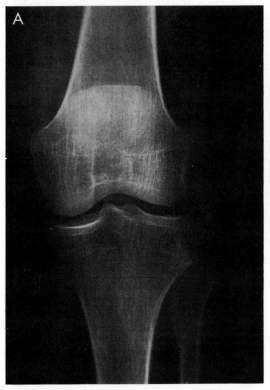

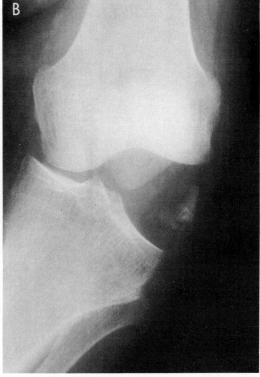

Fig 10–13. — **A,** anteroposterior roentgenogram of an injured knee. When a stress is applied **(B),** the true significance of the injury becomes apparent.

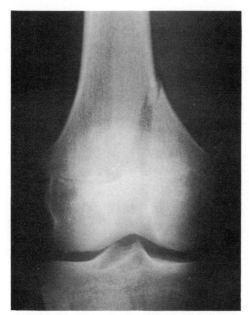

Fig 10–14.—Roentgenogram of the knee revealing an epiphyseal fracture of the lower femur that may be misdiagnosed as a ligamentous injury clinically.

tion. The extremity is placed in a long leg cast for six weeks with the joint closed on the side of the injury. After removal of the cast, a progressive knee rehabilitation program is begun, consisting of range-of-motion and hamstring and quadriceps-strengthening exercises.

Early surgical repair is indicated when the rupture is complete. Restoration of stability can only be accomplished by accurate suture of the ruptured ligament followed by casting for eight weeks. Postoperatively, exercises are begun and continued for several months after cast removal. The knee is often protected during this period of time by a specially constructed brace (Fig 10–15).

Chronic ligamentous instability usually requires reconstructive surgery in order to prevent further joint deterioration. A well-constructed brace may provide an alternative to surgery in the active individual.

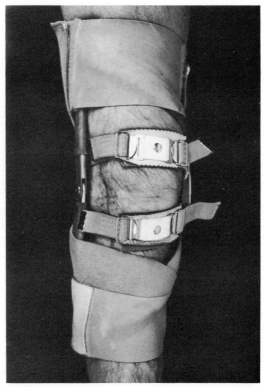

Fig 10–15.—The Lenox Hill brace is made from a cast impression of the injured knee. Most other braces of elastic or leather with hinges are of only limited value.

Pellegrini-Stieda Disease

Occasionally, a sprain of the medial collateral ligament is followed by the formation of a calcified mass at the site of the ligament injury (Fig 10–16). This area of dystrophic calcification may remain tender and swollen for an extended period of time. Ossification of the mass may even occur. The symptoms gradually subside, and symptomatic treatment is usually all that is necessary. The mass rarely needs to be removed.

DISORDERS OF THE EXTENSOR MECHANISM

The extensor mechanism of the knee is made up of the quadriceps muscles, the

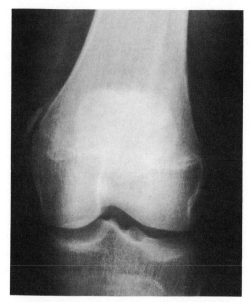

Fig 10–16. — Pellegrini-Stieda disease.

patella, and the patellar tendon. Several painful disorders may alter its function.

Chondromalacia of the Patella

Chondromalacia of the patella is a degenerative process of unknown cause that frequently occurs in young adults. It is one of the most common causes of knee pain in this age group. Several factors play a role in its formation.

Any injury or anatomical abnormality that predisposes to an irregular pattern of movement of the patella can lead to chondromalacia. Meniscus injuries frequently alter normal tibiofemoral motion, which, in turn, alters patellofemoral motion and can lead to pain. Recurrent subluxation of the patella, quadriceps imbalance, and angular deformities about the knee may cause an increase in pressure on the articular cartilage of one side of the patella. Direct trauma, such as that which occurs with a fall or a dashboard injury to the patella, may also predispose to continued patellofemoral pain.

Degenerative changes of varying degrees are seen in the articular surface of the patella. Grossly, the cartilage loses its normal smooth, glistening appearance and becomes fibrillated and frayed. It may even be completely denuded, thereby exposing the underlying subchondral bone.

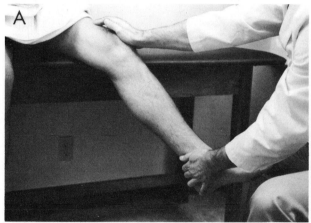
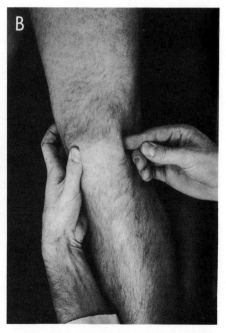

Fig 10–17. — Examination for retropatellar pain. **A,** with the knee slightly flexed, pressure against the patella as the knee is actively extended may produce typical pain. **B,** with the knee extended, the patella is displaced medially or laterally. Pain is reproduced by digital pressure under either the medial or lateral patellar facet.

CLINICAL FEATURES

The majority of patients are teenagers or young adults. Pain beneath the patella is the most common symptom. It is characteristically aggravated by walking up and down stairs, an activity that puts the greatest force against the patella. Squatting and prolonged sitting with the knee in flexion are also uncomfortable. This discomfort is often relieved by extension of the knee. Symptoms of giving way, crepitus, or locking may be present, and a history of previous trauma is common. The disease is frequently bilateral and may be confused with a meniscus injury.

Examination will reveal local tenderness, particularly under the medial facet of the patella. Direct pressure against the patella may be painful, and contraction of the quadriceps against patellar pressure is often uncomfortable (Fig 10–17). Swelling and crepitus may also be present, although there is no direct correlation between the presence of crepitus and the pain. The roentgenograms are usually normal.

TREATMENT

Treatment is directed toward the underlying cause, if any is present. Otherwise, aspirin, moist heat, and intensive quadriceps exercises in extension are usually helpful. Many cases recover spontaneously. If symptoms persist, surgery may be indicated. It usually consists of excision of the affected articular cartilage combined with realignment of the extensor mechanism to prevent abnormal patellar motion. Significant improvement is obtained in most cases.

Recurrent Subluxation of the Patella

Recurrent subluxation of the patella is a common disorder that is often undiagnosed because the symptoms are similar to other "internal derangements" of the knee. The patella usually subluxes or dislocates laterally. The condition may follow an acute patellar dislocation that fails to heal properly. The disorder is frequently bilateral and is one of the most common causes of internal derangement in the athlete.

CLINICAL FEATURES

The symptoms are pain, swelling, and a sensation of the knee giving out. Acute dislocation may even occur but, more commonly, the symptoms are due to recurrent subluxation.

Physical examination usually reveals local tenderness over the medial facet of the patella and in the soft tissue medial to the patella. The patella appears laterally displaced and may also appear higher than normal when the knee is slightly flexed (patella alta). Passive hypermobility with lateral displacement is often not-

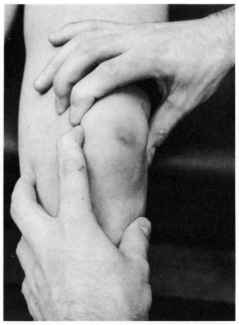

Fig 10–18.—The "apprehension" test. Abnormal lateral hypermobility may be noted when attempting to displace the patella laterally with the knee relaxed and slightly flexed. The patient may even become apprehensive and grab the examiner's arm to prevent further displacement.

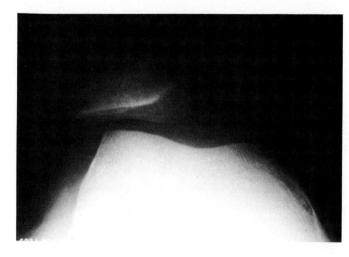

Fig 10–19. – "Sunrise" view of the knee revealing abnormal lateral displacement of the patella.

ed when pressure is applied against the patella with the knee relaxed (Fig 10–18). A joint effusion and mild quadriceps atrophy may be present.

Roentgenographic studies are frequently helpful. A "sunrise" view taken with the knee relaxed in slight flexion will often reveal lateral displacement (Fig 10–19).

TREATMENT

Treatment is directed at improving extensor muscle tone. Quadriceps exercises in extension are begun, and aspirin and moist heat are prescribed as necessary. Frequently, the vastus medialis portion of the quadriceps will strengthen enough to prevent further lateral subluxation from occurring.

Surgery may be indicated to reconstruct the extensor mechanism in order to prevent recurrence. A variety of procedures are available. All of them attempt to realign the patella either at the patella itself or distally at the patellar tendon insertion in order to prevent abnormal lateral excursion from occurring.

Acute Dislocation of the Patella

A sudden valgus strain to the knee or a direct blow against the medial aspect of the patella may cause the patella to dislo-

cate laterally. The deformity is usually obvious, with the patella displaced in the lateral position and the knee held in slight flexion. Roentgenographic examination should always be performed in order to rule out any associated osteochondral fracture.

Reduction is easily accomplished by lifting the heel of the extremity off the table. This extends the knee and flexes the hip, thereby relaxing the entire quadriceps mechanism. Gentle pressure against the patella may be necessary to complete the reduction. The knee is immobilized for six weeks by a cylinder cast applied with the knee in slight flexion. Exercises are begun as soon as the cast is removed.

Traumatic dislocation is always accompanied by a partial rupture of the medial retinaculum and supporting structures of the patella. This may lead to recurrent episodes of subluxation or dislocation. If it does, surgical reconstruction of the extensor mechanism may be necessary.

Ruptures of the Extensor Mechanism

The extensor mechanism is occasionally ruptured as a result of trauma. The rupture may take place in the quadriceps muscle or the patellar tendon. Active extension is immediately lost but pain may be minimal, especially in the older patient with chronic degeneration of the muscle-tendon unit.

CLINICAL FEATURES

Clinically, hemorrhage and a palpable sulcus are present in the area of the rupture. Extension of the knee is markedly weakened or even completely absent.

A lateral roentgenogram taken with the knee in 90° of flexion will usually reveal proximal displacement of the patella when the rupture has occurred in the patellar tendon (Fig 10–20). Roentgenograms are usually not helpful when the rupture has occurred proximal to the patella in the quadriceps mechanism.

TREATMENT

The treatment is immediate surgical repair followed by cast immobilization for six to eight weeks.

Osgood-Schlatter Disease

Osgood-Schlatter disease is a disorder that involves the growing tibial tuberosity of adolescents. The cause is unknown, but the disorder is generally considered to be a traumatically produced lesion that occurs at the attachment of the patellar tendon to the tibial tuberosity. It is a self-limited condition that ends with closure of the upper tibial epiphyseal plate. The disorder usually becomes manifest between the ages of 8 and 15 and is frequently bilateral. Males are affected three times as often as females.

CLINICAL FEATURES

Local pain, swelling, and tenderness over the tibial tubercle are characteristic clinical features. The pain is accentuated by activity. Stair walking and squatting on the knees may be especially uncomfortable. The pain is also increased by extension of the knee against resistance.

A lateral roentgenogram of the upper tibia with the leg slightly internally rotated usually reveals variable degrees of separation and fragmentation of the upper tibial epiphysis. Occasionally, the fragmented area fails to unite to the tibia and persists into adulthood (Fig 10–21).

Fig 10–20. — Rupture of the patellar tendon with marked proximal displacement of the patella.

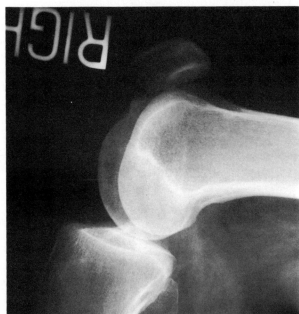

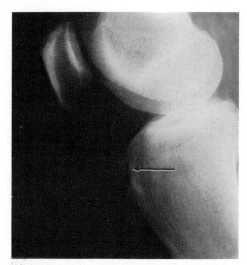

Fig 10–21. — Osgood-Schlatter disease *(arrow)*.

TREATMENT

Removing the stress on the tendon is usually sufficient treatment. Simple abstinence from physical activity will re-

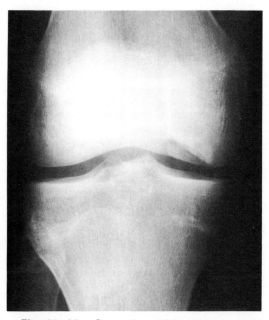

Fig 10–22. — Osteochondritis dissecans of the knee. The "tunnel" view is frequently helpful in visualizing the defect. This fragment may become detached and form a loose body. This area should not be confused with the normal irregularity of the distal femoral epiphysis in young children.

lieve the symptoms in most cases. Temporary immobilization in a cylinder cast or knee splint for four to six weeks may be necessary in resistant cases. Surgery is rarely indicated. The prognosis for complete restoration of function and relief from pain is excellent.

OSTEOCHONDRITIS DISSECANS

Osteochondritis dissecans is a condition of unknown cause in which a segment of subchondral bone undergoes avascular necrosis. This segment of bone, with its overlying articular cartilage, may separate or become detached from the joint surface, producing a loose body. The knee is the most common joint affected, and the lateral surface of the medial femoral condyle is the area that is usually involved. The condition is primarily a disorder of young adults, but it may also be seen in children. Males are more commonly affected, and the disorder may be bilateral.

CLINICAL FEATURES

The symptoms consist of pain, stiffness, and swelling that are worsened with activity. A painful limp is frequently present, and locking may even occur if the fragment has become detached.

Diminished motion, swelling, and medial joint tenderness are usually present. This tenderness may be well localized and is best elicited by deep local pressure over the affected area with the knee flexed 90°.

The roentgenogram is usually diagnostic (Fig 10–22). A fragment of avascular bone is seen that is demarcated from the adjacent femur by a radiolucent line. Occasionally, a loose body may be present.

TREATMENT

Undisplaced lesions in children are treated conservatively. The joint is protected from weight bearing by the use of crutches. A plaster cylinder cast with the knee in slight flexion may also be necessary. Several months are required for complete healing.

In the older child, the lesion is less likely to heal and surgery is frequently indicated. Simple drilling of the undetached fragment to encourage the ingrowth of blood vessels into the avascular segment is usually all that is necessary. In any age group, detached fragments should be replaced if the weight-bearing surface is involved, but they may be removed if the joint surface is not involved.

LOOSE BODIES

Loose bodies, commonly referred to as "joint mice," are often found in the knee joint. They may be present as the result of osteoarthritis, osteochondral fractures, osteochondritis dissecans, or secondary to primary disease of the synovium.

CLINICAL FEATURES

Loose bodies may cause swelling and intermittent locking of the joint. There is frequently a feeling of weakness and instability. The loose body is occasionally palpable and freely movable.

The roentgenogram is usually diagnostic. A primary lesion such as osteochondritis dissecans may be detected, but frequently no joint abnormality other than the loose body is visualized.

TREATMENT

The treatment is surgical. Because of the mechanical interference with motion and resultant wear on the articular surface, most loose bodies should be removed. Any underlying abnormality is corrected at the same time.

DEGENERATIVE ARTHRITIS

The knee is the joint most commonly affected by osteoarthritis. Although the cause is unknown, obesity, trauma, liga-

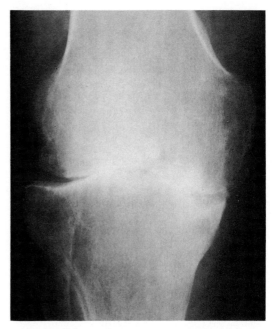

Fig 10–23.—Degenerative arthritis of the knee. The joint space is severely narrowed.

mentous instability, and malalignment of the lower extremity all play significant roles. The pathologic features have been described elsewhere (chapter 9).

CLINICAL FEATURES

The symptoms are similar to those that occur with osteoarthritis in any other joint. Pain with activity that is relieved by rest is characteristic. Morning stiffness that is relieved by activity is also usually present. A chronic effusion is not uncommon. Crepitus and grating are also frequent complaints. Restriction of motion, joint swelling, local tenderness, and deformity are common clinical findings.

The roentgenographic features consist of joint space narrowing, osteophyte formation, and sclerosis in the subchondral region (Fig 10–23).

TREATMENT

Symptoms are often relieved by conservative treatment consisting of weight loss, rest, salicylates, and quadriceps exercises. A cane is frequently helpful to relieve the weight-bearing stress. An intra-articular injection of steroid may be indicated in the older patient to relieve the acute inflammatory response. When pain is diminished, gentle range-of-motion exercises are begun in order to overcome contractures.

Surgical treatment involves elimination of the painful weight-bearing articulation. Arthrodesis in the active young adult will eliminate the pain, but the patient may find the permanent stiffness disturbing. Realignment osteotomy and joint replacement are indicated in older patients.

BURSITIS

Bursa sacs are present wherever soft tissue, such as muscle or tendon, moves over a bony prominence. One such bursa that is frequently symptomatic in the knee is the anserine bursa. This bursa is located deep to the insertions of the semitendinous, gracilis, and sartorius tendons (Fig 10–24). Local measures, including moist heat, rest, and the injection of a steroid/lidocaine mixture into the tender bursa, are usually curative. Salicylates are given to control pain and inflammation.

The prepatellar bursa lies between the skin and the patella. It frequently becomes irritated from recurrent trauma, especially kneeling (housemaid's knee). It is also occasionally involved in infection. Chronic traumatic changes may occur with permanent thickening of the bursa, which makes it more prone to recurrent injury.

Acute traumatic prepatellar bursitis usually responds to rest and moist heat. If infection occurs, open drainage, followed by the appropriate antibiotic coverage, is indicated. The chronic, swollen bursa that is vulnerable to repeated injuries should be excised. Complete excision with elimination of all dead space will usually result in a prompt cure.

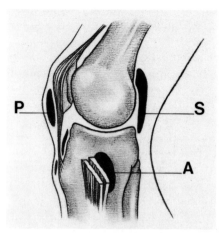

Fig 10–24. — Bursae of the knee: *A* = anserine bursa; *P* = prepatellar bursa; *S* = semimembranous bursa that may become enlarged and form Baker's cyst.

TENDINITIS

Several tendons adjacent to the knee joint may become chronically inflamed. The patellar tendon, quadriceps tendon, and flexor tendons are the ones most commonly involved. Pain with activity and local point tenderness are characteristic clinical features. As in most cases of tendinitis, the pain is aggravated by passive stretching of the tendon as well as by forceful contraction of the muscle-tendon unit against resistance.

The treatment is symptomatic with rest, heat, and anti-inflammatory medication. Steroid injections may be helpful, but the patellar tendon should never be injected. Temporary cast immobilization is occasionally necessary in resistant cases.

ARTHROSCOPY

Endoscopic examination is becoming an increasingly valuable tool in the diagnosis of disorders of the knee. The procedure is safe and relatively minor, with virtually no morbidity. It may be performed on an outpatient basis, with ambulation being possible shortly after the procedure. It is frequently done prior to routine arthrotomy of the knee in order to more adequately visualize the internal structures.

Its diagnostic accuracy exceeds 90% and its use frequently prevents needless surgery. Newer arthroscopes are being developed for minor intra-articular surgery.

Among its common uses is the detection of unsuspected lesions that may require a more complete surgical correction. It is frequently indicated in adults with Baker's cysts to determine if any intra-articular abnormality is present that needs treatment instead of removal of the cyst. It is also helpful in difficult diagnostic problems in those symptomatic knees with vague symptoms and few physical findings.

BIBLIOGRAPHY

Aegerter, E., and Kirkpatrick, J. A.: *Orthopedic Diseases* (3d ed.: Philadelphia: W. B. Saunders Co., 1968).

Brantigan, O. C., and Voshell, A. F.: The mechanics of the ligaments and menisci of the knee joint, J. Bone Joint Surg. 23:44, 1941.

Childress, H. M.: Popliteal cysts associated with undiagnosed posterior lesions of the medial meniscus, J. Bone Joint Surg. 52A: 1487, 1970.

Crosby, E. B., and Insall, J.: Recurrent dislocation of the patella, J. Bone Joint Surg. 58A:9, 1976.

Dandy, D. J., and Jackson, R. W.: The impact of arthroscopy on the management of disorders of the knee, J. Bone Joint Surg. 57B: 346, 1975.

Dinham, J. M.: Popliteal cysts in children, J. Bone Joint Surg. 57B:69, 1975.

Ficat, R. P., and Hungerford, D. S.: *Disorders of the Patello-femoral Joint* (Baltimore: Williams & Wilkins Co., 1977).

Goodfellow, J., Hungerford, D. S., and Woods, C.: Patello-femoral joint mechanics and pathology: Chondromalacia patellae, J. Bone Joint Surg. 58B:291, 1976.

Goodfellow, J., Hungerford, D. S., and Zindel, M.: Patello-femoral joint mechanics and pathology: Functional anatomy of the patello-femoral joint, J. Bone Joint Surg. 58B:287, 1976.

Helfet, A. J.: *Disorders of the Knee* (Philadelphia: J. B. Lippincott Co., 1974).

Hughston, J. C., et al.: The classification of knee ligament instabilities: I. The medial compartment and cruciate ligaments, J. Bone Joint Surg. 58A:159, 1976.

Hughston, J. C., et al.: The classification of knee ligament instabilities: II. The lateral compartment, J. Bone Joint Surg. 58A:173, 1976.

Insall, J., Falvo, K. A., and Wise, D. W.: Chondromalacia patellae, J. Bone Joint Surg. 58A:1, 1976.

Laurin, C. A., et al.: The abnormal lateral patellofemoral angle: A diagnostic roentgenographic sign of recurrent patellar subluxation, J. Bone Joint Surg. 60A:55, 1978.

Lipscomb, P. R., Jr., Lipscomb, P. R., Sr., and Bryan, R. S.: Osteochondritis dissecans of the knee with loose fragments, J. Bone Joint Surg. 60A:235, 1978.

Nicholas, J. A.: The five-one reconstruction for anteromedial instability of the knee, J. Bone Joint Surg. 55A:899, 1973.

O'Donoghue, D. H.: *Treatment of Injuries to Athletes* (3d ed.; Philadelphia: W. B. Saunders Co., 1976).

Slocum, D. B., and Larson, R. L.: Rotatory instability of the knee: Its pathogenesis and a clinical test to demonstrate its presence, J. Bone Joint Surg. 50A:211, 1968.

Wolfe, R. D., and Colloff, B.: Popliteal cysts, J. Bone Joint Surg. 54A:1057, 1972.

11 / The Ankle and Foot

THE ANKLE AND FOOT perform two major roles: they support the body and propel it forward. In the process of performing these functions, several painful conditions may develop. Most of these develop in the forefoot, and many of them are caused by poorly fitted shoes.

ANATOMY

The ankle is a hinge joint composed of the articular surfaces of the lower tibia, talus, and medial and lateral malleoli (Fig 11–1). The stability of this joint or "mortise" is maintained by the malleoli and their ligaments, which grasp the talus and prevent medial and lateral dis-

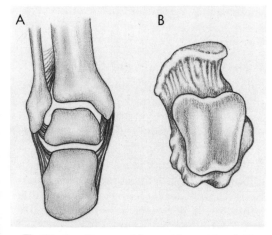

Fig 11–1. — Bones of the ankle and heel. The talus is held in position in the mortise by the malleoli and ankle ligaments **(A).** Its articular surface is wider anteriorly than posteriorly **(B).** The ankle is, therefore, more stable in neutral or slight dorsiflexion when the wider anterior portion of the talus fits in the mortise. It is unstable in plantar flexion. Wearing high-heeled shoes, therefore, may lead to chronic ankle and calf pain. Eversion and inversion movements take place in the subtalar (talocalcaneal) joint.

placement. The talus and socket are both broader in front, an arrangement that provides maximum stability when the ankle is in dorsiflexion or neutral, and prevents posterior displacement. Only movements of dorsiflexion and plantar flexion occur at the ankle.

The foot is composed of 26 bones, 12 of which are components of the medial and lateral longitudinal arches (Fig 11–2). Strong fascial supports maintain these arches and prevent collapse (Fig 11–3). Eversion and inversion movements of the foot take place in the hindfoot at the subtalar joint. Injury or disease that affects this joint will cause pain in the region of the heel when walking on uneven or irregular surfaces. Abduction and adduction movements occur in the midfoot or midtarsal joints.

FLATFOOT

Flatfoot is a common disorder that is defined as a depression or loss of the medial longitudinal arch of the foot usually combined with valgus or eversion of the heel and abduction of the forefoot. An apparent flatfoot is present in many children up to the age of 2. This is due to the presence of a fat pad in the area of the longitudinal arch. As the fat pad atrophies with weight bearing, the normal arch usually becomes visible. Flatfoot is usually one of two types, flexible or rigid.

Flexible Flatfoot

Flexible or hypermobile flatfoot is a disorder frequently seen in both adults and children. The condition is often hereditary and varies in severity. It is fre-

143

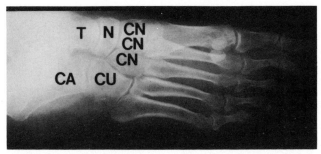

Fig 11–2.—Roentgenogram of the foot: *N* = navicular; *T* = talus; *CA* = calcaneus; *CU* = cuboid; *CN* = cuneiforms medial, intermediate, and lateral. The foot is divided into the forefoot (phalanges and metatarsals), midfoot (tarsals), and hindfoot (talus and calcaneus).

quently associated with a tight Achilles tendon (heel cord). The tight heel cord tends to hold the heel in eversion. With growth, stretching of the medial ligaments of the foot and ankle may occur.

CLINICAL FEATURES

The symptoms consist of pain, burning, and easy fatigability. With weight bearing, the heels are everted and the forefoot appears pronated and abducted (Fig 11–4). When it is not bearing weight, the foot often looks normal. Absence of the medial arch is apparent and the foot is mobile without any fixed deformity. A mild genu valgum (knock-knee) or internal tibial torsion may be present. With the heel inverted, passive dorsiflexion of the ankle will be limited if the heel cord is tight.

A lateral roentgenogram taken with the foot bearing weight will reveal loss of the normal arch and plantar flexion of the talus (Fig 11–5). Some secondary bony changes may be present in the adult.

TREATMENT

The treatment of flexible flatfoot is controversial. Many mild deformities improve spontaneously with maturity. Symptoms are rare during childhood and uncommon even in the adult with moderately severe deformity. Actually, most foot pain in young adults is due to an abnormally high rather than an abnormally low arch. Shoe corrections for this condition have never been scientifically proved to be of benefit. The standard treatment has always been to prescribe heel wedges and scaphoid cushions in order to correct the heel eversion and give support to the arch. In spite of wearing these shoes for several years, however, most children will still have a true flatfoot, both clinically and roentgenographically. Heel cups appear to offer some improvement over previous methods of treatment. They keep the heel in

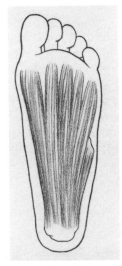

Fig 11–3.—The plantar fascia. It may be affected by Dupuytren's contracture similar to the hand.

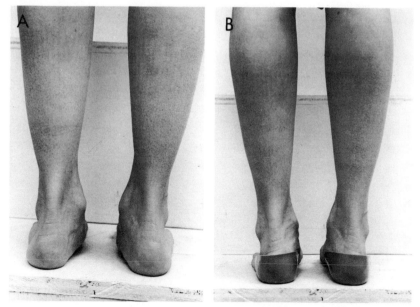

Fig 11–4. – **A,** flatfoot deformity with eversion of the heels and loss of the normal longitudinal arch. **B,** correction with heel cup.

the neutral position, correct the plantar flexion of the talus, and restore the longitudinal arch. Many cases will be permanently improved in two to three years. Exercises are of doubtful value, except for those that stretch the tight heel cords (Fig 11–6). These exercises will cure many cases associated with heel cord contractures. Surgery is reserved for symptomatic cases but is rarely indicated.

Rigid Flatfoot

Rigid or peroneal spastic flatfoot differs from flexible flatfoot in that the deformity is not passively correctable. This condition is usually secondary to a tarsal coalition or arthritis in the hindfoot. Tarsal coalitions are congenital cartilaginous or bony bridges that may be found between the two bones of the hindfoot or between either of these bones and the navicular.

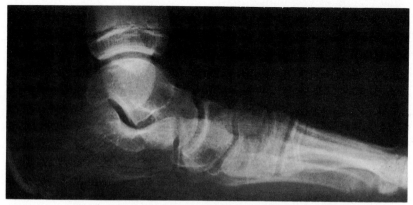

Fig 11–5. – Lateral weight-bearing roentgenogram revealing plantar flexion of the talus.

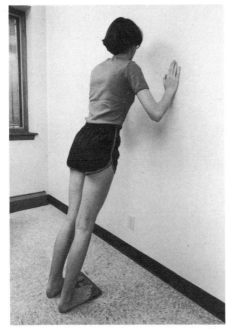

Fig 11–6.—Heel cord stretching exercises. The legs are internally rotated, the forefeet are placed on a 2.5-cm board, and the patient leans forward.

The resultant loss of motion in the hindfoot leads to local irritation and protective spasm in the peroneal muscles.

CLINICAL FEATURES

The onset of the disorder is usually gradual and begins in early adolescence if it is due to a coalition. Stiffness and a painful limp are the most common initial symptoms. Tenderness and pain may be present over the peroneal tendons or in the hindfoot. The heel is frequently everted, and midtarsal and subtalar motions are limited and painful. The forefoot may be abducted. Passive stretching of the peroneal tendons by forefoot adduction and inversion frequently reproduces the pain. Swelling will be present if the disorder is secondary to a rheumatoid process.

Roentgenograms may reveal arthritic changes in the hindfoot or the presence of a coalition (Fig 11–7).

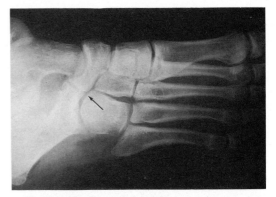

Fig 11–7.—Tarsal coalition. An incomplete calcaneonavicular bar is present *(arrow)*. The anterior process of the calcaneus is abnormally prolonged.

TREATMENT

Symptomatic treatment is indicated in early cases. Rest, heat, and salicylates are usually helpful. A short walking cast may be worn intermittently to relieve symptoms. Surgery is frequently necessary, however. If the disorder is secondary to arthritis, arthrodesis of the hindfoot and navicular is indicated. When a tarsal coalition is present, the bony or cartilaginous bar may be resected. If this does not alleviate the symptoms, arthrodesis is usually performed.

CLUBFOOT

Congenital clubfoot or talipes equinovarus is a fixed deformity that is present at birth. It is frequently bilateral and a hereditary factor is often present. The cause is unknown.

CLINICAL FEATURES

The deformity consists of three major components, none of which is passively correctable. This distinguishes clubfoot from other common foot deformities. The three components are equinus of the ankle and forefoot, varus of the heel, and adduction of the forefoot (Fig 11–8). The medial border of the foot is concave and the lateral border is convex.

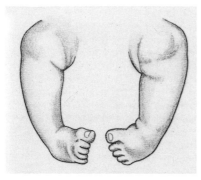

Fig 11–8. — Bilateral clubfeet (talipes equino-varus).

TREATMENT

The treatment consists of manipulation of the foot, in order to stretch the contracted soft tissues, followed by the application of a corrective cast. The cast is changed at weekly intervals and the foot is further manipulated until complete correction is obtained. Six to eight weeks are usually required. This method of treatment will frequently succeed if it is begun at an early age.

Approximately 50% of all cases of clubfoot will require some sort of corrective surgery. The procedures range from simple heel cord lengthening to wide soft tissue releases. The most common indication for surgery is resistance to correction by the usual casting methods.

Following full correction, a night brace or splint is worn for one to two years to maintain the correction and prevent relapse of the deformity. In addition, passive stretching exercises are performed by the patients on a daily basis.

CALCANEOVALGUS

Talipes calcaneovalgus is a common congenital deformity characterized by excessive eversion of the foot. The cause is unknown, but positional compression in utero is likely. In contrast to clubfoot, the deformity is not fixed and may be easily overcorrected.

CLINICAL FEATURES

The deformity is easily diagnosed shortly after birth. Marked laxity of the ligaments of the foot and ankle is obvious, and the foot can often be dorsiflexed so that the toes touch the anterior aspect of the tibia (Fig 11–9). The heel cord may appear to be severely stretched.

TREATMENT

Mild cases require no treatment. More severe cases respond well to passive stretching exercises. Corrective casts may be necessary for a short period of time. A mild flatfoot deformity may persist that could require corrective appliances when the child begins ambulation.

KÖHLER'S DISEASE

The tarsal navicular may undergo avascular necrosis similar to that which occurs in other bones. The cause of all of these disorders is not completely understood, but interference with the circulation to the bone is thought to be the usual cause of the ischemia.

The onset of this disorder is about the age of 5. A painful limp is the usual initial complaint. Local pain, tenderness, and swelling over the navicular bone are frequently present.

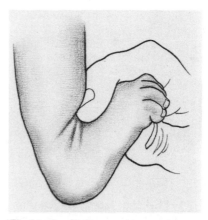

Fig 11–9. — Talipes calcaneovalgus.

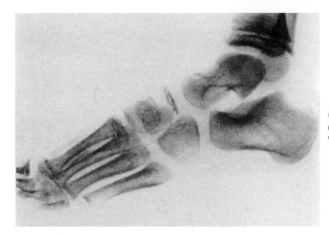

Fig 11–10.—Köhler's disease. (From Blount, W. P.: *Fractures in Children* © 1955 by Williams & Wilkins Co.)

The roentgenographic appearance is usually characteristic. Flattening, sclerosis, and irregularity of the navicular are usually present (Fig 11–10).

Protection from excessive trauma, usually by the use of a short walking cast for seven to eight weeks, is sufficient treatment in most cases. Spontaneous recovery is the rule, and complete reossification of the navicular usually occurs within two to three years.

ANKLE SPRAINS

The ankle sprain is the most common of all ankle injuries. Most of these injuries occur to the lateral ligaments as the result of an inversion and plantar flexion force that stretches or tears these ligaments (Fig 11–11).

CLINICAL FEATURES

The symptoms will depend on the severity of the injury. Mild sprains may be associated with only slight loss of function, but, in more severe injuries, swelling and pain are significant and prohibit further use of the extremity.

TREATMENT

The treatment will depend on the severity of the injury. Although some disagreement exists regarding the treatment of the severe injury with complete ligamentous disruption, mild and moderate sprains are always treated nonoperatively.

Initially, all of these injuries are elevated and packed in ice to prevent further swelling. A bulky compression dressing is applied for comfort and to assist in the control of swelling.

Mild sprains are then treated by early motion and exercise after the initial pain has subsided. Moderate sprains without instability should be treated by the application of a short walking cast that is maintained for approximately four weeks. The heel is placed in slight eversion and the ankle is placed in the neutral position.

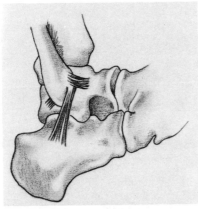

Fig 11–11.—The lateral ankle ligaments, anterior and posterior talofibular and calcaneofibular.

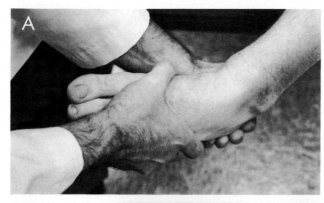

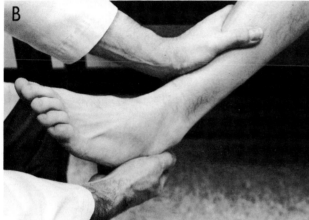

Fig 11–12.—Tests for ankle instability. **A,** inversion stress test. **B,** anterior drawer test with the foot slightly plantar flexed.

Severe sprains with obvious instability may be treated either by casting or by open surgical repair. The continuity of the lateral ligament can be determined by observing the amount of displacement

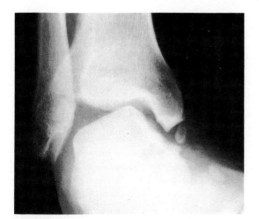

Fig 11–13.—Stress roentgenogram of the ankle revealing severe lateral instability.

or tilting that occurs when an inversion stress is applied to the heel (Fig 11–12). If significant disruption is present, the talus may also sublux anteriorly (anterior drawer test). The instability may be confirmed by stress films (Fig 11–13).

Ankles that are chronically unstable because of lateral ligamentous laxity may benefit by the application of a 0.3-cm lateral heel and sole wedge to prevent inversion. Continuing symptoms require surgical reconstruction of the lateral ligaments to prevent traumatic arthritis from occurring.

TARSAL TUNNEL SYNDROME

Nerve entrapment may occur in the foot by compression of the posterior tibial nerve beneath the flexor retinaculum at the ankle. This retinaculum arises from the medial malleolus and inserts into the

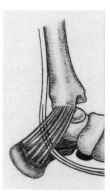

Fig 11–14.—The tarsal tunnel. The posterior tibial nerve runs beneath the flexor retinaculum.

medial aspect of the calcaneous (Fig 11–14). Space-occupying lesions, traction injuries, fibrosis secondary to fractures, or deformities of the heel and foot can all compromise the tunnel and cause pressure on the posterior tibial nerve.

CLINICAL FEATURES

The symptoms include a burning pain, numbness, and tingling in the sole of the foot. The exact location of these symptoms is variable. They are frequently worse with activity. The pain may even radiate into the calf. Sensory loss and intrinsic muscle weakness are occasionally present. Tinel's sign may be positive over the tarsal tunnel.

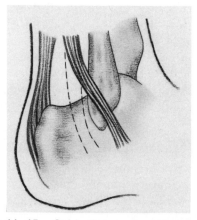

Fig 11–15.—Subluxing peroneal tendons.

TREATMENT

The preferred method of treatment is surgical release of the entrapment. A medial heel wedge or heel seat may be used in an attempt to remove traction from the nerve by inverting the heel.

SUBLUXING PERONEAL TENDONS

Sudden, forceful dorsiflexion of the foot accompanied by contraction of the peroneal muscles may cause a tear in the retinaculum that holds these tendons in their groove behind the lateral malleolus. This may allow the tendons to acutely or chronically sublux over the lateral malleolus (Fig 11–15).

CLINICAL FEATURES

The diagnosis is usually easily made. The tendons are seen or felt lying over the lateral malleolus. The subluxation can often be reproduced by the patient in chronic cases.

TREATMENT

Acute cases are treated by reduction and immobilization in a short leg walking cast for four weeks or open repair of the retinaculum. Chronic cases are usually treated surgically by reconstruction of the retinaculum.

OSTEOCHONDRITIS DISSECANS OF THE TALUS

This condition is characterized by the formation of a small area of necrotic bone on the articular surface of the talus. The cause is usually traumatic, and the medial aspect of the talus is the area most commonly involved.

CLINICAL FEATURES

The onset is gradual, and a history of the injury is frequently absent. The disorder usually occurs during adolescence or

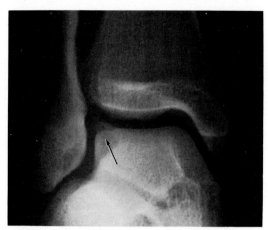

Fig 11–16.—Osteochondritis dissecans of the talus.

early adulthood. A painful limp and chronic swelling in the ankle with activity are common complaints. Examination of the ankle with the foot in plantar flexion may reveal an area of point tenderness over the articular surface of the talus. Ankle motion is frequently restricted.

Roentgenographic examination usually reveals the characteristic lesion (Fig 11–16). The necrotic fragment may even become detached into the joint cavity.

TREATMENT

The undisplaced fragment is treated by prolonged abstinence from weight bearing until the lesion heals. Cast immobilization is frequently indicated. Persistent symptoms or detachment of the fragment requires surgical removal of the necrotic piece of bone.

DISORDERS OF THE HINDFOOT

Plantar Fasciitis

The plantar fascia extends from the calcaneus to the proximal phalanges of each toe and plays an important role in gait. Inflammation of this fascia is a common occurrence and leads to pain on the plantar aspect of the heel. The pain may be present anywhere along the plantar fascia, but it is frequently found near the heel and along the medial longitudinal arch. It is a nonspecific inflammation that is probably secondary to repetitive strain. Both heels are frequently affected. This bilateral involvement may be an early symptom of other inflammatory disorders, such as ankylosing spondylitis, rheumatoid arthritis, or gouty arthritis.

CLINICAL FEATURES

The pain is usually felt directly beneath the calcaneus but may be present in the area of the medial arch. The discomfort is usually worse in the morning and after weight-bearing activities.

Examination reveals local point tenderness in the area of involvement. The pain may be aggravated by direct pressure or by maneuvers that place the fascia under a strain, such as dorsiflexing the toes and ankle.

The roentgenogram is usually normal but may reveal a traction spur on the os calcis that is directed distally (Fig 11–17). The significance of this spur in the etiology of symptoms is unknown. It may be a response to muscle tension and is frequently found in the asymptomatic foot.

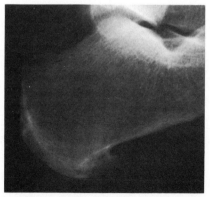

Fig 11–17.—Roentgenogram of the os calcis showing the distally directed spur on its inferior aspect.

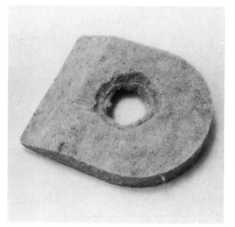

Fig 11–18. – Relief pad used in the treatment of the painful heel.

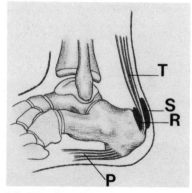

Fig 11–19. – Bursae of the heel: S = superficial calcaneal bursa; R = retrocalcaneal bursa; T = Achilles tendon; and P = plantar fascia.

TREATMENT

The treatment consists of padding the heel of the shoe or placing a relief pad around the area of tenderness (Fig 11–18). The pad is cut out around the tender area. A cup that redistributes the weight bearing on the heel may also be beneficial. A heel lift or high-heeled shoe will often help transfer some of the weight forward, away from the heel to the ball of the foot. Oral anti-inflammatory medication is used as necessary. Many patients will benefit from local infiltration of the tender area with a steroid/lidocaine mixture. The injection may be repeated three to four times. When conservative treatment fails, release of the plantar fascia at its attachment to the os calcis and excision of the bony spur are indicated.

Achilles Tendinitis

Chronic overuse of the calf muscles may result in inflammation of the Achilles tendon. This disorder is frequently seen in the athlete. Pain, swelling, and a dry crepitus may be present. Passive stretching of the tendon by dorsiflexion of the ankle typically aggravates the pain.

The treatment consists of rest, heat, and anti-inflammatory medications. A short leg walking cast may be necessary. Local steroid injections should be avoided as they diminish the normal pain response. In the absence of this response, the patient's return to normal activity may be too rapid and tendon rupture may result.

Bursitis

Two bursae are consistently present near the insertion of the Achilles tendon (Fig 11–19). The superficial bursa is often irritated by the constant rubbing of the counter of the shoe. The retrocalcaneal bursa may be irritated by a prominent posterosuperior angle of the calcaneus (Haglund's disease).

The treatment of both conditions is similar. Relief pads, heat, and elevation of the heel of the shoe with a soft cushion are usually sufficient. Occasionally, the bursa and any underlying bony prominence may have to be resected.

Calcaneal Apophysitis

A low-grade inflammatory reaction at the insertion of the Achilles tendon is frequently seen in association with irregular ossification and sclerosis of the cal-

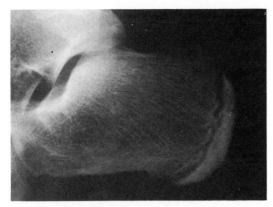

Fig 11–20.—Roentgenogram of the heel in Sever's disease.

caneal apophysis (Fig 11–20). This disorder, sometimes referred to as Sever's disease, usually occurs in boys between the ages of 8 and 14. Local pain, tenderness, and swelling that are aggravated by activity are common. Passive stretching of the heel cord may reproduce the pain.

The roentgenographic changes seen in this disorder are probably not related to the presence of pain in the heel as these same findings are frequently found in the normal, asymptomatic foot.

The treatment includes local heat and the avoidance of activity. A 1.25-cm heel lift may diminish the stress on the heel cord. A short leg walking cast applied with the foot in slight equinus may also be necessary in resistant cases. The disease is always self-limited.

Achilles Tendon Rupture

Spontaneous rupture of the heel cord is an uncommon injury that usually results from degeneration of the tendon or excessive force. The rupture usually occurs 2.5 to 5 cm from the insertion of the tendon into the os calcis.

CLINICAL FEATURES

The injury frequently occurs during an activity that puts great stress on the tendon, such as jumping. Following the injury, the patient walks flatfooted and is unable to stand on the ball of the foot. Tenderness and hemorrhage are present, and a sulcus is usually palpable at the site of the rupture. This sulcus may be obscured, however, by organizing clot if the examination is delayed. Although active plantar flexion is usually lost, some function occasionally remains because of the activity of the other posterior compartment muscles. Thompson's test is usually positive (Fig 11–21). Excessive passive dorsiflexion of the foot will be present on the injured side.

TREATMENT

The best results of treatment are obtained by immediate surgical repair. Nonoperative treatment by applying a short leg cast with the foot in equinus will also allow healing in many cases. Recurrence of the rupture is not uncom-

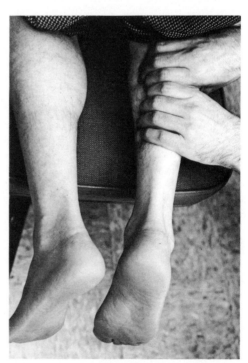

Fig 11–21.—Thompson's test. The normal foot will automatically plantar flex when the calf is squeezed. This movement is absent when the heel cord is ruptured.

mon regardless of treatment, and protection from excessive activity must be maintained for up to one year. Competitive athletes are rarely able to perform as well as before the injury.

Plantaris Tendon Rupture

The plantaris tendon lies medial to the heel cord in the calf and may occasionally rupture with activity. A sudden sharp pain will be felt in the calf, but there is no loss of strength. The treatment is symptomatic but differentiation from Achilles tendon rupture is important.

DISORDERS OF THE FOREFOOT

Morton's Neuroma

A common cause of pain in the forefoot is the interdigital neuroma. This lesion results from perineural fibrosis of the plantar nerve where the medial and lateral plantar branches communicate (Fig 11–22). The condition is probably secondary to repetitive trauma, and the fibrosis results in a painful fusiform swelling of the nerve. Females are more commonly affected.

CLINICAL FEATURES

The clinical picture is one of severe burning pain in the region of the third web space that is accentuated by activity. The pain may radiate into the third and fourth toes. Tight shoes aggravate the discomfort, and the pain is often relieved by removing the shoe and massaging the foot. Numbness may be present in the affected toes.

The examination is usually unremarkable except for exquisite tenderness on digital pressure between the third and fourth metatarsal heads. Compression of the forefoot transversely may also reproduce the pain. Some decrease in sensation may be present on the opposing surfaces of the two affected toes.

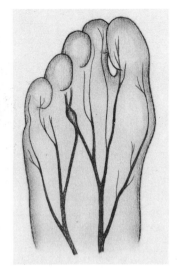

Fig 11–22. – Morton's neuroma.

TREATMENT

Surgical removal of the neuroma is usually indicated. A pad that separates the heads of the third and fourth metatarsals may be helpful, but conservative treatment usually does not provide permanent relief. A local injection of a steroid/lidocaine mixture into the tender area and the avoidance of tight-fitting shoes may also give temporary relief.

Metatarsalgia

Pain beneath the metatarsal head is referred to as metatarsalgia. A variety of abnormalities may be responsible for the pain, including an abnormally high arch, improper shoe wear (especially the high-heeled shoe), and a tight Achilles tendon. The disorder is frequently associated with hammer toes, clawed toes, and a hallux valgus deformity.

CLINICAL FEATURES

The symptoms consist of a typical burning or cramping pain in the region of the metatarsal heads, usually the middle ones. These symptoms are worse with activity and relieved by rest. Tender calluses frequently develop under the metatarsal heads. Variable degrees of dorsal contractures of the metatarsophalangeal joints may be present.

TREATMENT

The object of treatment is to transfer the weight-bearing pressure away from the affected metatarsal heads onto the metatarsal neck and shaft. The calluses that form secondary to the abnormal pressure will usually disappear with time. Trimming or paring them will only provide temporary relief if the pressures are not removed from the affected metatarsal heads. A low-heeled shoe with sufficient room in the forefoot is worn. A metatarsal bar may be added to transfer the weight behind the metatarsal heads (Fig 11–23). Warm soaks are prescribed as necessary. Surgery is reserved for those cases that fail to respond to conservative treatment.

Freiberg's Disease

Freiberg's disease is a disorder of unknown cause in which aseptic necrosis occurs in one of the metatarsal heads, usually the second. The condition is most common in adolescence.

CLINICAL FEATURES

The disease appears as pain, swelling, and restriction of motion of the metatarsophalangeal joint. The metatarsal head is usually palpably enlarged.

The roentgenographic examination reveals widening and irregularity of the metatarsal head (Fig 11–24). Loose bodies may be present.

TREATMENT

The inflammation is treated with salicylates, warm soaks, and local steroid injections. An anterior metatarsal bar will frequently relieve pressure on the metatarsal head. Persistent pain necessitates arthroplasty of the involved joint.

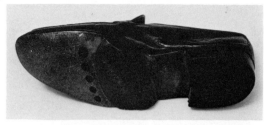

Fig 11–23.—The anterior metatarsal bar. It is placed behind the metatarsal heads so that weight is transferred to the metatarsal necks.

Hallux Valgus

Hallux valgus is a lateral deviation of the great toe at the metatarsophalangeal joint. This is usually associated with bony and soft tissue enlargement over the medial aspect of the first metatarsal head that is referred to as the bunion. Females are most commonly affected. The cause is unknown but heredity and improper shoe wear play important roles.

CLINICAL FEATURES

Pain and deformity are the main initial symptoms. The soft tissue over the prominence may become inflamed and tender. Painful calluses frequently develop on

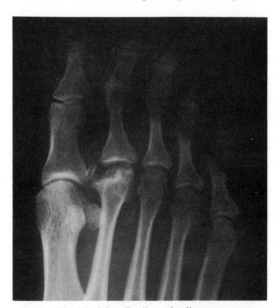

Fig 11–24.—Freiberg's disease.

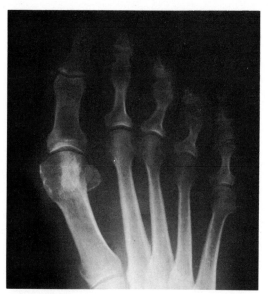

Fig 11–25.—Hallux valgus with bunion exostosis.

the second toe, which is forced into hyperextension by the deviated great toe.

The roentgenographic findings include lateral displacement of the proximal phalanx and the presence of a medial exostosis (Fig 11–25). Degenerative changes may also be present in the metatarsophalangeal joint.

TREATMENT

Conservative treatment is directed at relieving the pressure over the painful bunion prominence. Properly fitted, low-heeled shoes with the toe portion stretched to accommodate the bunion are effective. A splint that separates the first and second toes may also be beneficial. Local measures, such as rest and moist heat, are indicated when acute pain is present. Disabling pain and deformity are indications for surgery. Excision of the exostosis and realignment of the great toe are usually performed.

Hallux Rigidus

Hallux rigidus is a painful condition affecting the metatarsophalangeal joint of the great toe characterized by restriction

of motion. It is usually secondary to traumatic osteoarthritis. The condition may develop at any age but is most common in the third and fourth decades.

CLINICAL FEATURES

Gradually increasing pain and stiffness are typical. They are often precipitated by a minor injury. The pain occurs with ambulation, especially when the toe is dorsiflexed as the patient comes up on the ball of the foot.

Examination reveals swelling, tenderness, and restricted motion of the metatarsophalangeal joint. Attempts at passive motion, especially dorsiflexion, are painful. The toe is held in a protective position of slight flexion and, as the patient walks, more weight is borne on the outer metatarsal heads and lateral border.

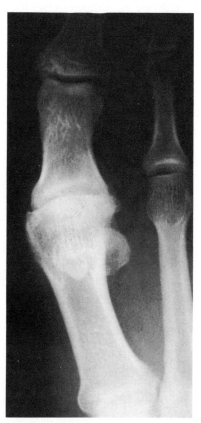

Fig 11–26.—Hallux rigidus. Narrowing and sclerosis are present at the metatarsophalangeal joint of the great toe.

The roentgenogram usually reveals typical findings of degenerative arthritis with joint narrowing and spur formation (Fig 11–26).

TREATMENT

Symptomatic relief can be obtained by rest, moist heat, and anti-inflammatory medication. An intra-articular injection of steroid may provide additional relief. A shoe with sufficient room in the forefoot is worn, and an anterior metatarsal bar is applied to the shoe. Arthroplasty or arthrodesis of the metatarsophalangeal joint is indicated in resistant cases.

Hallux Varus

Hallux varus is a deformity, usually seen in children, in which medial angulation of the great toe occurs at the metatarsophalangeal joint. It is usually congenital and associated with other foot deformities, but may be seen in adults following surgical overcorrection of a hallux valgus deformity.

Mild cases in children may respond to passive stretching exercises and proper shoe wear. More severe cases in both adults and children usually require surgical correction.

Congenital Overlapping Fifth Toe

This is a common familial deformity, frequently bilateral, in which the small toe is dorsiflexed and may come to lie on the top of the fourth toe (Fig 11–27). The capsule and extensor tendon on the dorsum of the metatarsophalangeal joint are shortened and do not allow passive correction of the deformity. Calluses may develop on the dorsum of the toe secondary to chronic irritation by the shoe.

Passive stretching of mild deformities is indicated but usually does not completely correct the problem. Surgical realignment or even amputation may be necessary in symptomatic cases.

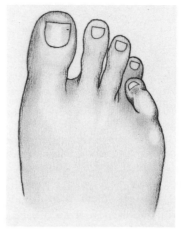

Fig 11–27. – Congenital overlapping fifth toe.

Hammer Toe

The hammer toe is one in which a flexion deformity develops at the proximal interphalangeal joint, causing the tip of the toe to be depressed downward (Fig 11–28). A mild hyperextension deformity at the metatarsophalangeal joint may be present. Painful calluses develop over the tip of the toe, the dorsum of the proximal interphalangeal joint, and under the metatarsal heads. The second toe is most commonly affected, and the disorder is frequently seen in association with a hallux valgus deformity of the great toe. The cause is frequently improperly fitted, tight shoes.

Mild deformities may be corrected by manipulating and taping the toe in the corrected position. Resistant cases usually require surgical correction.

Corns and Calluses

Corns and calluses develop in response to abnormal pressures against the skin of the foot. External pressure due to improper shoe wear combined with internal pressure from abnormal bony protuberances will frequently lead to the production of thickened, painful, hard skin over the bony prominence. In areas where moisture and perspiration collect, the skin becomes macerated and a soft corn (clavus mollum) develops.

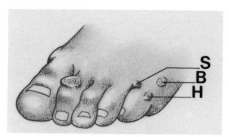

Fig 11–28.—Hammered second toe with a dorsal callus. Also shown are the soft corn *(S)*, bunionette *(B)*, and hard corn *(H)*.

Hard corns (clavus durum) are most commonly found on the dorsolateral aspect of the proximal interphalangeal joint of the fifth toe, while soft corns are most common in the fourth web space. The tailor's bunion or bunionette occurs on the dorsolateral aspect of the metatarsophalangeal joint of the fifth toe. Calluses are frequently seen under the weight-bearing portion of the metatarsal heads or sesamoid bones of the great toe.

Removal of the external pressure is essential in the conservative management of all of these soft tissue lesions in the forefoot. A low-heeled shoe with adequate width in the forefoot is worn. Relief pads and metatarsal bars are usually helpful. Warm soaks in soapy water followed by the application of a keratolytic medication such as salicylic acid salve will help eliminate the callus or corn. The normal skin should be avoided when applying the salve. The salve should remain in place for three to five days covered by adhesive tape. After the tape is removed, the hard callus or corn may be shaved in layers. This procedure is frequently helpful, but deep excision of any corn or callus should be avoided as an infected ulcer may result. Soft corns may be eliminated in one to two weeks, but hard calluses may take longer. A cotton ball may be worn between the toes if a soft corn is present, and a doughnut-shaped pad is always worn around a hard corn or callus. The toes should be kept as dry as possible at all times.

Surgical correction may be advised in resistant cases to eliminate the bony prominence.

Plantar warts also occur near the metatarsal heads but usually not directly on the weight-bearing surface. The wart is generally surrounded by a callus. Characteristic papillary tips are usually present. Paring or curettage of the wart and the use of salicylic acid salve will frequently effect a cure. Relief pads are worn as necessary. The lesion has a high incidence of spontaneous disappearance.

Disorders of the Toenail

A common condition that affects the great toe is the ingrown toenail. In this disorder, the nail does not actually grow into the soft tissue but, instead, the soft tissue overgrows and obliterates the nail sulcus. The cause is a combination of improperly fitted, tight shoes and incorrect nail trimming. A small nail spike may be formed that continues to grow and irritates the soft tissue (Fig 11–29). A chronic infection is usually the end result.

In most mild early cases, soaks, antibiotics, and proper shoe wear are curative. The nail edge should be kept elevated with a soft cotton wad or metal shield until it grows out beyond the soft tissue reaction. Proper transverse trimming of the nail will prevent recurrences. Surgi-

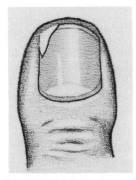

Fig 11–29.—The ingrown toenail frequently results from improper trimming, which produces a nail spike. The nail should always be trimmed transversely.

cal removal of part or all of the nail with curettage of the granulation tissue is indicated in resistant cases.

Two other common conditions, the hypertrophied nail and the ram's-horn nail, may result from poor local hygiene. Both are most common in the elderly. The hypertrophied nail is usually caused by a low-grade fungus infection. The affected nail is thickened, and a yellow, powdery substance is present beneath it. The ram's-horn nail is characterized by massive overgrowth. The nail may even curl over to the plantar aspect of the toe. Both disorders will usually respond to soaks and proper local care. Removal of the entire nail is occasionally required.

ACCESSORY BONES

Many accessory and sesamoid bones are present in the normal foot (Fig 11–30). Most are asymptomatic. An unusually large accessory navicular bone,

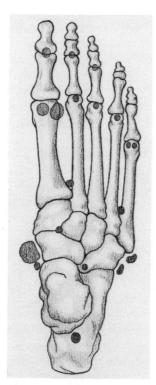

Fig 11–30. — Accessory and sesamoid bones of the foot.

however, may cause pain from local pressure. It is frequently associated with weakness in the longitudinal arch and a mild flatfoot deformity. Relief pads may eliminate symptoms, but surgical excision of the accessory bone is sometimes necessary to completely relieve the pain.

BIBLIOGRAPHY

Bleck, E. E.: The shoeing of children: Sham or science? Dev. Med. Child Neurol. 13: 188, 1971.

Bleck, E. E., and Berzins, U. J.: Conservative management of pes valgus with plantar flexed talus, flexible, Clin. Orthop. 122:85, 1977.

Cowell, H. R.: Talocalcaneal coalition and new causes of peroneal spastic flat foot, Clin. Orthop. 85:16, 1972.

DuVries, H. L.: *Surgery of the Foot* (2d ed.; St. Louis: C. V. Mosby Co., 1965).

Eckert, W. R., and Davis, E. A., Jr.: Acute rupture of the peroneal retinaculum, J. Bone Joint Surg. 58A:670, 1976.

Furey, J. G.: Plantar fasciitis: The painful heel syndrome, J. Bone Joint Surg. 57A:672, 1975.

Greenfield, G. B.: *Radiology of Bone Diseases* (Philadelphia: J. B. Lippincott Co., 1969).

Helfet, A. J.: A new way of treating flat feet in children, Lancet Feb. 11:262, 1956.

Inglis, A. E., et al.: Ruptures of the tendo Achilles: An objective assessment of surgical and non-surgical treatment, J. Bone Joint Surg. 58A:990, 1976.

Keats, T. E.: *An Atlas of Normal Roentgen Variants That May Simulate Disease* (Chicago: Year Book Medical Publishers, Inc., 1977).

Lea, R. B., and Smith, L.: Non-surgical treatment of tendon Achilles rupture, J. Bone Joint Surg. 54A:1398, 1972.

Milgram, J. E.: Office measures for relief of the painful foot, J. Bone Joint Surg. 46A: 1095, 1964.

Sarmiento, A., and Wolf, M.: Subluxation of peroneal tendons, J. Bone Joint Surg. 57A: 115, 1975.

Staples, O. S.: Ruptures of the fibular collateral ligaments of the ankle: Result study of immediate surgical treatment, J. Bone Joint Surg. 57A:101, 1975.

Tachdjian, M. O.: *Pediatric Orthopedics* (Philadelphia: W. B. Saunders Co., 1972).

Turco, V. J.: Surgical correction of the resistant club foot, J. Bone Joint Surg. 53A:477, 1971.

12 / Infections of Bone: Osteomyelitis

OUR DISCUSSION OF skeletal infections of bone will be limited to osteomyelitis and septic arthritis. This chapter will concern itself with osteomyelitis, and septic arthritis will be included in chapter 13.

Osteomyelitis remains a challenge to the physician because a high index of suspicion and early recognition will lead to appropriate diagnostic procedures and institution of antimicrobial therapy as a means to prevent the chronic refractory form of this disease. Osteomyelitis is, by definition, an acute or chronic inflammation of the bone and bone marrow. It may be classified in general according to the mechanism of introduction of the bacterial agent, or on the basis of microbial causes.

Primary osteomyelitis is a result of direct implantation of the microorganisms into the bone, and is likely to be localized at the site of the inoculation. Compound fractures, penetrating wounds, especially from firearms, and surgical operations on bone commonly provide the access for the microbial invasion. Occasional infections may be caused by intramedullary aspiration or by injection of medication. The majority of cases of primary osteomyelitis require surgical treatment, and the appropriate antimicrobial drug is the principal adjunctive therapy.

The route of infection of secondary osteomyelitis is usually hematogenous. Exceptions are spread through veins, particularly the bones of the pelvis and spine, and by direct extension from neighboring articular soft tissue infections, such as those of the skin.

Cause

Most cases of acute hematogenous osteomyelitis are caused by *Staphylococcus aureus;* however, there is no single bacterial cause. The prevalence of *S. aureus* as a cause has dropped from approximately 80% to 50%. In infants and children, important causes are nonhemolytic streptococci and *Hemophilus influenzae.* Gram-negative bacilli are particularly important causes of osteomyelitis involving the vertebral bodies in adults. There is a higher incidence of osteomyelitis in socioeconomically deprived individuals, caused primarily by *Staphylococcus* and tuberculosis. Tuberculous and fungal causes of osteomyelitis can usually be traced to the pulmonary system. Blacks afflicted with sickle cell disease have a particularly high susceptibility to *Salmonella* osteomyelitis. Osteomyelitis may follow any type of surgical manipulation, particularly colorectal surgery or infections of the genitourinary or biliary tracts. With the current higher incidence of intravenous drug abuse, there is a much higher incidence of osteomyelitis that is predominantly spondylitis, or intervertebral disc infection, secondary to this drug abuse. Particular involvement of the lumbar vertebrae or sacroiliac joints is peculiar to this type of development of osteomyelitis, and the organism causing the infection becomes the unusual rather than the usual, for example, *Klebsiella aerobacter* and *Pseudomonas aeruginosa.*

In general, acute hematogenous staphylococcal osteomyelitis occurs primarily in late infancy and also at puberty. In about half of these cases, the source of the *Staphylococcus* can be discovered by inspection of the skin, and not uncommonly a furuncle is found to be the primary source of spread.

Hemophilus influenzae is particularly virulent as a cause of osteomyelitis from infancy to approximately 6 years of age. In this age group *H. influenzae* can and does appear as a soft tissue cellulitis, and its presence should alert the physician to the possibility of underlying osteomyelitis. One should not forget that *H. influenzae* is not necessarily a disease only of children, because there is an increased incidence of this organism in aged individuals as well.

Overall, the incidence of osteomyelitis shows a predominance in men over women. Usually a single bone is involved, with bones of the lower extremities being affected more often than those of the upper extremities. A history of trauma to the bone is obtained in less than one third of the cases, but this should not lead the physician astray in keeping the possible diagnosis in mind.

It is clear that the physician must have a high index of suspicion in order to properly assess the patient's condition and to entertain the possibility of osteomyelitis as the cause of the patient's pain and/or systemic symptoms. Without this suspicion, the patient's primary problem might go undiagnosed and the patient would be left with the chronic form of the disease, which is generally difficult to treat and has a poor prognosis.

Fever, chills, malaise, and diaphoresis are the usual systemic complaints of acute hematogenous osteomyelitis; pain, tenderness, swelling of soft tissue, and limitation of joint motion are apparent on physical examination. Cultures of the blood or of the lesion are essential to determine the exact etiologic agent and to institute the proper antimicrobial thera-

py. Acute osteomyelitis is often preceded by signs of systemic disease and/or general sepsis. Anorexia, nausea, malaise, irritability, and fever are present, usually during the acute phase. This stage of the disease may last for several days, or as long as one to two weeks before bone pain and local overlying inflammation appear.

In infants, the disease may be alarming and life-threatening in its onset and may show overall symptoms of generalized sepsis. The involved area will usually show limitation of motion, and there may be tenderness in the region of the involved bone well before swelling and redness occur. In children, although the usual course is that of high fever, chills, and malaise, an altering of this presentation may occur, particularly when the underlying infection has been partially treated with antibiotics that were instituted earlier for an upper respiratory tract or skin infection. The physician may see only soft tissue swelling and some limitation of the involved portion of the skeleton or joint, and few systemic symptoms.

In the adult, the onset is usually less acute and more insidious. Constitutional symptoms may be considerably less marked, or even absent. In the older child and the adult, it is not uncommon for the first symptoms of osteomyelitis to be those of bone involvement. Again, the physician must be particularly suspicious in those cases where the patient complains of localized pain and has soft tissue swelling, with or without obvious bone involvement. Usually there will be limitation of joint motion, especially if the osteomyelitis involves the spine or if the primary lesions are particularly close to joint spaces where sympathetic effusions may occur in the joint nearest the involved bone. Tuberculous, fungal, rickettsial, and viral causes of osteomyelitis generally have a chronic, insidious onset. These diseases are more common in pa-

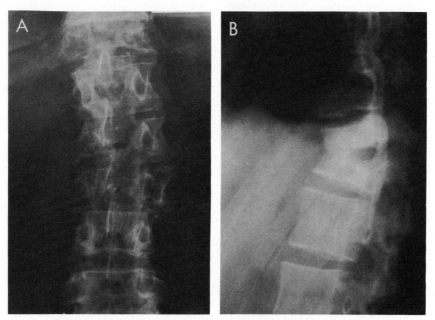

Fig 12–1. — Pott's disease. Angulation is present on both the anteroposterior **(A)** and the lateral **(B)** views.

tients who are immunologically depressed or who have other chronic underlying diseases, such as chronic alcoholism; those of the lower socioeconomic group; or those whose immune systems have been altered by immunosuppressive therapy. As was previously mentioned, the primary source of these infections is often pulmonary, and one should look for a low-grade fever, weight loss, anorexia, and chronic cough or sputum production. Tuberculous osteomyelitis may involve the vertebral column, with pathologic fractures of the involved vertebrae. This usually results in angular kyphosis of the spine, or so-called Pott's disease (Fig 12–1).

CLINICAL MANIFESTATIONS
OF OSTEOMYELITIS

Although osteomyelitis in the past has been looked on as primarily a disease of children and young adults, there has been a shift to the older age groups over the last few years. The femur and the tib-

ia are the most commonly involved sites, but in patients over the age of 50, the spine becomes the most common site. Often these older patients have a history of genitourinary disease and/or manipulation, and the onset of symptoms is chronic and insidious and occurs before the diagnosis is established.

Although the essentials of diagnosis for the child still remain fever, chills, and pain in a guarded limb, a number of patients with minimal temperature elevation, subcutaneous swelling, and a primary complaint of localized pain have been described. Usually laboratory evaluations can be of benefit insofar as leukocytosis and elevated sedimentation rate are concerned. However, it is not uncommon to see no leukocytosis at all and only an elevated sedimentation rate. The drug-abuse patient who presents with onset of back pain that is aggravated by moving, coughing, sneezing, or straining at stool, and who is afebrile, should be quickly examined for pyogenic spondylitis and gram-negative osteomyelitis should be suspected as the underlying cause. Roentgenographic changes are usually of little value in diagnosing adult osteomyelitis until at least 50% of bone resorption has occurred, which is generally two to four weeks into the illness, when periosteal elevation and irregularities of the cortex may first be noted (Fig 12–2). The usual onset of these roentgenographic changes in infants is seven to ten days. Roentgenographic changes may indicate not only destruction of disc space and adjacent vertebral end-plates above and below the primary site, but also evidence of soft tissue swelling and, particularly in children, adjacent calcification. Late changes occur as new bone forms, and sclerosis with fusion of vertebrae or obliteration of intervertebral spaces may be particularly noted in adults. In the majority of cases in children, blood cultures are positive in identifying the offending etiologic agent; it is not uncommon to find less than 50% of adults having positive blood cultures, or having completely negative blood cultures on multiple sampling.

Brodie's abscess should be mentioned, primarily for definition. It is a subacute pyogenic osteomyelitis, localized in the metaphysis, and it appears on roentgenograms as a lucent lesion with some surrounding sclerosis. The primary symptom is pain, with fever and leukocytosis being rare. The offending organism is usually *S. aureus*, or *S. albus*, but occasionally gram-negative organisms have been identified. This disease is usually insidious in onset, and it lacks the systemic symptoms of hematogenous osteomyelitis.

DIAGNOSIS AND DIFFERENTIAL DIAGNOSIS

In order to establish the diagnosis, a thorough history must be obtained from the patient, and this must be correlated with clinical and laboratory evidence of infection. The patient must be examined carefully for the presence of bone pain, soft tissue swelling, guarded extremities, and decreased range of motion of the spine. The physician cannot afford to wait

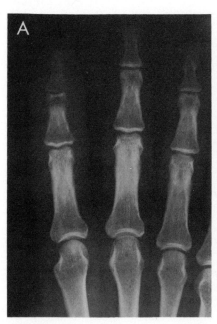 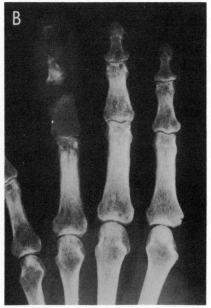

Fig 12–2.—Osteomyelitis. **A,** marked soft tissue swelling is usually present in the early case. **B,** the disease has progressed to destruction of bone.

for the roentgenographic changes to become apparent as the disease may progress into the chronic, less treatable form. In addition to the essentials of diagnosis that we have previously mentioned, the sedimentation rate is usually accelerated and the complete blood cell count (CBC) usually shows leukocytosis. Blood cultures should be obtained and, if possible, needle biopsy of the affected area should be done. Gram's stains of the aspirated material, as well as appropriate cultures and sensitivity, should be obtained. Although roentgenographic abnormalities would be helpful in confirming the presence of infection, often the physician has to make a presumptive diagnosis about osteomyelitis since the bone changes may not become apparent for at least five to seven days in the infant, or as long as two to three weeks in the adult. Of course, the physical examination should also be thorough enough to point to the primary cause of the hematogenous spread, such as a furuncle, or to evidence of chronic underlying disease, such as cirrhosis or carcinoma, to indicate an altered immune state and higher susceptibility.

Scans utilizing radioisotopes may be particularly beneficial in confirming a diagnosis. Since changes take place in blood flow long before they do in bone in osteomyelitis, the particular scanning material is readily picked up by the abnormal area. The use of technetium diphosphonate ^{99m}TC will usually point to a lesion early in the disease, be it in the spine or in the long bones. The scanning then is particularly of benefit in the adult, where there may be little if any clinical evidence to point to spinal disease.

Differential diagnosis must include acute suppurative arthritis, rheumatic fever, and cellulitis. In acute septic arthritis, the most common cause of the disease in young adults is *Neisseria gonorrhea*, while *S. aureus* is the major cause of septic arthritis in older adults. Also, in the older population septic arthritis is usually superimposed on some other bone disease, most commonly rheumatoid arthritis. In general, the clinical manifestations of septic arthritis are variable and related to the type of organism causing the underlying infection. Most patients with gonococcal septic arthritis have prominent prodromal symptoms, such as fever, chills, headaches, anorexia, and malaise, followed by the development of monoarticular septic arthritis. In gonococcal arthritis, an important portion of the diagnosis lies in the history of a migratory polyarthralgia. One also sees a tenosynovitis, but cultures from this involved synovium usually are sterile; however, the skin lesions and small joint effusions are generally positive for the offending organism. The arthritis seen in

TABLE 12–1.—MODIFIED JONES CRITERIA°

Major Criteria
    Carditis
    Polyarthritis
    Chorea
    Subcutaneous nodules
    Erythema marginatum
Minor Criteria
    Fever
    Arthralgia
    Prolonged P-R interval in the ECG
    Increased ESR, WBC, or presence of C-reactive protein
    Preceding β-hemolytic streptococcal infection
    Previous rheumatic fever or inactive rheumatic heart disease

°The presence of two major or one major and two minor criteria is highly suggestive of rheumatic fever.

gonococcal disease is that of involvement of the large joints, primarily the knee, followed by the wrists, ankles, and elbows.

The clinical picture of patients with acute rheumatic fever, gout, and rheumatoid arthritis, or just trauma to a joint, may mimic that seen in acute septic arthritis. Synovial fluid examination is helpful to differentiate these three underlying causes. The diagnosis of acute rheumatic fever is still best obtained by adhering to the Jones criteria of major and minor manifestations (Table 12–1). Again, a high index of suspicion is the only method by which the physician may perceive the necessary diagnostic steps in order to come to a conclusion regarding a particular patient, and those underlying predisposing factors that are so important to the development of osteomyelitis can easily be obtained from the patient's past medical history.

COMPLICATIONS

The most common complications of acute secondary osteomyelitis are soft tissue abscess formation, septic arthritis from extension to the adjacent joints, and metastatic infections from the initial focus. The most common chronic complication is the development of chronic osteomyelitis. If extensive bone destruction does occur, pathologic fractures may be seen. This is particularly noted in people with osteomyelitis secondary to mycobacterium tuberculosis.

TREATMENT

The institution of appropriate treatment for osteomyelitis is based on obtaining the precise etiologic organism, and the sensitivity of this organism to appropriate drugs. Since the majority of cases of acute hematogenous osteomyelitis are caused by S. *aureus*, it is appropriate to initiate a penicillinase-resistant semisynthetic penicillin intravenously. Usually, oxacillin or cloxacillin is the drug of choice because both of these drugs are nearly as active as penicillin G against non-penicillinase-producing S. *aureus* and *Streptococcus pyogenes* group A. These drugs are usually given in daily doses of 8 to 16 gm intravenously in the adult. Treatment should be maintained for at least four to six weeks, or three to four weeks after abatement of symptoms. In children of appropriate age range, besides utilizing surgical drainage of the area, one should begin treatment with intravenous ampicillin. Intravenous ampicillin would also be the drug of choice in those patients with sickle cell anemia, in whom the incidence of *Salmonella* osteomyelitis is much more common.

The selection of specific antibacterial agents for treatment of osteomyelitis caused by gram-negative bacteria is a much more difficult decision. It must be based on the results of the cultures and the susceptibility of these organisms to specific antimicrobial agents. Certain antibiotic agents, such as ampicillin and gentamicin, must be the first in the mind of the physician and are appropriate for institution of therapy.

It is unfortunate that even after acute hematogenous osteomyelitis has been properly diagnosed and treated it can clinically recur. This recurrence can be as much as 30 to 40 years later and is usually due to the same organisms. In general, the recurrences are related to recent trauma, and the history should again alert the physician to the possible underlying cause of the patient's complaint of pain.

In general, the prognosis for acute osteomyelitis is good. If the diagnosis is made early and appropriate antimicrobial therapy is instituted, the infection can usually be eradicated with no deformity. However, if the diagnosis is delayed and treatment is not instituted, the physician and the patient may be faced with the problem of chronic osteomyelitis, which is rarely eradicated, even by long-term antimicrobial therapy. If chronic osteomyelitis has become established, the necrotic bone and tissue must be surgically removed before healing will occur. This adds to the morbidity and the development of residual deformities in the patient. If linear bone growth becomes interrupted, a variety of orthopedic surgical procedures and/or appliances may become necessary to restore function to the involved area.

Osteomyelitis may also be due to infection gaining entrance to a bone from a compound fracture, or through a surgical procedure, such as a total knee replacement. One may also see osteomyelitis developing secondary to dental problems, such as root abscesses, or as a result of radiation, particularly in the facial bone area. Infection can also occur in the frontal and ethmoid sinuses. As a complication of a frontal sinusitis, one may see the development of the so-called Pott's puffy tumor, which represents a collection of pus under the periosteum of the bone, causing swelling and edema over the forehead.

In general, if one is entertaining the diagnosis of osteomyelitis secondary to a contiguous infection, the best method of diagnosis is needling of the suspected lesion, or open surgery. Of course, it is obvious that when a prosthetic device is being used by the patient, it may be necessary to remove it before the infection can be controlled.

Infections of the bones of the feet and of the toes are particularly common in diabetic patients, who have particular difficulty with coincidental peripheral vascular disease. The diabetic patient may have pain and swelling in the infected limb and painless ulcers secondary to the polyneuropathy. One may also see fractures in the feet and toes of a diabetic patient with prolonged hyperemia and swelling, which is normal in his healing process but which may be viewed by the physician as the development of possible osteomyelitis. Although these particular patients may have an elevated sedimentation rate, the CBC is usually normal, and there are no systemic complaints, such as fever or chills. If the peripheral vascular disease is the main underlying problem, the response by the diabetic patient to antimicrobial agents is generally poor and amputation is usually the treatment of choice.

BIBLIOGRAPHY

Emmons, C. W., Binford, C. H., and Utz, J. P.: *Medical Mycology* (2d ed; Philadelphia: Lea & Febiger, 1970).

Green, M., Nyhan, W. L., Jr., and Fausek, M.D.: Acute hematogenous osteomyelitis, Pediatrics 16:368, 1956.

Hoeprich, P. D.: *Infectious Diseases* (Hagerstown, Md.: Harper and Row, 1972).

Holzman, R. S., and Birkko, F.: Osteomyelitis in heroin addicts, Ann. Intern. Med. 75:693, 1971.

Rutstein, D. D., et al.: Jones criteria (modified) for guidance in diagnosis of rheumatic fever, Mod. Concepts Cardiovasc. Dis. 24:291, 1955.

Schmid, F. R.: Principles of Diagnosis and Treatment of Infectious Arthritis, in Hollander, J. L., and McCarty, D. J., Jr. (eds.): *Arthritis and Allied Conditions* (8th ed.: Philadelphia: Lea & Febiger, 1972).

Vu Quoc, D., Nelson, J. D., and Holtalin, K. C.: Osteomyelitis in infants and children, Am. J. Dis. Child. 129:1273, 1975.

Warsman, A. D., Bryon, D., and Siemsen, J. K.: Bone scanning in the drug abuse patient: Early detection of hematogenous osteomyelitis, J. Nucl. Med. 14:647, 1973.

13 / The Arthritides

DISORDERS OF THE JOINTS are common and may cause considerable pain and disability. They are frequently classified as either noninflammatory, inflammatory, or infectious. This chapter will review the more common joint affections.

THE SYNOVIUM

A synovial lining encloses the joint space of all diarthrodial joints. This membrane is also present in bursae and tendon sheaths. It is normally one to three cells thick and is constructed of multiple villi. It will reflect not only local disturbances but also systemic disease and is responsible for the production of joint fluid.

Synovial fluid is a clear, slightly yellow liquid that is present only in small amounts in the normal joint. Its main functions are those of lubrication and nutrition. Its characteristic viscosity is due to the presence of high concentrations of hyaluronic acid, which is produced by the synovial lining cells. This mucopolysaccharide also contributes a portion of the matrix of the synovial lining and is partially responsible for the filtering properties of the synovium.

Joint fluid is a dialysate of blood plasma; that is, crystalloids are present but colloids are not. Normal joint fluid does not clot because many of the coagulation factors are absent. Glucose is present in concentrations 10 mg/dl lower than serum. This difference increases to 30 mg/dl in rheumatoid and other inflammatory types of arthritis and may approach 70 mg/dl in infectious arthritis. Normal fluid also contains complement, lipids, and proteins in amounts much lower than the serum level. The WBC count is usually under 200/cu mm, with the majority being mononuclear. Inflammation increases the cell count and the percentage of polymorphonuclear leukocytes.

A great deal of information can be obtained from the examination of a joint aspirate (Table 13–1). This examination is not indicated in every joint effusion, however, and should be limited to those diagnostic problems that are not secondary to trauma. The joint is usually aspirated from the extensor side under sterile conditions. Three test tubes are sufficient for most determinations: (1) a plain tube for gross examination, clotting, and the mucin clot test; (2) one EDTA-treated tube for cell and crystal analysis; and (3) one heparinized tube for bacteriologic study. Five milliliters of fluid is placed in each tube.

A quick bedside assessment of the fluid can be made prior to the more extensive laboratory analysis. The color and clarity of the sample are estimated by merely observing the fluid in the syringe. The viscosity can be roughly determined by the thread test. A drop of the fluid is placed between the apposed thumb and index finger. The fingers are gradually spread apart, and the length of the thread the fluid forms before it breaks is measured. Normal and osteoarthritic fluid may "string" out 2.5 to 5 cm before breaking, but the dilute fluid of inflammation will string very little.

The Mucin Clot Test

This determines the amount of hyaluronate in the fluid. Acetic acid is added to the tube and the sample is observed for

TABLE 13–1.—SYNOVIAL FLUID ANALYSIS

DISEASE	APPEARANCE	VISCOSITY	MUCIN CLOT	WBC, % POLYMORPHONUCLEAR LEUKOCYTES	OTHER FINDINGS
Noninflammatory					
Normal	Clear, yellow	High	Good	Under 200, under 10%	
Traumatic arthritis	Cloudy, straw to red	High	Good	Under 2,000, under 25%	Cartilage debris
Osteoarthritis	Straw, yellow, clear	High	Good	Under 5,000, under 25%	Cartilage debris
Inflammatory					
Rheumatoid	Cloudy, green/gray	Low	Fair/ poor	15,000, 50%–80%	Glucose difference 10–25 mg/dl, R A cells
Gout	Cloudy, white, flaky	Decreased	Fair/ poor	10,000, 25%–75%	Sodium urate crystals
Pseudogout	Cloudy	Decreased	Fair/ poor	5–15,000, 25%–75%	Calcium pyrophospate crystals
Systemic lupus erythematosus	Cloudy, yellow	High	Good/ fair	5–10,000, under 25%	Lupus erythematosus cells
Infectious					
Bacterial	Cloudy, purulent	Low	Poor	50–200,000, over 90%	Glucose difference over 50 mg/dl, culture +

clot formation. A "poor" mucin clot indicates a decrease in hyaluronate. This results from dilution, depolymerization, and loss of filter function from either inflammation or infection. A "good" clot is present in normal fluid and osteoarthritis.

Crystal Analysis

Reliable crystal examination requires the use of polarized light. The sodium urate crystals present in gout are needle-shaped and negatively birefringent. The calcium pyrophosphate crystal in pseudogout (chondrocalcinosis) is rhomboid-shaped and positively birefringent.

OSTEOARTHRITIS

The most common type of noninflammatory arthritis is degenerative or osteoarthritis. This condition is characterized by articular cartilage deterioration and bony overgrowth of the joint surface.

The cause is unknown, but trauma, heredity, and the normal aging process are all factors. Pathologically, the cartilage loses its normal glistening appearance and becomes roughened and irregular. Eventually, the cartilage becomes completely worn away, thus exposing the subchondral bone. Secondary synovitis and osteophytic spur formation are common. The clinical course is slowly progressive.

CLINICAL FEATURES

Pain is the most common initial symptom. This frequently occurs with motion or activity and is relieved by rest. Joint stiffness typically occurs with rest and improves with activity.

The physical findings include crepitus, swelling, restriction of motion, and joint enlargement from spur formation. In the hands, these osteophytic overgrowths are termed Heberden's nodes when they are

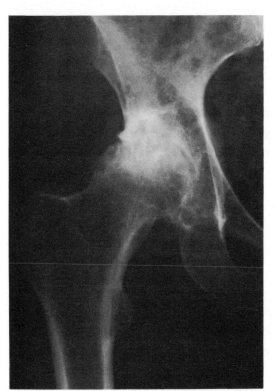

Fig 13–1.—Degenerative arthritis of the hip. Joint space narrowing, sclerosis, and subchondral cyst formation are present.

present at the distal interphalangeal joint and Bouchard's nodes when they occur at the proximal interphalangeal joint. Pain is usually present on joint motion. Disuse atrophy of the adjacent musculature may develop rapidly, thus increasing the disability and pain.

The roentgenographic findings consist of joint space narrowing, spur formation, sclerosis, and subchondral cyst formation (Fig 13–1). The laboratory findings and synovial analysis are normal except for occasional flakes of cartilage in the joint fluid.

TREATMENT

The main objectives of treatment are the relief of pain and prevention of progression. As with any joint disorder, the patient should not be told that arthritis is present unless the physical and laboratory findings are consistent with the diagnosis. The stigma of "arthritis" should not be attached to any condition merely to explain vague or nonspecific symptoms. Once the diagnosis is established, however, the patient should be made to realize that while miracles cannot be expected, there is almost always something that can be done to relieve the pain and deformity, regardless of the cause.

For osteoarthritis, the treatment begins with rest of the involved joint. This will help reduce inflammation and pain. Weight loss and temporary abstinence from weight bearing by the use of a cane or crutch will lessen the pressure on the involved lower extremity. Removable splints or braces are also helpful.

The joint should be passed through a full range of motion several times daily to reduce joint stiffness. The local application of moist heat is beneficial during the acute painful stage and may be especially helpful prior to exercise. Exercises designed to combat stiffness and restore muscle strength are important because the weakness will contribute to joint instability and disability. Anti-inflammatory agents, especially aspirin, in combination with the heat and rest are also effective. Intra-articular cortisone injections will frequently relieve a great deal of the pain, but their effect is only temporary.

The surgical procedures most commonly employed are arthrodesis and arthroplasty (Fig 13–2). Each is effective in eliminating the painful articulation. Realignment of faulty weight-bearing joints by osteotomy may also be beneficial.

GOUT

Gouty arthritis is an inherited metabolic disease characterized by a disturbance in purine metabolism in which crystals of sodium urate are deposited in various soft tissues. These crystals and the resultant symptoms are due to an increase in the serum uric acid, a normal end product of purine metabolism.

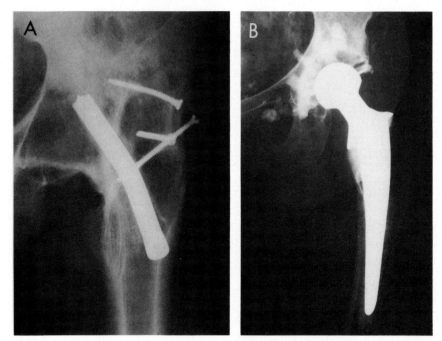

Fig 13–2. – **A,** arthrodesis, and **B,** total hip arthroplasty.

The majority of patients are men in the third and fourth decades. The disorder is uncommon in women and rare before the menopause. Secondary gout may follow hyperuricemia from many causes, including leukemia, hemolytic anemia, and other blood dyscrasias.

CLINICAL FEATURES

The initial attack usually occurs in a single joint in the lower extremity. The metatarsophalangeal joint of the great toe is classically the first site of involvement. The pain and inflammation are usually severe and may be precipitated by exercise, dietary indiscretion, and physical or emotional stress. The typical attack begins at night.

Swelling, heat, redness, and other signs of inflammation are usually present. The physical findings may even simulate cellulitis. The area is often tender to even the slightest touch. Fever, tachycardia, and other constitutional symptoms may accompany the attack. The initial episode may be followed by polyarticular involvement. Eventually, deposits of urate crystals, termed tophi, may form in the subcutaneous tissue.

Early in the disease, the roentgenogram is normal. Later, erosive changes appear that have a characteristic punched-out appearance (Fig 13–3). Destruction and degeneration of the articular cartilage frequently follows.

Laboratory findings include a mild leukocytosis, elevated sedimentation rate, and hyperuricemia. The synovial aspirate is usually cloudy and mildly inflammatory in nature. Urate crystals are usually demonstrable.

TREATMENT

The treatment will depend on the stage of the disease. The objectives in management are to terminate or prevent the acute attack, encourage mobilization of tophaceous deposits, and reduce the serum uric acid.

Patients with asymptomatic hyperuri-

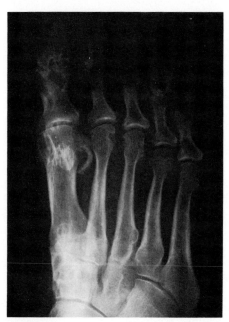

Fig 13–3.—Gouty arthritis. Multiple punched-out lesions are present.

cemia (over 9 mg/dl) should probably be treated to prevent the acute attack and complications of elevated uric acid level. For the initial acute episode, colchicine is the drug of choice. Two 0.5-mg tablets are given initially, followed by 1 tablet every hour up to 12 tablets until the symptoms subside or diarrhea ensues. This is accompanied by rest, elevation, and moist heat. Disappearance of symptoms with the colchicine therapy also helps to confirm the diagnosis. Future acute attacks are treated with phenylbutazone.

Between attacks, prophylaxis is maintained by one of two agents, probenecid or allopurinol. Probenecid is a uricosuric agent; that is, it increases the renal excretion of uric acid. It should not be used in the presence of renal disease. Probenecid is also effective in reducing the size of tophaceous deposits. Allopurinol is a xanthine oxidase inhibitor that prevents formation of uric acid from xanthine and hypoxanthine. It is especially valuable in the patient who forms urate stones be-

cause it directly decreases the production of uric acid.

Surgery is usually limited to excision of large tophi and, occasionally, arthroplasty.

PYOGENIC ARTHRITIS

Pyogenic or septic arthritis may occur in any age group but is more common in the young. The hip and knee joints are most frequently involved. The offending organism is usually *Staphylococcus aureus*, but a variety of other bacteria may be causative. Entrance to the joint is usually gained by direct extension from an adjacent infection or by hematogenous spread.

On invasion of the joint by the pathogenic bacteria, the synovial membrane becomes swollen and hyperemic. It begins to produce large amounts of joint fluid that distends the joint capsule. Frank pus eventually accumulates, and destruction of the articular cartilage may even occur.

CLINICAL FEATURES

The onset is usually acute, with pain being the most common early symptom. A history of infection elsewhere is frequently obtainable. If a weight-bearing joint is involved, ambulation is usually difficult and may become impossible because of the pain. Fever and other signs of systemic infection are usually present.

The examination generally reveals a warm, swollen, diffusely tender joint. The joint is usually held in slight flexion because, in this position, the intracapsular pressure is decreased and discomfort is thereby minimized. Attempts at passive motion tend to be extremely painful.

The roentgenographic findings early in the disease process are usually minimal and consist primarily of distention of the joint capsule. The peripheral WBC count is markedly elevated as a rule, and blood cultures may be positive.

Confirmation of the diagnosis is best made by joint aspiration under sterile conditions. Most joints are best aspirated on the extensor side, except the hip, which may be aspirated from the anterior or lateral aspect. Because the joint is usually distended, aspiration is ordinarily not difficult. The fluid is initially cloudy and thin but may be purulent. The joint glucose level is decreased and the WBC count is markedly increased as a rule. A Gram's stain is performed and cultures are taken.

TREATMENT

The treatment should begin immediately in order to prevent joint destruction and, in the case of the hip joint, dislocation. Rest, moist heat, and traction will diminish the pain. The definitive antibiotic therapy will depend on the Gram's stain and culture. The intravenous route should always be used. Intra-articular injection is unnecessary as most antibiotics readily pass through the synovial membrane. Direct instillation may even provoke an inflammatory synovitis.

Surgical drainage of the affected joint is usually indicated. This is especially true of the hip. Surgery may be delayed if a dramatic clinical response occurs with conservative treatment, but if such a response is not forthcoming, drainage should be performed immediately. Surgery will diminish the intra-articular pressure, allow evacuation of the thick fibrous exudate, and prevent the articular destruction that may occur in pyarthrosis.

PSEUDOGOUT (CHONDROCALCINOSIS)

Pseudogout is a condition that resembles gout in its clinical manifestations except that large rather than small joints are more commonly involved. It is characterized by the deposition of crystals of calcium pyrophosphate in the joint cartilage and capsule.

CLINICAL FEATURES

The symptoms are similar to those of chronic gouty arthritis. Intermittent acute episodes occur, but the joint most commonly involved is the knee rather than the great toe. The condition is frequently familial and is occasionally associated with diabetes, renal disease, and other systemic conditions.

In addition to the gout-like symptoms, calcification of the cartilage of the knee, especially the meniscus, is common (Fig 13–4). Calcification of the anulus fibrosus, radioulnar disc, and symphysis pubis may also be seen. Synovial fluid analysis reveals typical rhomboid-shaped crystals that exhibit positive birefringence under polarized light. There are no specific changes in blood or urine.

TREATMENT

Aspiration and cortisone injections are often effective in the acute phase. A short course of phenylbutazone or indomethacin may also be beneficial.

RHEUMATOID ARTHRITIS

Rheumatoid arthritis is a systemic disorder of unknown cause characterized by joint inflammation. In contrast to many of the other arthritides, it is a potentially crippling disease. The condition

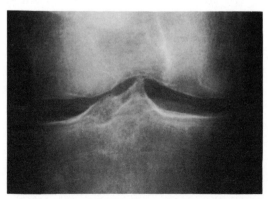

Fig 13–4. — Calcification of the meniscus.

is most common in women between the ages of 25 and 45.

Pathologically, the synovium becomes thickened, inflamed, and hypertrophic. Infiltrating granulation tissue from the synovium (pannus) typically spreads over the joint cartilage. Eventually, erosion and destruction of the articular surface results from the chronic inflammatory process.

CLINICAL FEATURES

The onset is usually gradual. Weakness, fatigue, and anorexia are common prodromal symptoms. Eventually joint involvement becomes apparent, with stiffness, swelling, heat, and redness. Most cases initially present with multiple symmetric joint involvement, most often in the hands and feet. Remissions and exacerbations are common, but the condition is chronically progressive in the majority of cases.

The physical signs are due to the inflammation of the synovial membrane. Joint effusions, tenderness, and restriction of motion are usually present early in the disease. Eventually, the characteristic deformities appear, consisting of subluxations, dislocations, and joint contractures.

In addition to the joint manifestations, extra-articular findings are common. Tendon sheaths and bursae are frequently affected by the chronic inflammation. Tendon rupture may even occur. Rheumatoid nodules are present in 25% of cases and are most common over bony prominences such as the elbow and shaft of the ulna. Splenomegaly, pericarditis, and vasculitis may also occur.

The roentgenogram usually reveals soft tissue swelling and osteoporosis early in the disease. Eventually, joint space narrowing, erosion, and deformity become visible as the result of continued inflammation and cartilage destruction (Fig 13–5).

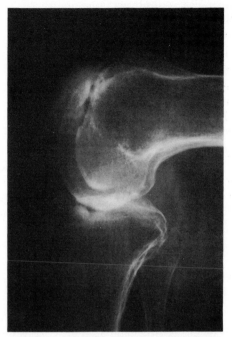

Fig 13–5.—Rheumatoid arthritis of the knee. Osteoporosis and severe joint space narrowing are present.

The laboratory findings consist of a mild anemia, leukocytosis, and elevated sedimentation rate. The rheumatoid factor is positive in approximately 75% of cases. The joint fluid is usually turbid and forms a poor mucin clot. The cell count is elevated, with an increase in polymorphonuclear leukocytes.

TREATMENT

Proper management requires close cooperation among primary physician, therapist, and orthopedist. Rest is beneficial in reducing inflammation. When combined with an exercise program, moist heat, and splinting, joint deformities can frequently be prevented or corrected.

Aspirin remains the drug of choice for most patients. The usual dose is two to three tablets every three to four hours. Although it is not curative, it will suppress the symptoms and many of the objective signs of articular inflammation. When salicylates fail to alleviate the symptoms, several other drugs, including gold, steroids, antimalarial and other anti-inflammatory agents, have been used with varying success.

Among the surgical procedures that are helpful are synovectomy, soft tissue releases, arthroplasty, and arthrodesis. The soft tissue procedures are most beneficial early in the disease before significant fixed deformity or subluxation appears. The results of synovectomy in particular are better when it is performed before irreversible articular damage occurs.

Juvenile Rheumatoid Arthritis (Still's Disease)

The rheumatoid arthritis that occurs in youth differs in many respects from that which occurs in the adult. The main differences are the systemic toxicity that occurs in children and the tendency for fewer joints to be involved. The juvenile variety is frequently difficult to differentiate from other childhood diseases, especially rheumatic fever.

CLINICAL FEATURES

Juvenile rheumatoid arthritis is usually one of three types: (1) systemic (20%), (2) pauciarticular (30%), or (3) polyarticular (50%). Systemic or acute febrile juvenile rheumatoid arthritis is characterized by extra-articular manifestations, especially spiking fevers and a typical rash. The rash frequently appears in the evening and may be elicited by gently scratching the skin in susceptible areas (Koebner's phenomenon). Splenomegaly, generalized lymphadenopathy, pericarditis, and myocarditis may also occur. The articular findings are often minimal and are usually overshadowed by the systemic symptoms. The morbidity from this form is usually from chronic arthritis, however.

The pauciarticular or oligoarticular form usually involves the larger joints, such as the knees, elbows, and ankles. Systemic features are often minimal and only one to three joints are usually involved. The joint disease rarely causes impairment, but iridocyclitis develops in approximately 30% of cases with this form and permanent loss of vision will develop in a high percentage of these patients. Frequent ocular examinations, early detection, and treatment are therefore indicated. In this form of juvenile rheumatoid arthritis, accelerated growth of the affected limb from chronic hyperemia may result in a temporary leg length discrepancy that eventually equalizes in most cases on control of the inflammation.

Polyarticular juvenile rheumatoid arthritis resembles the adult rheumatoid disease in its symmetrical involvement of the small joints of the hands and feet. Cervical spine involvement is not uncommon and may produce marked restriction of motion. Early closure of the ossification centers of the mandible may produce a markedly receding chin, a characteristic of this form. Systemic manifestations are similar to the febrile variety but are not as dramatic.

The roentgenographic findings in juvenile rheumatoid arthritis are the same as those in the adult, except that joint destruction is less frequent (Fig 13–6). The laboratory findings are also similar, except that the peripheral WBC count may be very high and the rheumatoid factor is rarely demonstrable in the serum of children.

TREATMENT

The treatment is similar to that given the adult except that phenylbutazone and indomethacin should not be used.

NEUROARTHROPATHY

The neuropathic or Charcot's joint is one that results from a disturbance in the

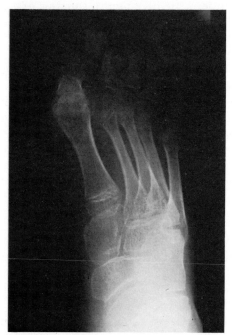

Fig 13–6.—Juvenile rheumatoid arthritis. Osteoporosis is present, but joint destruction is minimal.

sensation to the joint. It is usually associated with central or peripheral nerve lesions. The most common causes are tabes dorsalis, diabetic neuropathy, and syringomyelia. The loss of sensation leads to extreme destruction, new bone formation, and instability of the joint.

CLINICAL FEATURES

The foot is usually involved in diabetes, the shoulder and elbow joint in syringomyelia, and the vertebrae and lower extremities in tabes dorsalis. Gradual enlargement and instability of the affected joint are common complaints. Pain is usually present, but tends to be relatively mild compared to the severity of the joint destruction.

The examination is characterized by swelling and hypermobility. Palpation frequently reveals overgrowth of bone, crepitus, and loose bodies.

Variable degrees of joint destruction and disintegration with exuberant osteophyte formation are usually present on roentgenographic examination. Later, subluxation and deformity may be seen (Fig 13–7).

TREATMENT

Ordinary conservative and surgical treatment, including arthrodesis, are usually unsuccessful. Immobilization and protection of the affected joint with braces is sometimes effective.

SYSTEMIC LUPUS ERYTHEMATOSUS

Systemic lupus erythematosus is an inflammatory disease that affects the vas-

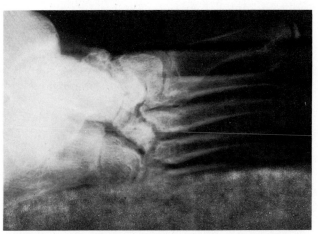

Fig 13–7.—Diabetic neuroarthropathy of the foot. Severe destructive changes are present in the midtarsal joints.

cular and connective tissue of many organ systems but commonly appears with joint pain and swelling similar to that seen in rheumatoid arthritis. It should always be considered in the differential diagnosis of systemic arthritis. It is most common in women in the third and fourth decades and affects the joints in 90% of patients. The joint involvement is usually accompanied by the other characteristic features of the disease, namely, the butterfly rash on the face and hematopoietic, renal, and cardiac involvement. Lupus erythematosus cells and antinuclear antibodies are usually present in the serum.

OCHRONOSIS

Alkaptonuria is an uncommon inherited disorder that results from a failure to properly synthesize homogentisic acid oxidase. Homogentisic acid is thus excreted in the urine, causing it to turn black on oxidation. Ochronosis is the result of alkaptonuria and is characterized by the deposition in the soft tissue and cartilage of a pigment derived from homogentisic acid.

The arthropathy of ochronosis primarily involves the spine, hips, knees, and shoulders. Typical calcifications appear in the intervertebral discs and menisci. Eventually, the peripheral joint changes become indistinguishable from osteoarthritis while the spine involvement resembles ankylosing spondylitis.

No specific treatment is available. The peripheral arthritis is treated as osteoarthritis.

REITER'S SYNDROME

Reiter's syndrome is characterized by (1) urethritis, (2) conjunctivitis, and (3) arthritis. The cause in unknown, but the disorder is probably transmitted by sexual contact.

The arthritis is usually polyarticular. Large joints are most commonly affected, with joint involvement occurring two to three weeks after the urethritis. The patient may be febrile and the joint is often warm and tender.

The disorder is self-limited. Symptoms usually resolve in six to eight weeks and complete recovery is the rule. No treatment is available, but because of the similarity of the disorder to gonococcal arthritis, penicillin should probably be administered until the diagnosis is clarified.

PSORIATIC ARTHRITIS

Psoriasis may occasionally be accompanied by a form of arthritis that is clinically similar to adult rheumatoid arthritis. The skin disorder usually precedes the arthritis by several years.

The arthritis is usually progressive and initially involves the distal interphalangeal joints of the fingers and toes. Its activity tends to parallel the activity of the skin disease. Severe bone destruction and ankylosis are not uncommon, especially in the hands.

PALINDROMIC RHEUMATISM

Palindromic rheumatism is an uncommon benign condition characterized by episodic attacks of arthritis. The small joints of the hands are typically involved. The attacks may last only a few hours or days and are usually followed by complete remission. The condition is believed by many to represent an atypical form of rheumatoid arthritis.

SJÖGREN'S SYNDROME

Sjögren's syndrome is a fairly common disorder characterized by (1) dry eyes (keratoconjunctivitis sicca), (2) dry mouth (xerostomia), and (3) chronic arthritis. The chronic arthritis is usually polyarticular in nature and occurs in two thirds of cases. The patients typically are middle-aged women.

The joint involvement resembles rheumatoid arthritis in its pathologic, clinical, and roentgenographic appearance. It commonly precedes and may be accompanied by rheumatoid nodules. The rheumatoid factor is positive in almost 100% of patients. Treatment of the arthritis is the same as for rheumatoid arthritis.

BIBLIOGRAPHY

Aegerter, E., and Kirkpatrick, J. A.: *Orthopedic Diseases* (3d ed.; Philadelphia: W. B. Saunders Co., 1968).

Bjelle, A., and Sunden, G.: Pyrophosphate arthropathy: A clinical study of 50 cases, J. Bone Joint Surg. 56B:246, 1974.

Decker, J. L. (ed): Primer on the rheumatic diseases, J.A.M.A. 190:127–140, 425–444, 509–530, 741–751, 1964.

Flatt, A. E.: *The Care of the Rheumatoid Hand* (2d ed.; St. Louis: C. V. Mosby Co., 1968).

Gutman, A. B.: Views on the pathogenesis and management of primary gout—1971, J. Bone Joint Surg. 54A:357, 1972.

Hollander, J. L., and McCarty, D. J. (eds.): *Arthritis and Allied Conditions* (8th ed.; Philadelphia: Lea & Febiger, 1972).

Jaffe, H. L.: *Metabolic, Degenerative, and Inflammatory Diseases of Bones and Joints* (Philadelphia: Lea & Febiger, 1972).

Katz, W. A.: *Rheumatic Diseases, Diagnosis, and Management* (Philadelphia: J. B. Lippincott Co., 1977).

King, B. G., Jr., Galveston, S. N., and Evans, E. B.: Palindromic rheumatism: An unusual cause of the inflammatory joint, J. Bone Joint Surg. 56A:142, 1974.

Laskar, F. H., and Sargison, K. D.: Ochronotic arthropathy, J. Bone Joint Surg. 52B:653, 1970.

Laurin, C. A., et al.: Long-term results of synovectomy of the knee in rheumatoid patients, J. Bone Joint Surg. 56A:521, 1974.

14 / Fracture Treatment

MOST FRACTURES are easily recognized both clinically and roentgenographically (Fig 14–1). A satisfactory end result in the treatment of these injuries will depend not only on the reduction of the fracture and the maintenance of that reduction, but also on the restoration of the function of the injured extremity. These goals are reached by appreciating both the bony and soft tissue structures involved.

TERMINOLOGY

Fracture: a break in the continuity of a bone
   Open ("compound"): fracture in which there is an open wound of the skin and soft parts that leads into the fracture
   Closed ("simple"): fracture that does not have an open wound in the skin
   Comminuted: fracture with multiple fragments

Impacted: fracture whose ends are driven into each other
Displaced: fracture whose ends are separated
Greenstick: an incomplete fracture that usually occurs in children
Pathologic: fracture that occurs because the bone is weakened by some abnormal condition
Intra-articular: fracture that involves the joint surface of a bone
Fatigue: fracture that results from repeated minor stresses
Apposition: the amount of end-to-end contact of the fracture
Alignment: rotational or angular position
Nonunion: failure of bony healing
Malunion: healing in an unsatisfactory position

GENERAL CONSIDERATIONS

Initial Care

All major long bone fractures should be splinted before the patient is transported. Careless handling of the extremity that further damages the soft tissue should be avoided, but it is wise to correct any significant rotational or angular malalignment before applying a splinting device. This is done by gentle traction in the long axis of the limb. Do not, however, pull the protruding bone ends of an open fracture back into the wound.

A variety of splinting devices are available that make transfer of the patient to the hospital more comfortable (Fig 14–2). Their use should be only temporary, however, until the diagnosis is confirmed roentgenographically. If definitive treatment of the fracture is to be delayed, a

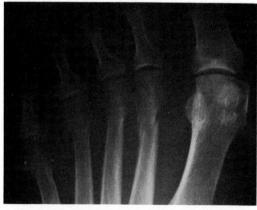

Fig 14–1.—Fracture of the second metatarsal neck and a bipartite tibial sesamoid. The fracture is distinguished from the bipartite sesamoid or accessory bone by its sharp, pointed edges and irregular margin.

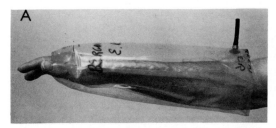

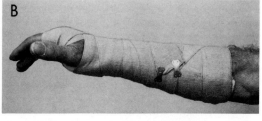

Fig 14–2.–**A,** temporary splint used for transfer. **B,** well-padded bulky dressing reinforced with plaster splints that should be applied as soon as possible. An elastic bandage alone should never be used. It does not immobilize nor does it "reduce" swelling. It may, in fact, do more harm by further compressing the already compromised lymphatic and venous drainage systems.

well-padded plaster splint is then applied for immobilization, and the extremity is elevated and ice is applied to prevent swelling. The neurologic and circulatory function of the extremity distal to the site of the injury should always be checked and recorded. If immediate treatment is contemplated, adequate anesthesia can usually be obtained by direct infiltration of the fracture hematoma, under sterile conditions, with 5 to 10 ml of a local anesthetic.

Definitive Fracture Care

The ability to reduce and maintain the reduction of many fractures is dependent on several factors, one of which is the surrounding soft tissue. Whenever displacement of the fragments is present, the soft tissue on the concave side of the fracture usually remains intact (Fig 14–3). This soft tissue can be utilized to reduce the fracture by guiding the fragments into place. It will also maintain the reduction and prevent overreduction from occurring.

In general, the first step in fracture reduction is restoration of the length of the extremity by steady traction and countertraction along the axis of the limb. Excessive force is usually unnecessary. Rotation is then corrected and the distal fragment is placed in apposition to the proximal fragment. The angular deformity is then corrected, and while the assistant maintains tension on the soft tissue

hinge, the extremity is immobilized in a well-molded circular plaster cast (Fig 14–4). The cast itself will not completely immobilize the fracture, but if it is used properly it will keep enough tension on the soft tissue structures so that sufficient relative immobilization of the extremity will be obtained and the reduction will be held in position.

Once the fracture has been reduced

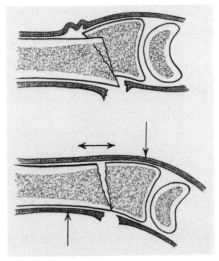

Fig 14–3.–**A,** typical fracture of the distal radius. **B,** the fracture is reduced by traction and manipulation using the soft tissue and periosteum on the concave side to "guide" the fragments into place. Pressure is then applied at the appropriate points *(arrows)* on the cast to keep tension on the soft parts and maintain the reduction. (Adapted from Charnley, J.: *The Closed Treatment of Common Fractures* [3d ed.; Edinburgh: Churchill Livingstone, 1970].)

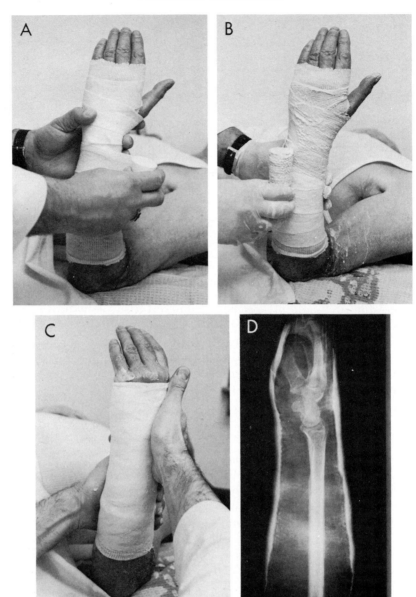

Fig 14–4.—The plaster cast. **A,** stockinette and cast padding are applied. The padding is overlapped by one-half with each turn and need only be two layers thick. **B,** the cast is then applied, moving continuously up and down the extremity. The plaster should be kept on the extremity and is rolled away rather than toward the physician. The cast should be of uniform thickness and 0.6 cm thick. It should not be any thicker over the fracture site than at the ends. **C,** the cast is then molded, applying the proper forces to hold the reduction and maintain tension on the soft parts and periosteum. **D,** roentgenogram showing the proper thickness and snug fit of the cast. Casts should not extend beyond the distal palmar crease in the hand unless specifically indicated. Fractures of the distal third of the forearm are immobilized in pronation, fractures of the middle third in neutral, and fractures of the proximal third in supination.

and immobilized, the extremity is elevated and ice is applied. The patient is closely observed for signs of circulatory obstruction (pain, pallor, paralysis, and pulselessness). Hospitalization may even be necessary in some cases. Strict, detailed instructions regarding care of the extremity are given to the patient, and the cast is split at the earliest sign of any circulatory embarrassment. The entire cast, cotton, and stockinette must be split completely along one side of the cast down to the skin. Even a small tight band of stockinette is sufficient to cause Volkmann's ischemic paralysis (Fig 14–5).

Roentgenograms are repeated at weekly intervals for two to three weeks to assess the state of the reduction and the progression of healing. The length of time required for complete healing varies with the age of the patient, the nature and site of the fracture, and the specific bone involved. As a rule, fractures in children and fractures near the ends of the bone (metaphysis) heal more rapidly than do those in the relatively avascular midshaft (diaphysis).

The determination as to when a cast may be removed is not made on the basis of the roentgenogram alone. Roentgenographic evidence of complete healing may lag several weeks behind true clinical union. In general, however, the cast may be removed when sufficient time has passed for the particular bone under treatment to heal. This varies with each bone. A clinical and roentgenographic assessment is made after the cast has been removed. If the fracture has no motion and is not tender to palpation, pressure, or stress, then sufficient healing has probably occurred to allow the cast to be left off. If any doubt exists, a removable protective splint may be applied for another two to three weeks and gradual resumption of limited activity is allowed. If motion or tenderness is present, another circular cast is applied and the fracture is reassessed in two to three weeks.

Rehabilitation

Rehabilitation is actually begun on the day of the injury. By preventing excessive soft tissue swelling from occurring, scar formation is diminished and a more functional extremity is the end result once the fracture has healed. After the initial pain and swelling have subsided, the patient is encouraged to use any joints that are not immobilized and to perform some meaningful tasks at home or at work.

Following cast removal, active mobilization of joints that were immobilized by the cast is begun. A repetitive exercise that the patient may perform at home is

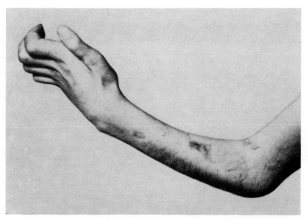

Fig 14–5. — Volkmann's ischemic contracture.
(From Blount, W. P.: *Fractures in Children* © 1955 by Williams & Wilkins Co.)

preferable to most forms of physical therapy. Exercise in a swimming pool is an excellent method of restoring strength and mobility following many injuries. Most extremities are able to regain most of their motion and strength by four to six weeks after the cast has been removed, but it is not uncommon for some stiffness and weakness to persist even longer.

Additional Principles

1. Always obtain comparison roentgenograms of the opposite extremity whenever a questionable fracture is present.

2. Always obtain roentgenograms in at least two planes and include a joint above and below the fracture.

3. When one bone of a two-bone set (forearm, lower leg) is fractured and shortened or angulated, always look for injury to the other bone.

4. Be certain to correct both rotational and angular malalignment in the reduction.

5. Painful pressure sores may develop rapidly under a cast. The skin tends to become insensitive after necrosis has occurred. These pressure sores should be treated quickly before necrosis occurs. If a "window" must be cut in the cast, the window should always be replaced to prevent the soft tissue from swelling out through it.

6. The measure of success is the usefulness of the extremity and not just the roentgenographic appearance.

FRACTURES IN CHILDREN

Fractures in children differ from those in adults in many respects. They are usually less complicated and, with a few exceptions, are always treated by closed methods. Nonunion is rare due to the active periosteum and abundant blood supply surrounding the bone of the growing child. The principles of treatment are similar to those in adults. However, the fact that in children the bone continues to grow after the fracture has healed will allow for some correction and remodeling of minor deformities.

Principles of Treatment

1. Mild angular deformities will frequently correct with growth. The amount of correction depends on the amount of angulation, the age of the child, and the distance of the fracture from the end of the bone. The closer the fracture is to the end of the bone and the younger the patient, the greater the amount of angulation that is acceptable. Correction is also more complete if the angulation is in the same plane of motion as the nearest joint. Angular deformities that are not in the same plane of motion as the nearest joint will persist, however.

2. Rotational malalignment will persist.

3. Apposition and mild shortening are of little importance in the young child. Bayonet (side-to-side) apposition is perfectly acceptable in long bone fractures in boys under 12 and girls under 10. Slight shortening with reduction may actually be desirable because acceleration of growth occurs following a displaced fracture. The tibia and humerus may overgrow up to 1 cm following a displaced fracture. Thus, some slight overlapping of these bones is desirable.

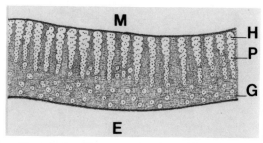

Fig 14–6. — The growth plate: *M* = the metaphyseal side; *H* = zone of hypertrophic cartilage; *P* = zone of proliferating cartilage cells; *G* = germinal cell layer; and *E* = epiphyseal or joint side of the growth plate.

4. Physical therapy after the fracture has healed is usually unnecessary and may even be unwise in the child. Forceful manipulation of the extremity will only cause more swelling and stiffness.

The Epiphyseal Plate

Two types of epiphyses exist in growing bones: the pressure epiphysis and the traction epiphysis (apophysis). Pressure epiphyses occur at the ends of long bones and contribute to the longitudinal growth of the bone. Traction apophyses, such as the iliac crest and trochanters of the hip, contribute primarily to the contour of the bone and little to actual longitudinal growth. They are present at the origin of major muscles and respond to traction rather than to pressure.

The epiphyseal plate itself consists of several zones or layers (Fig 14–6). The zone nearest the joint is the germinal cell layer. Moving away from the joint are the zone of proliferation, the zone of hypertrophic cartilage, and the zone of provisional calcification. Epiphyseal fractures may be categorized according to the type of injury, the relationship of the fracture line to the germinal cell layer, and the prognosis. Salter's classification is commonly used.

Most epiphyseal fractures occur irregularly through the weakest zone, the zone

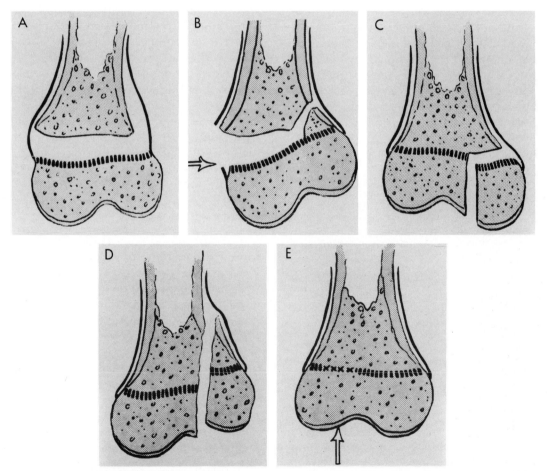

Fig 14–7.—Epiphyseal fractures. **A,** type I; **B,** type II; **C,** type III; **D,** type IV; **E,** type V crushing fracture. (From Salter, R. B., and Harris, W. R.: J. Bone Joint Surg. 45A:609, 1963.)

of hypertrophic cartilage. They are usually transverse and do not travel vertically across the germinal cell layer. These fractures are classified by Salter as type I or type II fractures, and the prognosis for normal healing is good (Fig 14–7). Manipulative reduction is usually successful. Overzealous attempts to correct minor persistent deformities during the reduction should not be made as these mild deformities will usually correct with growth. Further damage to the growth plate may be caused by overaggressive treatment.

Fractures that do traverse the growth plate vertically may disturb the growth so that angular deformity will result from continued growth. Cross-union may occur across the epiphyseal plate. These fractures are also frequently intra-articular in nature and accurate reduction is mandatory to prevent growth disturbance from occurring and to restore the joint surface. Surgery is usually necessary in order to accomplish these goals. Type V fractures are crush injuries that have a poor prognosis (Fig 14–8). Frequently, no definite fracture line is visible.

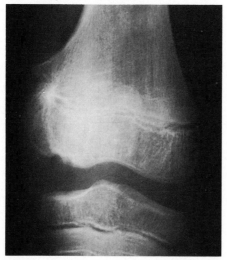

Fig 14–8.—Salter type V crush fracture that resulted in a complete bony bridge being formed in the medial aspect of the lower femoral epiphysis.

INJURIES OF THE SHOULDER

Fracture of the Clavicle

The clavicle is the only rigid bony connection between the shoulder and the chest, and it functions to hold the shoulder upward and backward. It may be injured by a fall on the outstretched hand (Fig 14–9).

Reduction is obtained by manipulating both shoulders upward, outward, and backward in order to reestablish the length of the clavicle (Fig 14–10). Infiltration of the fracture site with a local anesthetic will usually eliminate the pain. The reduction is maintained by a figure-of-eight dressing for four to five weeks in the child and five to six weeks in the adult. A prominence at the fracture site will often persist in the adult, but it usually disappears in the child a few months after remodeling of the bone has occurred. If undue pressure on the axillary vessels and nerves occurs during use of the dressing, pressure can be relieved by allowing the patient to lie down and temporarily abduct the shoulders. Open reduction is never indicated in the child and only rarely in the adult.

Fractures of the Scapula

Fractures of the scapula usually result from a direct blow or fall (Fig 14–11). Fractures that do not involve the articular surface of the glenoid cavity require little treatment. A sling or shoulder immobilizer may be used for one to two weeks until the pain subsides. Gentle motion of the shoulder is encouraged as soon as possible, and the results are usually excellent. The rare fracture that involves the shoulder articulation may require more extensive surgical treatment.

Fractures of the Upper Humerus

Undisplaced or impacted fractures of the surgical neck of the humerus are

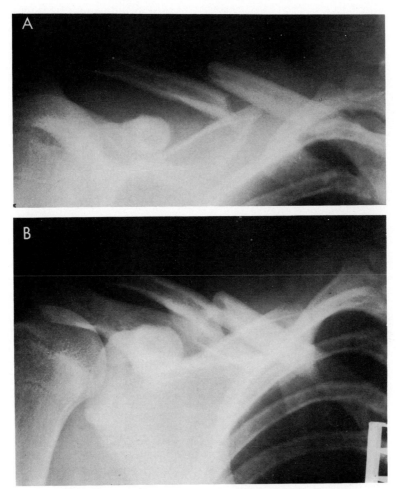

Fig 14–9. – **A,** fracture of the clavicle with overriding.
B, the length has been restored by manipulation.

common in elderly patients (Fig 14–12). Slight degrees of malalignment should be accepted in this age group.

The treatment consists of a dressing that immobilizes the arm and forearm to the chest and abdomen. This is continued for approximately two weeks and is followed by a sling for two more weeks. Pendulum exercises are performed in the sling. All immobilization is discontinued after four weeks. A hanging cast should not be used in these fractures as it may disimpact the bony fragments. The disability in this injury results not from the fracture itself, which usually heals readily, but from the secondary stiffness that develops in the shoulder, especially in elderly patients. It is not uncommon for some permanent loss of abduction to result from this injury, and full range of motion may take several months to return.

Displaced fractures of the surgical neck may require manipulative reduction and a hanging long arm cast. If closed methods fail, open reduction is occasionally indicated.

Fractures of the tuberosities of the upper humerus may occur from a fall or in association with a shoulder dislocation (Fig 14–13). Undisplaced fractures require only a sling for seven to ten days,

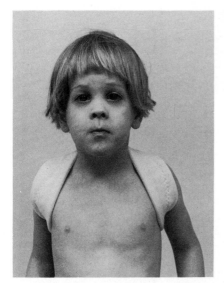

Fig 14–10. — After restoring the length to the clavicle, the fracture is immobilized by a figure-of-eight dressing. The dressing should remain snug and may have to be tightened by the parent.

followed by early range-of-motion exercises. Fractures that are displaced over 5 to 10 mm frequently require open reduction and internal fixation. If this is not performed, a bony impingement to abduction may result.

Fractures of the Shaft of the Humerus

Fractures of the shaft of the humerus usually heal well with nonoperative treatment. The function of the radial nerve should always be evaluated as it may be injured in its course around the humeral shaft.

Manipulative reduction with the patient under local anesthesia may be required, but distraction of the fracture fragments should be avoided. With the patient sitting on a stool and leaning forward, the weight of the arm will frequently reduce the fracture (Fig 14–14). The wrist is supported to overcome apprehension, but the elbow should hang free. Gentle traction and countertraction

are applied, and the fracture fragments are manipulated to correct any angulation. End-to-end apposition is tested by upward pressure on the elbow. If no "telescoping" of the fracture fragments occurs, apposition is usually secure. The fracture is immobilized by the application of a "U"-shaped plaster splint. Additional fixation may be obtained by strapping the humerus to the chest wall. After four to six weeks, gentle motion is encouraged. Healing is usually complete by eight to ten weeks (Fig 14–15).

INJURIES OF THE ELBOW

Fractures of the Head and Neck of the Radius

Fractures of the radial head and neck result from a fall on the outstretched hand with the elbow extended (Fig 14–16). All are characterized by tenderness over the radial head, local swelling, and pain on rotation or flexion of the forearm.

Undisplaced or minimally displaced fractures in adults and children are treated conservatively. If the swelling is extremely painful, the joint may be aspirated through the posterolateral triangle. A light posterior plaster splint and sling are applied with the elbow flexed 90°. The splint is removed in one to two weeks and early motion is encouraged. The sling is continued for another one to two weeks.

Displaced or comminuted fractures in adults are usually treated by early (24 to 48 hours) excision of the entire radial head. Otherwise, permanent restriction of joint motion and traumatic arthritis may result. Early removal is especially indicated in grossly comminuted and displaced fractures because the fracture fragments may act as a nidus for soft tissue calcification in the anterior elbow region, and myositis ossificans may result (Fig 14–17).

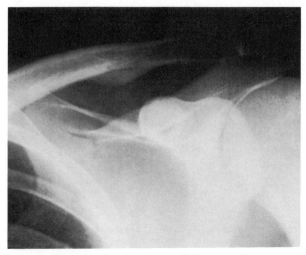

Fig 14–11.—Fracture of the scapula.

Children's fractures with less than 15° to 30° of angulation are treated as undisplaced fractures. Displaced fractures, or fractures that are angulated greater than 15° to 30°, are treated by closed or open reduction. The radial head is never removed in the growing child, however, as removal of the epiphysis will result in unequal growth of the forearm bones.

Regardless of the method of treatment, some loss of extension of the elbow is not uncommon. However, little functional impairment usually results.

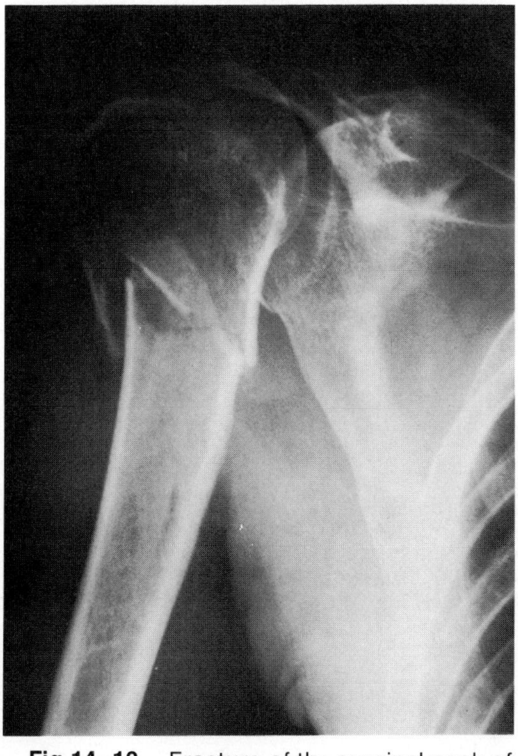

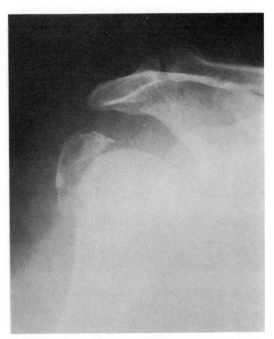

Fig 14–12.—Fracture of the surgical neck of the humerus.

Fig 14–13.—Displaced fracture of the greater tuberosity of the humerus.

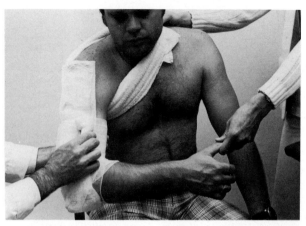

Fig 14–14. — Fracture of the humerus reduced by downward traction and countertraction. A "sugar-tong" or "U"-shaped splint is then applied and wrapped with gauze or elastic bandage. The splint begins in the axilla and ends over the shoulder. It may have to be tightened at intervals. A collar and cuff are added.

Fractures of the Olecranon

Fractures of the olecranon usually result from falls on the tip of the elbow (Fig 14–18). They are either displaced or undisplaced. The extensor mechanism is intact in undisplaced fractures and fur-

ther displacement is unlikely. The undisplaced fracture is easily treated with a molded posterior plaster splint for two weeks, followed by a sling and gradually increasing range-of-motion exercises.

Displaced fractures usually require

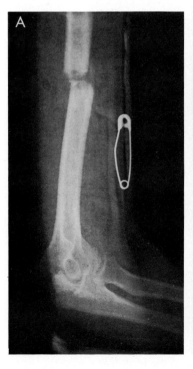

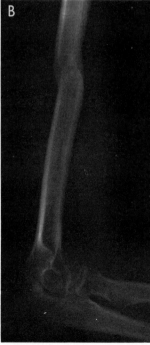

Fig 14–15. — **A,** transverse fracture of the humerus immobilized in a "U"-shaped splint. **B,** the end result.

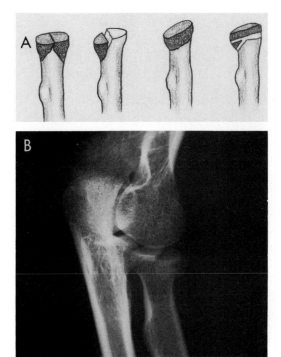

Fig 14–16.—**A,** various types of fractures of the radial head or neck that may be treated nonsurgically. **B,** typical head fracture in which full, pain-free motion was restored following conservative treatment.

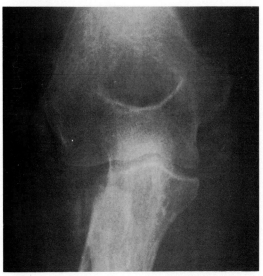

Fig 14–17.—Roentgenogram of the elbow following a comminuted radial head fracture showing multiple areas of ossification (myositis ossificans) in the adjacent soft tissue.

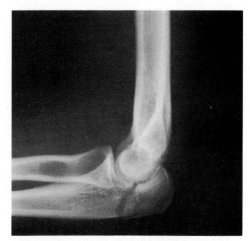

Fig 14–18.—Fracture of the olecranon.

open reduction and internal fixation in order to restore the bony alignment and repair the triceps insertion.

Monteggia's Fracture-Dislocation

This injury consists of a fracture of the proximal third of the ulna and a dislocation of the radial head (Fig 14–19). Closed treatment may suffice in the child, but open reduction with internal fixation is frequently necessary in the adult.

FRACTURES OF THE FOREARM

Fractures in Adults

Fractures that occur through both bones of the forearm in adults are usually shortened and displaced. Accurate reduction of these injuries by closed methods is difficult, and there is a strong tendency for these unstable fractures to angulate after swelling subsides in spite of a good reduction and cast immobilization. Strong muscular forces acting across the fracture fragments predispose to this loss of correction. Consequently, there is a high rate of nonunion. For these reasons, displaced fractures of both bones of the forearm in the adult are often treated by primary open reduction and internal fixa-

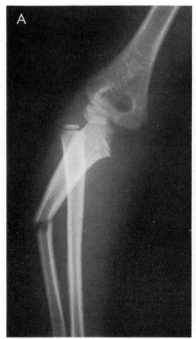

Fig 14–19.—A, Monteggia's fracture-dislocation of the elbow. Note the angulation of the ulna. Also, a line drawn through the shaft of the radius no longer passes through the capitellum. **B,** after reduction. It is always important to obtain a roentgenogram of the joint above and below any fracture.

tion (Fig 14–20). Closed treatment may be attempted, but if it is unsuccessful the first time, operative intervention is usually indicated. The length of immobilization is shorter with surgery and there is a more rapid return of function.

Isolated fractures of either the radius or the ulna are treated in a similar manner. If enough angulation is present to interfere with rotation, closed reduction is attempted. If it is unsuccessful, open reduction and internal fixation are indicated. Undisplaced fractures are treated with a long arm cast for eight to 12 weeks or until healing is complete.

Fractures in Children

Fractures in children differ from those in adults in that surgery is rarely necessary. Reduction is usually possible by manipulation with the patient under light anesthesia. Angulated fractures are re-

duced by traction and countertraction with manual correction of the angulation. It is often necessary to break the opposite cortex of the greenstick fracture in order to prevent reangulation from occurring in the cast (Fig 14–21). Displaced fractures are treated by reduction with traction and countertraction. Slight "bayonet" apposition is acceptable in young children if the alignment is satisfactory, because subsequent remodeling of growth will correct minor deformities. Children are examined at weekly intervals for three weeks in order to determine if any reangulation of the fracture is occurring after the swelling subsides. If angulation does recur before two weeks, it can usually be corrected manually. If more than two weeks passes, however, the healing is so rapid in children that the angulation may be permanent. The cast is continued for seven to eight weeks.

All forearm fractures in children and

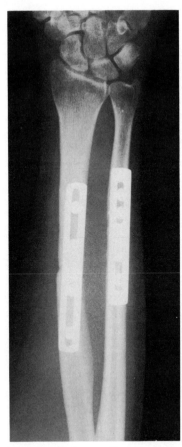

Fig 14–20.—Postoperative roentgenogram of a fracture of both bones of the forearm successfully treated by primary open reduction with internal fixation.

adults are immobilized by a long arm cast with the elbow flexed 90°. The forearm portion is always molded to prevent encroachment on the interosseous space (Fig 14–22).

INJURIES OF THE WRIST

Several common injuries occur in the region of the wrist joint: Colles' fracture, fracture of the distal radius in children, epiphyseal fractures of the distal radius, and fractures of the scaphoid. The treatment of all these injuries is very similar.

Colles' Fracture

Colles' fracture is the most common injury about the wrist. It usually results from a fall on the outstretched hand. The force of the fall fractures the distal radius and displaces it into the typical "silver-fork" position. In addition to the dorsal angulation, there is shortening and radial deviation of the distal fragment. There is usually an associated injury to the ulnar styloid or ulnar collateral ligament of the wrist (Fig 14–23).

The fracture can usually be reduced with the patient under local anesthesia if reduction is performed within a few hours. If more time passes, a general

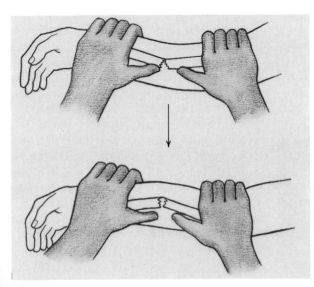

Fig 14–21.—Angulated greenstick fractures of both bones of the forearm should be manually broken through to prevent recurrence. The periosteum will remain intact. Reduction is then accomplished by simple traction.

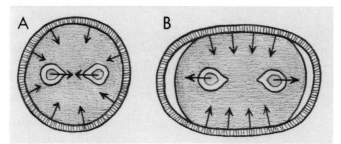

Fig 14–22. – **A,** cross section of an improperly molded forearm cast that may allow the forearm bones to move together. **B,** proper elliptical molding of the cast that prevents encroachment on the interosseous space. (From Charnley, J.: *The Closed Treatment of Common Fractures* [3d ed.; Edinburgh: Churchill Livingstone, 1970].)

anesthetic may be necessary as the local anesthetic may not diffuse through the clotted hematoma after several hours have passed. The tip of the ulna should also be injected.

With the assistant grasping the forearm for countertraction, the surgeon grabs the hand of the affected wrist (Fig 14–24). The thumb of the surgeon's other hand is placed over the distal fragment and the wrist is hyperextended to break up any impaction. Traction and countertraction are then applied and, using the thumb for pressure on the distal fragment, the rotation is corrected and the dorsal cortex of the distal fragment is forced onto the dorsal cortex of the proximal fragment. Ulnar and volar pressure over the distal fragment will then correct the radial and dorsal angulation. The radial styloid is palpated to determine if the length has been restored. With the assistant maintaining volar and ulnar tension on the hand, a well-molded cast is applied with the wrist slightly pronated. The cast is well molded over the dorsal and radial aspects of the distal fragment and the volar aspect of the proximal fragment in order to keep the dorsal soft tissue tight. A short arm cast is usually sufficient. Excessive volar flexion of the wrist should be avoided and is unnecessary if the cast is properly applied and molded. Excessive flexion of the wrist may cause median nerve compression. The base of the thumb should

be included to the interphalangeal joint to help prevent radial collapse.

If the reduction is satisfactory, the wrist is elevated and ice is applied for 48 to 72 hours. Active motion of the fingers is encouraged and the roentgenogram is repeated in seven to ten days. The fracture is immobilized for approximately five weeks.

After the cast is removed, some temporary stiffness should be expected for several weeks. This usually subsides gradually as the activity level is increased. A temporary splint that is removed several times a day for exercise is frequently helpful in the transition period between cast removal and full use of the extremity.

Occasionally, some loss of reduction may occur after the swelling subsides. This is particularly true if there is comminution of the dorsal cortex. In the elderly patient, this position should be accepted rather than attempting to remanipulate the fragments in order to improve the roentgenographic appearance. This would only lead to more swelling, stiffness, and loss of function. Accepting the minor cosmetic deformity caused by the slight malunion is preferable in the older patient.

Fracture of the Lower Radius in Children

In children and adolescents, a fracture may occur through the distal radial epiph-

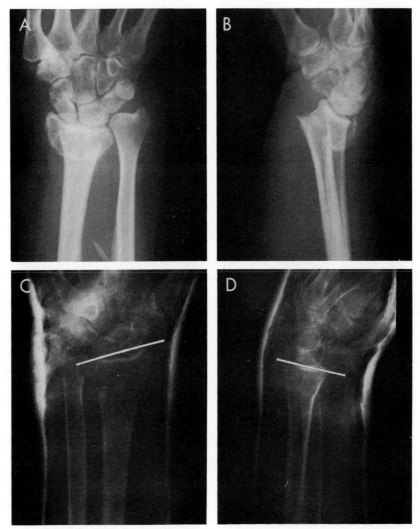

Fig 14–23. — **A** and **B,** typical Colles' fracture with dorsal and radial displacement. Normally, the tip of the styloid process of the distal radius extends 1 cm distal to the tip of the ulnar styloid. The articular surface of the lower ra- dius inclines 25° ulnarward and 10° volarward. **C** and **D,** following complete reduction, the length and these angular relationships are re- stored.

ysis. If it is displaced, it is reduced in the same manner as Colles' fracture and immobilized for five weeks. If it is undis- placed, the diagnosis may be difficult. It should be kept in mind, however, that sprains of the wrist are very rare in chil- dren. This is because the epiphyseal plate is weaker than the surrounding ligamen- tous structures, and trauma will usually produce an epiphyseal fracture rather than a ligamentous sprain. Clinical ten- derness over the epiphysis is highly suggestive of a fracture, and a short arm cast should be applied to these injuries for two weeks even though the roentgen- ogram may be normal. If healing callus is present at the end of two weeks, the cast is continued for an additional two weeks. If no callus is present, the cast is removed and the "sprain" has had excellent treat- ment.

Fractures of the distal radius also occur

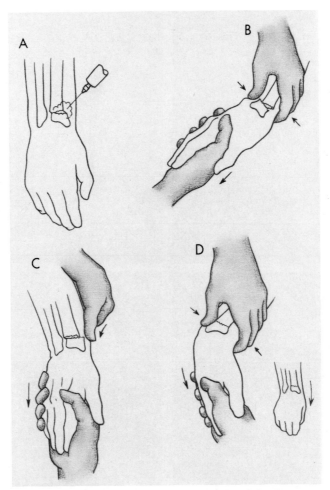

Fig 14–24. — Reduction of Colles' fracture. **A,** the needle is inserted dorsally into the fracture hematoma and 5 to 10 ml of local anesthesia is injected. **B,** the distal fragment is disimpacted and longitudinal traction is applied. Thumb pressure is then applied to the distal fragment to correct the dorsal displacement. **C,** the radial displacement is corrected by further digital pressure and ulnar deviation of the wrist. **D,** upward pressure on the proximal fragment and tension on the slightly flexed, ulnarly deviated hand will maintain the reduction. A cast is then applied and properly molded. (Adapted from Compere, E. L., Banks, S. W., and Compere, C. L.: *Pictorial Handbook of Fracture Treatment,* 5th ed., © 1963 by Year Book Medical Publishers, Inc., Chicago.)

in children approximately 2.5 cm above the wrist joint. They are treated in the same manner as Colles' fracture. Undisplaced or so-called torus fractures also occur in this area (Fig 14–25). No displacement occurs with this injury, but it should be immobilized in a short arm cast for three weeks.

Fractures of the Scaphoid

The scaphoid is the carpal bone that is most prone to fracture (Fig 14–26). This injury also occurs as the result of a fall on the outstretched hand.

The blood supply to this bone frequently enters the distal portion. Conse-

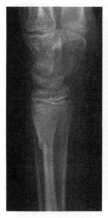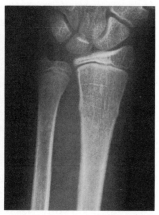

Fig 14–25.—The "buckle" or torus fracture of the distal radius.

quently, fractures that occur through the midportion of the bone may lead to avascular necrosis of the proximal fragment. Nonunion is also more frequent following this injury.

The diagnosis is sometimes difficult. It should be suspected, however, in any patient with a history of a "sprained wrist" who has persistent swelling and pain in the wrist. Clinically, tenderness and swelling in the anatomical snuffbox are characteristic findings.

The initial roentgenogram is often normal because there may be little or no displacement of the fracture fragments. The fracture usually becomes visible in two to four weeks, however, as decalcification around the fracture line occurs.

Whenever this injury is suspected, even if the roentgenogram is normal, a short arm cast including the thumb should be applied. The roentgenogram is repeated in two to three weeks. If a fracture is present, the immobilization is continued until the fracture has healed, which in this case may take from three to six months. A minimum of six weeks' immobilization is necessary. If there is any displacement of the fracture fragments, a long arm cast should be applied for six weeks, followed by a short arm cast for an additional six weeks.

INJURIES OF THE FINGERS

The principles of treatment of finger injuries are similar to other fractures, except that in the hand the reduction must be more accurate. With certain exceptions, manipulation and external immobilization constitute satisfactory treatment.

Principles of Treatment

1. Immobilize only the injured finger, if possible.

2. Avoid overimmobilization.

3. Be certain to correct rotational as well as angular malalignment.

4. Early surgery, in the form of open reduction and internal fixation, is often more "conservative" than overzealous manipulation and prolonged, improper splinting.

5. Fingers should be immobilized in

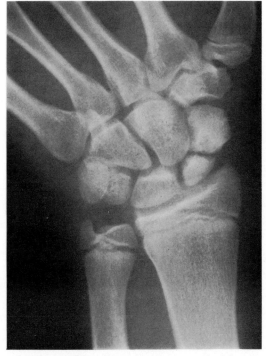

Fig 14–26.—The fractured scaphoid.

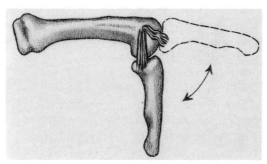

Fig 14–27.—Collateral ligaments of the metacarpophalangeal joint. These ligaments are normally lax in extension and tight in flexion. Prolonged splinting in extension may allow them to shorten slightly, making future flexion difficult.

the position of moderate flexion. Avoid splinting the finger joints in extension, especially the metacarpophalangeal joint (Fig 14–27).

6. Displaced intra-articular fractures involving greater than 25% of the joint surface are unstable and usually require open reduction and internal fixation.

7. In the position of grasping, the axes of all flexed fingers point to the navicular bone (Fig 14–28). Failure to appreciate this fact may result in rotational malunion.

Fractures of the Metacarpal

Fractures of the shaft of the finger metacarpal often present with dorsal angula-

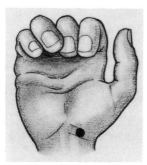

Fig 14–28.—Normally, the axes of the flexed fingers point to the navicular *(dot)*. Malunion with rotation will cause the fingers to overlap when a fist is made. The resultant functional disability may be great.

tion because of the action of the interosseous muscles (Fig 14–29). Fractures that are in good alignment and apposition will heal satisfactorily in four weeks. Slight shortening may be accepted. A short arm cast incorporating an aluminum splint and extending over the finger provides adequate immobilization.

Fractures of the neck of the metacarpal are common in the area of the small finger (Fig 14–30). These commonly occur in fist fights and are sometimes called "boxer's" fractures. Clinically, there is swelling over the fracture site and depression of the knuckle of the affected finger. Fractures with minimal angulation are treated with a compression dressing for one week, followed by gradually increasing active exercises. Fractures with angulation over 40° should be reduced. If closed reduction is successful, the finger is immobilized in a plaster cast and splint for four weeks. Even if fractures of the fourth and fifth metacarpal necks heal with a moderate amount of angulation, the functional result is usually good. Open reduction is occasionally indicated in severely angulated fractures.

Bennett's fracture is actually a fracture-dislocation that occurs at the carpometacarpal joint of the thumb (Fig 14–31). The metacarpal is usually dislocated proximally because of the pull of the long abductor muscle that inserts at its base. This injury requires exact reduction in order to avoid disturbing the function of this important joint. Most of these injuries are displaced and require reduction and internal fixation for the best overall results.

Fractures of the Phalanges

Fractures of the proximal phalanx usually angulate to the volar aspect of the hand (Fig 14–32). This angulation is produced by the pull of the intrinsic muscles. Oblique fractures of this bone are the most common cause of rotational deformity in the fingers. Reduction of the

require open reduction and internal fixation with elevation of the depressed plateau fragment.

Fractures of the Patella

Fractures of the patella usually result from a direct blow to the knee. They are classified as undisplaced or displaced (Fig 14–39).

Undisplaced fractures are easily treated nonoperatively. A compression dressing followed by a removable splint may be all that is necessary in the conscientious patient. Otherwise, a cylinder cast with the knee flexed approximately 5° is applied and maintained for five to six weeks. This is followed by an active exercise program to restore strength and mobility.

Displaced fractures usually require surgery. Comminuted fragments are removed, and the patellar fracture and extensor mechanism of the knee are repaired.

FRACTURES OF THE ANKLE

The talus is held in its position by bony and ligamentous structures and occupies a special position in the ankle joint. Any

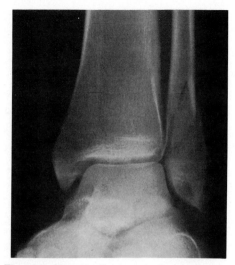

Fig 14–40.—Undisplaced fracture of the lateral malleolus.

deviation from that position through injury will inevitably result in traumatic arthritis if untreated. Undisplaced fractures of the ankle usually do not disturb the joint or "mortise," but displaced fractures with ligamentous injury frequently do and surgical repair is often necessary.

Fractures without Separation

Isolated, undisplaced fractures of either malleolus are usually stable and require only the application of a short leg walking cast with the ankle in the neutral position (Fig 14–40). Immobilization should be continued for seven to eight weeks. The fracture line of the lateral malleolus may persist roentgenographically for several months, but immobilization beyond eight weeks is usually unnecessary.

Undisplaced bimalleolar fractures are treated with a long leg cast to prevent motion and displacement of the fracture fragments. This cast is flexed 30° at the knee in order to prevent rotation of the lower leg. In four weeks, a short leg walking cast may be applied that is maintained for an additional four weeks.

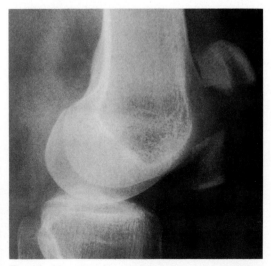

Fig 14–39.—Displaced fracture of the patella.

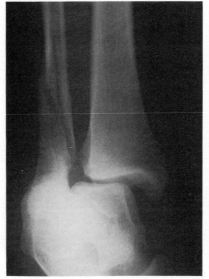 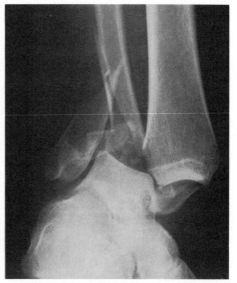

Fig 14–41 (left).—Displaced fracture of the lateral malleolus with widening of the ankle mortise.

Fig 14–42 (right).—Fracture-dislocation of the ankle.

Fractures with Separation

Fractures with significant displacement must be reduced, especially if any widening of the ankle joint is present (Fig 14–41). Isolated lateral malleolar fractures can frequently be treated nonoperatively, but bimalleolar and displaced medial malleolar fractures usually require surgery.

Fractures with dislocation of the talus should be reduced as rapidly as possible (Fig 14–42). If the dislocation is not promptly reduced, severe soft tissue injury with blistering and skin breakdown may result. Definitive surgical treatment of the fractures may also have to be delayed. The dislocation is reduced by traction and manipulation with the patient under local anesthesia. Following the reduction, the ankle is placed in a soft, bulky compression dressing reinforced with plaster splints. Any necessary surgery can then be performed on an elective basis.

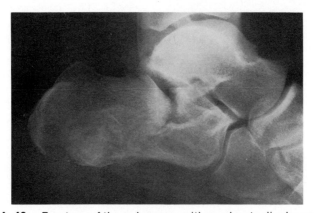

Fig 14–43.—Fracture of the calcaneus with moderate displacement.

FRACTURES OF THE FOOT

Fractures of the Calcaneus

A fracture of the calcaneus usually results from a fall on the heel. It is frequently associated with a compression fracture of the lumbar spine. The os calcis is usually crushed and the fragments are displaced in varying amounts (Fig 14–43).

Fractures of the os calcis are painful injuries characterized by severe swelling. The swelling may be so intense that blistering and even skin necrosis may occur. In order to control the swelling and hemorrhage, all calcaneus fractures are treated initially with a soft compression dressing, ice, and elevation. A cast is never applied immediately after the injury. The pain from the fracture and swelling is only intensified if a constricting circular cast is present over the heel.

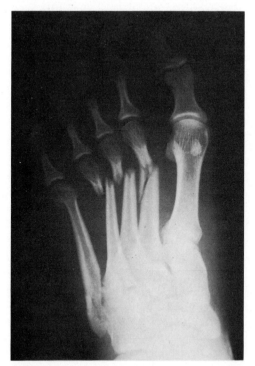

Fig 14–44. – Displaced fractures of the metatarsals that required open reduction and internal fixation.

Minimally displaced fractures are treated by cast immobilization for two to three weeks. The cast is removed as soon as possible in order to begin mobilization of the ankle and heel. Eversion and inversion movements are begun, but weight bearing is not allowed for six to eight weeks until the fracture has healed.

Displaced fractures are treated by either closed or open reduction. An attempt is made to elevate the depressed central articular fragment and reduce the widening of the heel.

Regardless of treatment, prolonged immobilization is inadvisable. Temporary disability following this injury may persist for one to two years, and some permanent impairment is common. Early motion without weight bearing appears to be most beneficial. Some restriction of eversion and inversion is usually permanent, which makes walking on rough, irregular surfaces difficult.

Fractures of the Metatarsals

Fractures of the necks or shafts of the metatarsals usually result from compression injuries of the foot. Undisplaced fractures require little treatment other than a compression dressing and crutches for four to six weeks. A short leg walking cast or hard-soled sandal may be preferable in a few days to allow the patient to discard the crutches.

Displaced fractures of the necks of the metatarsals should be reduced in order to prevent pain from developing under the metatarsal heads (Fig 14–44). Manipulation with the patient under anesthesia is sometimes effective, but maintenance of the reduction is frequently difficult. Open reduction with internal fixation is often necessary.

Fractures of the base of the fifth metatarsal are common and result from an inversion injury to the foot (Fig 14–45). They are usually undisplaced and require little treatment. A light compres-

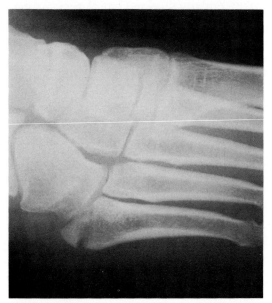

Fig 14–45.—Fracture of the base of the fifth metatarsal.

sion dressing and hard-soled sandal are usually sufficient. Crutches may be necessary for seven to ten days and healing is usually complete in five to six weeks.

Fractures of the Phalanges

Fractures of the toes are common and usually require little treatment. Undisplaced fractures may be treated by taping the injured toe to the adjacent toe for three to four weeks. Displaced fractures can usually be reduced with the patient under local anesthesia. Open reduction is

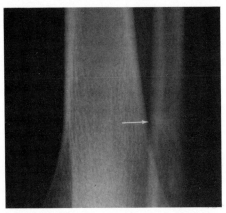

Fig 14–46.—Fatigue fracture of the lower fibula.

rarely necessary. Fractures of the proximal phalanx of the great toe, however, should be reduced accurately.

PATHOLOGIC FRACTURES

Pathologic fractures develop because of some abnormal local condition that causes the bone to become weakened. The most common causes are tumors that metastasize to bone. With the increase in the survival rate of cancer victims, there has also been an increase in the incidence of pathologic fractures. In order to maintain the highest possible level of function in such patients, aggressive management of these fractures is frequently indicated.

The treatment is usually surgical. Although radiation therapy may relieve the pain, it can actually impede fracture healing. By stabilizing the fracture, however, immediate use of the extremity is frequently possible. This is accomplished by curetting the tumor and filling the resultant cavity with methylmethacrylate cement. This is supplemented by the appropriate internal fixation device. The procedure may also be performed on a prophylactic basis.

FATIGUE FRACTURES

Fatigue or stress fractures are incomplete fractures that occur as the result of prolonged, repetitive strains. They may occur in any weight-bearing bone but are most common in the metatarsal ("march" fracture), neck of the femur, calcaneus, tibia, and fibula. Unconditioned athletes are prone to this injury. It is also common in military personnel who are subjected to long hikes or marching in their physical training program.

Clinically, a history of unusual stress with subsequent pain over a bone is common. Local tenderness and swelling over the affected bone are usually present.

The roentgenogram is usually normal early in the disorder. If this condition is suspected, treatment is instituted and roentgenograms are repeated at two-week intervals (Fig 14–46). A healing stress line is usually seen in two to four weeks. Exuberant periosteal bone formation may even simulate malignancy.

The treatment consists of protecting the bone from stress. Elimination of the offending activity is usually curative, although crutches are occasionally necessary. Gradual resumption of normal activity is allowed after the pain and tenderness subside.

FRACTURES REQUIRING SPECIAL CARE

Most of the fractures described in this chapter can be safely managed by the generalist using nonoperative means. There are, however, several common fractures, some previously mentioned, that are fraught with complications even when treated by one familiar with them. Many fractures will also require surgical intervention or specialized closed treatment. These fractures should always be referred to an orthopedic surgeon. Some of the more common injuries include the following: (1) All open fractures. These need meticulous cleansing and debridement to prevent osteomyelitis or gas gangrene. (2) Intra-articular fractures. These require accurate reduction to prevent the onset of traumatic arthritis. (3) All femur fractures, many of which will require prolonged traction, special casting, or surgery. (4) Most fractures of both bones of the lower leg in adults. In addition, there are several specific fractures in children and adults that should be treated only by an orthopedic surgeon (Table 14–1).

BIBLIOGRAPHY

Blount, W. P.: *Fractures in Children* (Baltimore: Williams & Wilkins Co., 1955).

Charnley, J.: *The Closed Treatment of Common Fractures* (3d ed.; Edinburgh: Churchill Livingstone, 1970).

Compere, E. L., Banks, S. W., and Compere, C. L.: *Pictorial Handbook of Fracture Treatment* (5th ed.; Chicago: Year Book Medical Publishers, Inc., 1963).

Flatt, A. E.: *The Care of Minor Hand Injuries* (3d ed.; St. Louis: C. V. Mosby Co., 1972).

Harrington, K. D., et al.: The use of methylmethacrylate as an adjunct in the internal fixation of malignant neoplastic fractures, J. Bone Joint Surg. 54A:1665, 1972.

Hunter, J. M., and Cowen, N. J.: Fifth metacarpal fractures in a compensation clinic population: A report on 133 cases, J. Bone Joint Surg. 52A:1159, 1970.

Marcove, R. C., and Yang, D. J.: Survival times after treatment of pathologic fractures, Cancer 20:2154, 1967.

McLaughlin, H. L.: *Trauma* (Philadelphia: W. B. Saunders Co., 1959).

Pool, C.: Colles' fracture, J. Bone Joint Surg. 55B:540, 1973.

Ryan, J. R., Rowe, D. E., and Salciccioli, G. G.: Prophylactic internal fixation of the femur in neoplastic lesions, J. Bone Joint Surg. 58A:1071, 1976.

TABLE 14–1.—COMMON FRACTURES AND THEIR COMPLICATIONS

FRACTURE	COMPLICATION
In Children	
Supracondylar fracture of the humerus	Volkmann's contracture, malunion
Lateral condylar fracture of the humerus	Nonunion, cubitus valgus, late ulnar nerve paralysis
Epiphyseal fractures III, IV, V	Growth disturbance
Radial neck and head fracture	Growth disturbance
In Adults	
Fracture of both bones of the forearm or displaced single bone forearm	Malunion, nonunion, restricted forearm rotation
Displaced malleolar or bimalleolar fracture	Nonunion, traumatic arthritis
Supracondylar, intercondylar fracture of the humerus	Traumatic arthritis, joint stiffness
Displaced olecranon fracture	Nonunion
Displaced radial head fracture	Traumatic arthritis, joint stiffness

15 / Special Topics

REFLEX SYMPATHETIC DYSTROPHY

REFLEX SYMPATHETIC DYSTROPHY is a syndrome of unknown cause that often follows a relatively minor injury. It has been called by several names: Sudeck's atrophy, causalgia, shoulder-hand syndrome, posttraumatic dystrophy, and others. The pathogenesis of the disorder is unclear, but a disturbance in the sympathetic nervous system apparently develops that leads to the characteristic symptoms and signs of pain and vasomotor disturbances.

CLINICAL FEATURES

Persistent pain that develops after an injury is the characteristic feature. It is frequently severe and often out of proportion to the amount of trauma. Initially, the pain is localized to the area of the injury, but gradually it spreads throughout the extremity. Hypersensitivity to light touch is also a frequent symptom. The extremity appears swollen and warm, and excessive perspiration may be present. Later, motion in the affected joints becomes restricted and the involved area becomes cool and atrophic. The skin appears dry and glossy. Stiffness and intractable pain may persist for several weeks or months.

The roentgenogram often reveals patchy osteoporosis (Fig 15–1).

TREATMENT

Reflex sympathetic dystrophy is best treated by prevention. All injuries should have immediate attention, and pain and swelling should be controlled. Early use of the extremity is also important. Once reflex sympathetic dystrophy develops, it is very difficult to treat. The most important aspect of therapy is restoration of motion by exercise. Active use of the extremity should be encouraged in spite of the pain. The edema may be controlled by elevation. Physical therapy in the form of passive range-of-motion exercises may be helpful but should not replace home treatment by the patient. Smoking should be discouraged. Repeated sympathetic blocks are frequently necessary. The treatment is often prolonged.

ROTATIONAL DEFORMITIES OF THE LEGS IN CHILDREN

Developmental abnormalities of the lower extremities are common and are frequently a source of concern to parents. The cause of these deformities is unknown, but heredity and persistent postnatal malpositioning play important roles.

In-toeing

The in-toeing gait pattern seen in young children is the most common rotational deformity and is usually secondary to one or more of the following causes: (1) internal rotation deformity of the hip secondary to contracture or excessive femoral anteversion, (2) internal (medial) torsion of the tibia, or (3) metatarsus varus (adductus) of the foot.

All three of these deformities are aggravated by positions or postures that are frequently assumed by the child or infant. Lying in the prone position with the legs extended and the feet internally rotated is often associated with in-toeing deformity. Sitting in the "reverse-tailor"

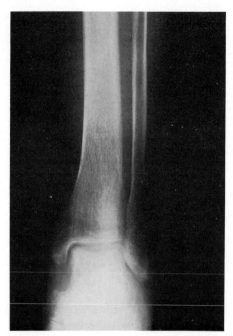

Fig 15–1.—Roentgenogram of the ankle several weeks following a relatively minor sprain. Severe osteoporosis (Sudeck's bone atrophy) of the lower tibia and fibula are present.

position with the feet internally rotated beneath the buttocks is directly related to persistent tibial rotation and adduction of the forefoot (Fig 15–2). Children may assume these positions for extended periods of time while sleeping, playing, or watching television.

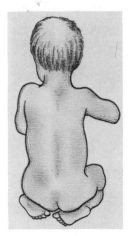

Fig 15–2.—The reverse-tailor position.

Children with internal rotation deformities have a high incidence of bowing of the lower extremities. This is frequently more apparent than real because the lower limb is never visualized in the true anteroposterior plane but rather in the oblique plane. The gait is often clumsy and the appearance may be unsightly.

INTERNAL FEMORAL TORSION

The diagnosis is made by clinical examination. It is helpful to mark the patellae and observe their position as the child walks. If the child toes in and the patellae face medially, excessive femoral anteversion or an internal rotation contracture of the hips should be suspected. If the child toes in and the patellae face straight forward, then the deformity is distal to the knee, either internal tibial torsion or metatarsus varus. Internal femoral torsion can also be measured with the patient prone, the hips extended, and the knees flexed 90° (Fig 15–3). External and internal measurements of hip motion are then made, with the tibia acting as a pointer. An internal rotation deformity exists at the hip when internal rotation exceeds external rotation by greater than 30°.

INTERNAL TIBIAL TORSION

An approximate measurement of tibial torsion can be obtained by having the patient sit on the examining table with the knees flexed 90° over the side. The tibial tubercle is palpated and directed straight forward. The malleoli are then grasped with the thumb and index finger and the position of the axis of the ankle joint is determined (Fig 15–4). Normally, approximately 20° to 30° of external tibial torsion is present in adults and the lateral malleolus will be posterior to the medial malleolus. In children with internal tibial torsion, the lateral malleolus will be anterior to the medial malleolus.

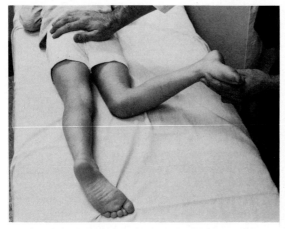

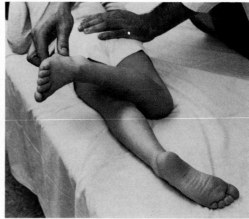

Fig 15–3. – Measuring femoral torsion. The tibia can act as a pointer. Internal femoral torsion is present when internal rotation **(left)** is 30° greater than external rotation **(right)**. External femoral torsion exists when external rotation exceeds internal rotation by the same amount.

METATARSUS VARUS

With the child in the same sitting position, the foot is examined for deformity. If metatarsus varus is present, the lateral border of the foot is convex and the medial border is concave (Fig 15–5).

TREATMENT

The treatment of internal rotation deformity of the hip is first directed at de-veloping proper sleeping and sitting habits. The child is encouraged to sleep on the side rather than in the prone position. The reverse-tailor position should be avoided. A stool or chair should be used for sitting rather than the floor. Passive stretching exercises of the hips are performed several times daily in the direction opposite the deformity, and the family is reassured that internal rotation deformity of the hips usually corrects spon-

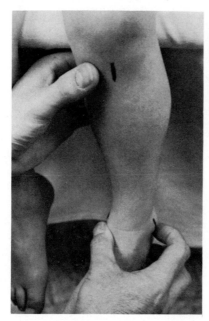

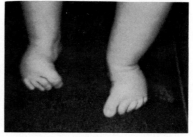

Fig 15–4 (left). – Measuring tibial torsion.
Fig 15–5 (above). – Metatarsus varus (adductus). The lateral border of the foot is convex.

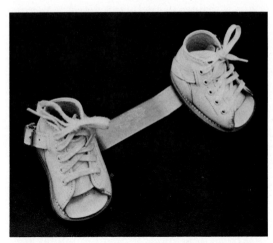

Fig 15–6.—The Denis Browne bar. It should not be wider than the width of the pelvis. Regular shoes may be used unless treatment is necessary for a deformity of the foot. The bar may be used full-time in the infant or at night only.

taneously by the age of 6. The Denis Browne splint may be helpful in these cases, but it should be used with some caution (Fig 15–6). Overaggressive attempts at correction of the hip deformity can result in ligamentous instability and angular deformity at the knee. Little actual corrective force can be applied to the hip by a device attached only to the feet. The splint should be used primarily to hold the feet in a neutral position. It may be used up to the age of 3, but it is usually not tolerated very well after that age. The splint is worn full time initially in the infant. After correction is obtained, it is used during naps and at night for several weeks to maintain the proper neutral alignment and prevent recurrence. Cable twisters may be of some benefit in the older child. The rare severe case that does not correct by the age of 8 may require surgery.

Tibial torsion is best treated by observation until the age of 12 to 18 months. Spontaneous correction usually occurs with growth. Improper sitting and sleeping habits should be corrected. Stretching exercises are of no value. The Denis Browne bar, used cautiously, is frequent-ly beneficial in cases that do not appear to be spontaneously correcting. It is used during naps and at night and should not be externally rotated more than 25° from the neutral position. The correction should be gradual in order to avoid damage to the ankle and knee joints. Over the age of 3, the cable twister is often helpful in internal tibial torsion. Shoes with corrective wedges or torque heels appear to be of little benefit in the treatment of in-toeing from femoral or tibial torsion.

The treatment of metatarsus varus will depend on whether the deformity is fixed or not. If the foot is flexible and the deformity easily overcorrectable, passive stretching exercises and a straight or reverse-last shoe are usually effective (Fig 15–7). If passive correction of the forefoot is not possible, early treatment with corrective casts is indicated. The correction should begin shortly after birth.

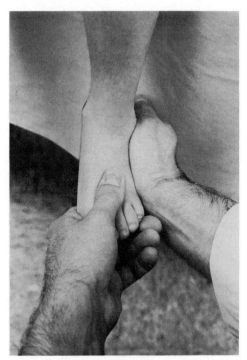

Fig 15–7.—Stretching exercises for metatarsus varus. The heel is firmly grasped. The forefoot is then passively manipulated into the corrected position and held for ten seconds. The exercise is repeated two to three times at regular intervals during the day.

When the disorder is seen after the age of 1 or 2, operative intervention is occasionally necessary. Early diagnosis is therefore important.

Out-toeing

External rotation deformity of the lower extremities is usually caused by the following: (1) external rotation of the hip secondary to soft tissue contracture or femoral retroversion (external femoral torsion), (2) external tibial torsion, or (3) calcaneovalgus or flat feet. Out-toeing is often associated with a genu valgum deformity and may be aggravated by sleeping in the prone position (Fig 15–8). The use of wide diapers or a children's "walker" with a wide pad will also potentiate an externally rotated gait.

If femoral retroversion is the cause, the examination will reveal that external rotation of the hips is significantly greater than internal rotation. External tibial torsion is diagnosed by the marked posterior position of the lateral malleolus as compared to the medial. The flatfoot deformity is frequently associated with eversion of the heels (chapter 11).

TREATMENT

Improper postural habits should be corrected. Wide diapers and walkers with wide canvas slings are avoided. Stretch-

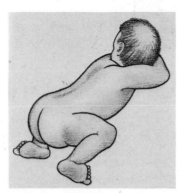

Fig 15–8.—The prone sleeping position, which frequently potentiates external rotation deformities.

ing exercises are begun for any hip deformity. The Denis Browne bar may be used for external femoral and tibial torsion, but only to hold the feet in the neutral position. Surgery is reserved for severe deformities.

ANGULAR DEFORMITIES OF THE LEGS IN CHILDREN

Genu Varum (Bowed Legs)

Genu varum with mild internal tibial torsion is a common, almost normal finding in early childhood. With growth and weight bearing, this developmental bowing spontaneously corrects in over 95% of patients. There is even a normal physiologic "swing" to a knock-knee deformity between the ages of 18 months and 3 years in many cases. The knock-knee deformity will then usually correct between the ages of 4 and 7.

The child is commonly seen because of the wide space between the knees and the mild in-toeing gait. Other possible causes of bowing (rickets, Blount's disease, and so on) can generally be ruled out by the child's history. There is usually no evidence of any intrinsic bone disease. The amount of genu varum can be determined by measuring the distance between the medial femoral condyles with the child standing and the medial malleoli touching.

Developmental genu varum is usually not severe and rarely requires any treatment. The family can be reassured that spontaneous correction will usually occur by the age of 3 years. Any associated metatarsus varus or tibial torsion should be appropriately treated, however. If improvement fails to take place by the age of 3 or 4, corrective braces may be necessary.

Genu Valgum (Knock-Knee)

Knock-knee may be due to a variety of disorders, including injury and metabolic disease. Most genu valgum, however, is present as one stage in the normal physiologic "swing" between developmental genu varum and normal alignment. It is usually bilateral and is most common between the ages of 2 and 4 years.

The severity of the deformity can be determined by measuring between the medial malleoli or Achilles tendons with the child standing, the medial femoral condyles touching, and the patellae facing forward (Fig 15–9).

Most patients need only reassurance and follow-up. Children with knock-knee who are under the age of 7 usually require no treatment as long as the intermalleolar distance is less than 8.75 cm. The rare case that persists beyond the age of 7 may require brace correction. If the deformity is excessive or unequal, a thorough search should be made for the underlying abnormality.

LEG LENGTH INEQUALITY

Limb length discrepancies in the lower extremities may result from several causes. The most common are fractures, os-

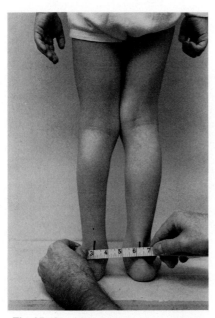

Fig 15–9. — Measuring genu valgum.

teomyelitis, neuromuscular disease, and vascular anomalies. Usually the affected limb is shorter, but occasionally the inequality is the result of overgrowth due to epiphyseal stimulation by inflammation or injury. Frequently, no cause is found. The inequality may cause a mild limp and compensatory scoliosis.

In children, a thorough search should be made to determine the cause. If any is found, the appropriate treatment is instituted. If no cause is noted, and the difference is less than 1 cm, the child is followed up by repeated careful measurements until mature to determine if the inequality is static or increasing. Both types of inequality require specialized care, and surgical correction of the asymmetry may be indicated. In children with growth remaining, equalization of the discrepancy may be accomplished either by lengthening the shortened extremity or by prematurely closing the epiphyseal plate on the longer extremity. The latter is more commonly performed.

In the adult, the amount of leg length discrepancy that is clinically significant is controversial, but it would appear that up to 2.0 cm of shortening is well tolerated. Chronic low back pain that may be accompanied by a leg length discrepancy should probably be treated with a shoe lift, however, to compensate for the difference. It is not known whether the leg length discrepancy actually causes the low back pain, but occasionally the pain will be relieved by the lift.

BRACES

Braces are appliances that allow partial movement of a joint. They perform several functions, including protection and stabilization. They are most commonly used to temporarily support and restrict motion in the treatment of painful disorders of the spine. The patient should also be encouraged to exercise and develop proper muscular tone, however, so that dependence on the support is avoided.

Cervical Collars

Cervical collars extend from the head to the thorax and are usually soft, although semirigid collars are also available (Fig 15–10). The soft collar is usually more comfortable but restricts motion less than the other collars. These appliances are all used in the treatment of degenerative disc disease and minor ligamentous or muscular injuries of the cervical spine.

Taylor Brace

This is a fundamental back brace useful in dorsal and lumbar spine disease (Fig 15–11). It is a high, semirigid brace that may be modified. Degenerative disc disease and minor fractures may be treated with this brace or one of its modifications (long Taylor, modified Taylor, short Taylor).

Knight Spinal Brace (chairback)

This is a rigid lumbar orthosis that is very useful in treating chronic low back pain when more support is required. It is also used in the treatment of disc disease and spondylolisthesis.

Jewett (hyperextension) Brace

This three-point brace provides pressure over the lumbar spine, sternum, and symphysis pubis. It is used in minor fractures of the dorsal spine when extension is desired. It is also useful in the treatment of epiphysitis.

Knight-Taylor Spinal Brace

This is a rigid high back brace used for fractures of the spine above L3. It may also be used for degenerative disc conditions throughout the entire spine.

Light Lumbar Supports

These supports are usually made of canvas and may be reinforced with metal stays. They are commonly used in the treatment of lumbar disc disease and chronic low back pain syndromes. They also function to increase the intra-abdominal pressure that aids in the support of the low back. They are more comfortable than the Knight spinal brace but provide less support.

DISABILITY RATING

The physician is frequently called on to determine the amount of disability that

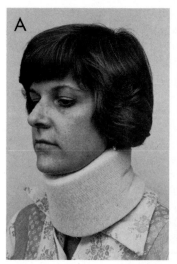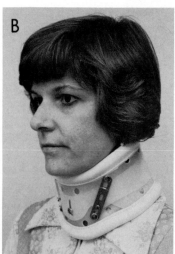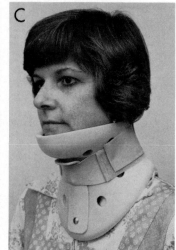

Fig 15–10.—Cervical collars. **A,** the soft foam collar. **B,** the adjustable collar. **C,** the Philadelphia collar.

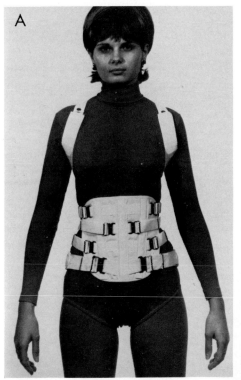

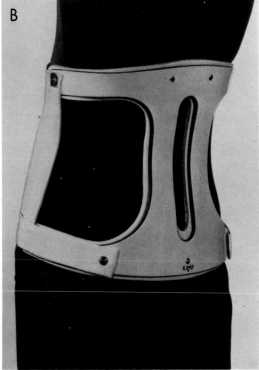

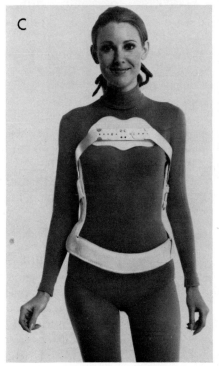

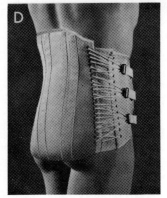

Fig 15–11.—Spinal braces. **A,** the Taylor brace. **B,** the Knight spinal (chairback) brace. **C,** the Jewett hyperextension brace. **D,** the lumbosacral support. (From Camp International, Inc., Jackson, Mich.)

is present as the result of musculoskeletal disease or injury. This determination is frequently used as the basis for settlement in workmen's compensation cases as well as personal injury litigation. It is usually, however, the "physical impairment rating" expressed as a percentage rather than "disability" that must be determined. It is not the duty of the physician to determine how this impairment affects the patient socially or economically. Frequently, however, it is the impairment rating that is used as the sole basis for the determination of disability by those administrators responsible for it.

Disability may be defined in various ways and is not a medical but rather an administrative term. Medically, it is physical impairment that prohibits the performance of normal physical function. Under Social Security, it means the inability to do any work for at least 12 months because of a physical impairment. Legally, it means permanent bodily injury for which restitution may be judged necessary. Under workmen's compensation statutes, disability is frequently divided into (1) temporary total disability during which period of time the patient is under care and unable to work, (2) temporary partial disability during which time recovery is sufficient that some employment may be begun, or (3) permanent disability, which is permanent loss of function after maximum recovery.

Physical impairment can usually be measured accurately on the basis of loss of physical function. A careful clinical history and physical examination are mandatory. Laboratory and roentgenographic analysis may also be necessary. In the evaluation of pain that may be present by history or during the examination, it is generally accepted that when no organic findings or clinical manifestations are found to substantiate its presence, it contributes little, if anything, to a physical impairment rating.

For the determination of specific ratings for each impairment, the following manuals are excellent: *Manual for Orthopedic Surgeons in Evaluating Permanent Physical Impairment,* "A guide to the Evaluation of Permanent Impairment of the Extremities and Back," and *Disability Evaluation Under Social Security.*

JOINT REPLACEMENT SURGERY

Great advances have been made in the past 15 years in the surgical treatment of degenerative and rheumatoid arthritis. These advances have been due primarily to improvements in the techniques of joint arthroplasty. This procedure is most commonly used for conditions of the hip and knee, but devices have been developed for use in almost every joint (Fig 15–12).

The basic purpose of these techniques is to implant a device into the joint that replaces the degenerated articular surfaces. Most of the procedures utilize a hard plastic, high-density polyethylene for the socket (Fig 15–13). This articulates with a metallic component, both components being fixed to the bone by a cementing compound, methylmethacrylate.

The goal of joint replacement surgery is to eliminate the disability that results from pain, loss of motion, and malalignment. The operation is indicated in adults with osteoarthritis and patients with rheumatoid arthritis at any age. It is suitable in patients with bilateral disease, and advanced age is no contraindication. It has been used successfully in almost every age group. Rehabilitation following a joint replacement is usually rapid. Motion and partial weight bearing are started within two to four days after surgery on the lower extremities. Progressive ambulation is allowed for the remainder of the hospitalization, which normally lasts 10 to 14 days. A home exercise program is continued for two

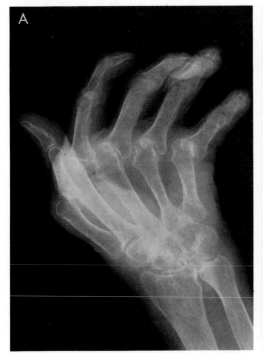
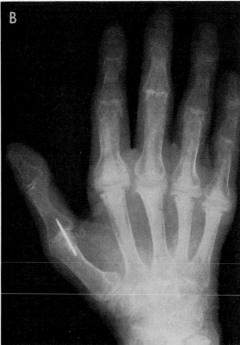

Fig 15–12. – **A,** severe rheumatoid arthritis of the hand with dislocations of the metacarpophalangeal joints. **B,** postoperative roentgenogram following metacarpophalangeal replacement. The alignment and function are markedly improved.

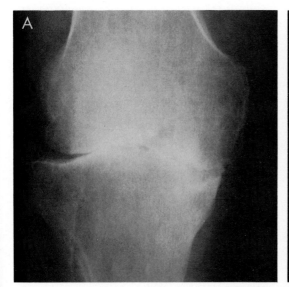
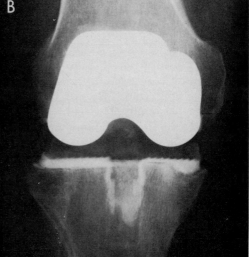

Fig 15–13. – **A,** degenerative arthritis of the knee.
B, postoperative roentgenogram following total knee replacement.

months after dismissal, and a cane or crutches may be necessary for that period of time.

Mechanical problems following total knee replacement are slightly more common than those following total hip replacement, but the results are uniformly good in both procedures. Over 90% of patients undergoing arthroplasty have excellent relief of pain and improvement in motion.

COMPARTMENT SYNDROMES OF THE LOWER LEG

Compartment syndromes are disorders of the extremities in which increased tissue pressure compromises the circulation to the muscles and nerves within the space. These conditions are most common in the lower leg, where four natural compartments exist (anterior, lateral, deep posterior, and superficial posterior). The anterior compartment is most commonly involved.

The disorder may be acute or chronic in nature. Chronic cases may be confused with stress fractures, tendinitis, and other forms of "shin splints." The acute case is associated with significantly greater morbidity.

CLINICAL FEATURES

The acute form may follow exercise, burns, trauma, or vascular injury. Pain, numbness, and weakness are the most common complaints. The pain is often severe because of muscle and nerve ischemia. The chronic case is usually related to exercise, and symptoms are generally mild.

Weakness, hypoesthesia, and pain on passive stretch of the involved muscle are usually present. The affected area may also be swollen and tense. The peripheral pulse is often diminished. There is usually an increase in intracompartmental tissue pressure that can be measured directly.

The roentgenogram is usually normal but should be obtained in the chronic case to rule out stress fracture.

TREATMENT

The chronic case usually subsides with rest, but fasciotomy is occasionally performed to prevent recurrence. The acute form requires immediate surgical decompression. Without treatment, necrosis of muscle and nerve may occur, resulting in permanent weakness, contracture, and nerve dysfunction similar to Volkmann's ischemic contracture in the upper extremity.

MYOSITIS OSSIFICANS

Myositis ossificans is a condition characterized by the formation of heterotopic bone in the soft tissues. It usually develops in muscle as the result of trauma (myositis ossificans circumscripta). A rare congenital form (myositis ossificans progressiva) may begin without trauma or shortly after birth.

The more common traumatic form usually follows a single injury or multiple blows to the same area. The mechanism of bone formation is unknown, but interstitial hemorrhage is thought to play a role. Eventually the hematoma becomes calcified and ossified.

CLINICAL FEATURES

The favorite sites of development are the quadriceps, brachialis, deltoid, and hamstrings. After the injury, a large hematoma usually forms. The area becomes swollen and tender and motion is gradually restricted. As the swelling and pain subside, a firm mass becomes palpable in the involved area. Motion may continue to be restricted because of obstruction by the mass or from inelasticity of the muscle.

The initial roentgenographic appearance is that of a poorly defined opaque mass in the soft tissue adjacent to the bone. As the mass matures, it becomes more clearly outlined and dense (Fig 15–14). Eventually, it will diminish slightly in size and become transformed into mature bone.

TREATMENT

Early aspiration of large, well-localized hematomas may prevent heterotopic bone formation. Ice, elevation, and rest will prevent further swelling. Once bone formation has begun, rest of the affected part is indicated. Moist heat and gentle exercise may be helpful to prevent stiffness, but physical therapy will only lead to more disability. If the heterotopic bone is locally painful or disabling, it may be removed, but excision is absolutely contraindicated until complete bony maturity is reached. This may take several months. Premature removal will only result in a recurrence that is often more extensive than the original mass.

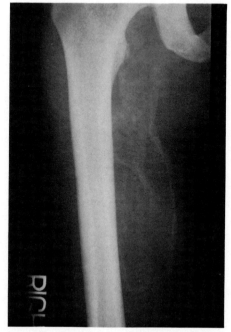

Fig 15–14.—Large ossifying hematoma (myositis ossificans) in the hamstrings.

INJECTION AND ASPIRATION THERAPY

Locally injected analgesics and steroids are frequently used in the treatment of musculoskeletal diseases. Their use in many specific affections has been described in previous chapters. This section will deal with their use in other common conditions.

In general, these compounds are used to relieve pain and improve function. The exact mechanism by which this is accomplished is unknown. An increase in the local blood flow and improvement in local tissue metabolism are common explanations. A placebo effect is undoubtedly present in some cases.

A variety of materials are available but the most commonly used are 1% plain lidocaine and various corticosteroids, either short- or long-acting. They may be injected separately or together. The use of a small amount of local anesthetic for skin infiltration may be necessary in the apprehensive patient. If a joint is to be entered that has a thick capsule, it should also be infiltrated. A 20- or 22-gauge needle is then used for the injection or aspiration. The patient should also be cautioned that a mild inflammatory reaction occasionally occurs following steroid injection and lasts for one to two days. It usually responds to ice, rest, and analgesics.

When employing these compounds, it is important not to rely solely on their use in the treatment of any disorder. They are used only as an adjunct to the appropriate treatment of the underlying abnormality. Sufficient knowledge of the relevant regional anatomy is also essential, and no more than four to six injections should be given over a six-month period.

General Principles

1. Maintain strict sterile technique.
2. Avoid injection and aspiration in the presence of local infection. A needle

passed into a joint through an area of cellulitis may spread the infection into the joint.

3. Avoid the injection of major weight-bearing tendons (patellar tendon, Achilles tendon) and joints. Such injections may mask the normal symptoms and allow a level of activity that could be locally harmful. An exception is for the temporary relief of the degenerated joint.

Soft Tissue Injection

Painful disorders of the soft tissue include such conditions as bursitis, tendinitis, tenosynovitis, trigger points, and so-called fibrositis. Most of these conditions have been previously described. Trigger points, fibrositis, and other similar syndromes are poorly understood disorders that present with pain and localized tenderness. A common site for the development of these tender areas is the spine, especially the interscapular and lumbosacral areas.

The depth of the injection varies from 1.25 to 5 cm and it may be necessary to inject several areas. The best relief is obtained when the area is well defined. If the area to be infiltrated lies directly over bone, it is usually safe to insert the needle until it touches bone. Fluid may be injected at this point and the needle is then retracted for further infiltration. Particular care should be exercised, however, when the injected area does not lie over bone but rather over soft structures such as viscera.

Joint Injection

There are occasional instances where intra-articular aspiration and injection are helpful. These are more easily performed when an effusion is present. Except for the shoulder and hip, most joints are entered on their extensor aspect. The major neurovascular bundle is usually found on the flexor side. Fluid will also usually distend the joint most in the direction of the extensor side, making entrance easier.

The knee is the joint most commonly entered. If fluid is present in the suprapatellar pouch, the joint may be entered through the area of maximum swelling. Otherwise, the medial or lateral surface is used so that the needle passes between the patella and femur with the knee extended. Relaxation of the extensor mechanism is necessary. Other joints, including the smaller joints, are entered in a similar manner.

BIBLIOGRAPHY

Bloomberg, M. H.: *Orthopedic Braces* (Philadelphia: J. B. Lippincott Co., 1964).

Charnley, J.: The long-term results of low-friction arthroplasty of the hip performed as a primary intervention, J. Bone Joint Surg. 54B:61, 1972.

Disability Evaluation Under Social Security (Chicago: American Medical Association, 1969).

Gross, R. H.: Leg length discrepancy: How much is too much, Orthopedics 1:307, 1978.

A guide to the evaluation of permanent impairment of the extremities and back, J.A.M.A. (special issue), Vol. 166, 1958.

Johnson, R. M., et al.: Cervical orthoses: A study comparing their effectiveness in restricting cervical motion in normal subjects, J. Bone Joint Surg. 59A:332, 1977.

Knight, R.: Developmental deformities of the lower extremity, J. Bone Joint Surg. 36A:521, 1954.

Manual for Orthopedic Surgeons in Evaluating Permanent Physical Impairment (Chicago: American Academy of Orthopedic Surgeons, 1959).

Matsen, F. A., and Clawson, D. K.: The deep posterior compartmental syndrome of the leg, J. Bone Joint Surg. 57A:34, 1975.

Morley, A. J. M.: Knock-knee in children, Br. Med. J. 2:976, 1957.

Salenius, P., and Vankka, E.: The development of the tibiofemoral angle in children, J. Bone Joint Surg. 57A:259, 1975.

Sheridan, G. W., and Matsen, F. A.: Fasciotomy in the treatment of the acute compartment syndrome, J. Bone Joint Surg. 58A:112, 1976.

Sherman, M.: Physiologic bowing of the legs, South. Med. J. 53:830, 1960.

Swanson, A. B.: Flexible implant arthroplasty for arthritic finger joints, J. Bone Joint Surg. 54A:435, 1972.

Tachdjian, M. O.: *Pediatric Orthopedics* (Philadelphia: W. B. Saunders Co., 1972).

16 / Radiologic Aspects of Orthopedic Diseases

DEAN F. TAMISIEA, M.D.

Contained within this chapter are a radiologist's viewpoints and suggestions regarding the interpretation of bone roentgenograms that hopefully will serve as a useful and practical guide for the busy family practitioner. Principles concerning roentgenographic positioning, anatomy, and pathology will be presented utilizing a regional anatomical approach.

GENERAL CONSIDERATIONS OF ROENTGENOGRAPHIC BONE ANATOMY

Before beginning a detailed discussion of regional roentgenographic anatomy and pathology, a consideration of pertinent radiologic bone anatomy is important. A bone can be evaluated according to its various components (Fig 16-1).

Epiphysis

The primary growth center of a bone is termed the epiphysis. It contributes to the growth in length of the bone. It, as well as the following components, can be affected and changed in appearance by congenital, metabolic, nutritional, traumatic, and other disease processes.

Physis

The radiolucent band between the epiphysis and metaphysis constitutes the physis or epiphyseal cartilage plate. It is formed in part by the zone of provisional calcification.

Metaphysis

The metaphysis characteristically is splayed or funnel-shaped. It is a favorite site for the development of benign as well as malignant lesions.

Diaphysis

The long tubular segment of bone forms the diaphysis. The constituent parts include the central medullary cavity and spongiosa and the dense cortex lined internally by the endosteum and covered externally by periosteum.

Apophysis

There are several apophyses found throughout the skeletal system, the best example being the greater trochanter of the proximal femur. They do not contribute to bone growth but are considered accessory ossification centers. They tend to appear later than the epiphyses in normal bone development, forming protrusions to which ligaments and tendons attach.

Epiphyses and apophyses occasionally fail to unite to the parent bone, resulting in unfused ossicles or accessory bones that are often misinterpreted as fractures. Most of these will be discussed under regional anatomical variations. When confronted with such problems as accessory bones, *An Atlas of Normal Roentgen Variants That May Simulate Disease* (Keats, 1974), and *Borderlands of the*

219

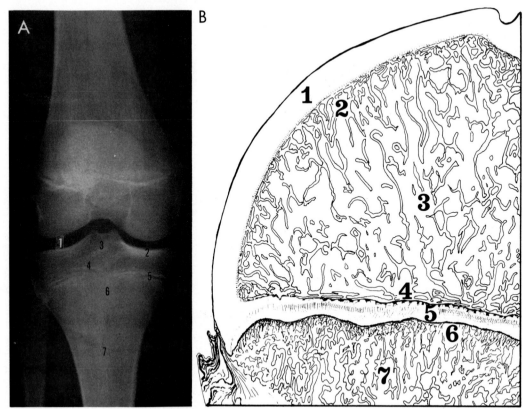

Fig 16–1.—Anatomy of a bone. **A,** radiologic terms: (1) articular cartilage does not show in film; (2) white outline of subarticular margin of epiphysis; (3) epiphysis; (4) increased density of terminal plate; inner bone margin of epiphysis; (5) epiphyseal line; strip of lesser density; epiphyseal plate; diaphyseal-epiphyseal gap (roentgenographically, these terms exclude the recently calcified cartilage, which appears as part of the metaphysis); (6) metaphysis; includes both calcified cartilage and newly formed bone; and (7) diaphysis or shaft. **B,** histologic terms: (1) articular cartilage; (2) compact bone of subarticular margin; (3) epiphysis, spongy bone; (4) terminal plate; (5) epiphyseal disc; growth cartilage (histologically, these terms include the calcified cartilage); (6) metaphysis; includes only newly formed bone of primary ossification; and (7) spongy bone of diaphysis. (From Pyle, S. I., and Hoerr, N. L.: *Radiographic Atlas of Skeletal Development of the Knee* [Springfield, Ill.: Charles C Thomas, Publisher, 1955].)

Normal and Early Pathologic in Skeletal Roentgenology (Kohler and Zimmer, 1968) are excellent reference sources.

In addition to the status of nonfusion, epiphyseal and apophyseal centers can be divided before they unite, causing further confusion with fractures. Sesamoid bones, as seen in the hands and feet, can also be divided.

Bone Vessels

There is only indirect evidence of the presence of blood vessels on roentgeno-grams, and they are the nutrient canals and foramina. They enter the medullary cavity by way of foramina, most often near the midshaft of a long bone, resulting in radiolucent channels. When viewed on the roentgenogram, one can be confused with a fracture.

Prominent nutrient canals frequently are seen in the diaphyses of the femur and tibia. Y-shaped nutrient canals occur in the midportion of the iliac bones of the pelvis and in the subspinous region of the scapulae.

ANALYTIC APPROACH
TO BONE CHANGES

General Considerations

Rather than going into a great deal of confusing anatomical and pathologic detail, some basic fundamentals and principles related to bone roentgenograms will be discussed. The first and foremost rule: every roentgenogram is abnormal until it is proved, after thorough examination, that everything is, indeed, normal. It may not work all of the time, but it encourages as complete a search of the film as possible. This results in two important objectives. First, it eliminates the method of instantaneous pattern recognition. Second, it prods the physician to search for even the slightest, most subtle change in bone roentgenographic patterns.

It is important to avoid tunnel vision, to look at the "whole thing" from the corners of the film to the center. Evaluate separately the soft tissues, the joints, bone density, architecture, and trabecular patterns. Scrutinize the medullary cavity and spongiosa as well as the cortex, periosteum, and endosteum.

In other words, attempt an analytic approach by evaluating each specific feature of bone. Visualize each detail separately. An obvious fracture catches one's attention, and the tendency is to forget the remainder of the picture, possibly missing an associated but unsuspected dislocation or even an early destructive tumor.

Two views of a bone at right angles is an important law in radiology. Never make a diagnostic interpretation on the basis of one view. One should not hesitate to obtain additional projections of the suspicious area if he is convinced that something is wrong. Comparative films of the opposite side are also often helpful, especially in younger patients whose growth centers cause more than enough confusion. And if the roentgenograms remain normal to the eye but clinical suspicion persists, have the patient return in seven to ten days for repeated films since it is not uncommon for a stress fracture, radial head fracture, or early osteomyelitis to have delayed appearances roentgenographically.

Once a bone lesion is discovered on an x-ray film, one is in the challenging position of forming a differential diagnosis. At first the spectrum of possibilities might be quite broad, but by correlating historical, physical, and laboratory findings with the roentgenographic discovery, the spectrum can be narrowed to a few diseases and will, in most instances, lead to the correct diagnosis.

To permit the most accurate diagnosis, the differential list should be based on certain, specific bone responses that are most characteristic of the disease process. There are various distinctive visible reactions that bone may have to singular disease entities, such as the pattern of bone destruction or production, the type of periosteal reaction, and soft tissue involvement, if any.

Unfortunately, there are more diseases affecting bone than there are responses that bone can create. Consequently, there are more roentgenographic similarities than differences among the various bony lesions. For example, the periosteal reaction usually associated with Ewing's sarcoma, characteristically described as "onion skin," quite often occurs with osteomyelitis.

Conversely, there are specific disease processes that produce more than one kind of predictable bone reaction. Such is the case with osteomyelitis, whose periosteal response can appear benign but can also mimic malignant changes.

Specific Parameters

There are certain specific parameters of bone that need careful attention. In the process of evaluating these, employing a systematic approach can lead to a logical conclusion. Among the criteria to be analyzed are increase or decrease in bone density, alterations in osseous texture (trabecular pattern), periosteal reactions, and the conditions of the cortex, endosteum, and medullary spongiosa.

If any changes of these are observed, then the abnormality should be studied in terms of its size and configuration and the sharpness of its margins (transition zone); the specific bone involved and the position of the lesion within that bone (epiphysis, metaphysis, or diaphysis) should be noted. For example, leukemia, metastatic neuroblastoma, a benign simple cyst, and Brodie's abscess have a predilection for the metaphysis, whereas a chondroblastoma typically involves the epiphysis.

This is a simple, general outline with many more particulars coming into play. But by developing this type of approach, the many clues offered will help to determine the nature of the pathologic process and place the lesion into a certain category (for example, benign, malignant, infectious, traumatic, or metabolic). In Table 16–1 some of the specific characteristics of different bone lesions have been listed.

Many noteworthy textbooks are available that cover this topic in greater detail (Edeiken and Hodes, 1967; Greenfield, 1975). However, there are two parameters that require more expanded discussion: types of bone destruction and periosteal reaction.

Patterns of Bone Destruction

Three roentgenographic patterns of bone destruction have been described according to Lodwick: geographic, moth-eaten, and permeative.

1. Geographic bone destruction is distinguished by single or multiple sharply marginated, relatively large, punched-out holes. Multiple myeloma and histiocytosis X (eosinophilic granuloma, Letterer-Siwe disease, and Hand-Schüller-

Christian disease) tend to fit this pattern.

2. Moth-eaten bone destruction involves a lesion containing multiple, coalescing holes of moderate size, suggesting a somewhat aggressive process. Osteomyelitis and less pathogenic tumors may exhibit this form of destruction.

3. Permeative bone destruction is seen when the bony alterations are characterized by multiple, tiny holes that become smaller and fewer in number near the periphery of the lesion, resulting in a wide transition zone from abnormal to normal bone. This will be seen in very aggressive tumors and poorly localized infections.

It is of interest that no matter what type of osseous resorption is taking place, as much as 50% of the bone must be destroyed before becoming evident roentgenographically. Radionuclide bone scans constitute a much more sensitive examination for determining the presence of bone replacement by tumor or infection. In one recent comparative study, the accuracy of isotope imaging with technetium Tc 99m phosphate complexes for skeletal lesion detection was 98%, as compared to 28% for standard roentgenography (Siberstein et al., 1973). Because of this fact, the use of skeletal roentgenographic surveys has declined in favor of nuclear scans. Nevertheless, although the sensitivity of scanning is high its specificity is low, and therefore roentgenographic studies of the abnormal isotope areas are mandatory.

Types of Periosteal Reactions

When the outer periosteal membrane of bone is irritated, its constituent osteoblastic cells react by producing new bone. This new bone can take on either a solid or an interrupted appearance, and the specific form can assist in identifying the inciting cause (Table 16–2).

Solid periosteal reactions are usually indicative of a benign process. The new

TABLE 16–1.—General Characteristics of
Different Bone Lesions

Characteristics of Benign Bone Lesions
   Sclerotic margins (narrow transition zone)
   Homogeneous periosteal reaction
   Expansion of an intact cortex
Characteristics of Solitary Malignant Bone Lesions
   Permeative or moth-eaten destruction (wide transition zone)
   Irregular sometimes spiculated periosteal reaction
   Preferential metaphyseal location
   Extraosseous extension with soft tissue mass and occasional
      fluffy calcifications
Characteristics of Metastatic Lesions
   Absence of periosteal reaction
   Moth-eaten destruction of medulla and cortex
   Preferential diaphyseal location
   Pathologic fractures
   Multiple bone involvement
Characteristics of Infection
   Often irregular periosteal reaction, no spiculation
   Bone destruction variable
   Diaphyseal involvement, often involving long segments
   Destruction of adjacent cartilage, crossing joints (majority of
      malignant neoplasms lack this ability)
   Sequestration and involucrum formation

bone is consistently uniform in density. As seen in Table 16–2, the thickness and marginal characteristics vary according to the precipitating factor.

The interrupted forms of periosteal reactions are more commonly found in malignant disease, although benign lesions are occasionally responsible. The classical spiculated or sunburst pattern of osteogenic sarcoma and the lamellated or onion-skin periosteal reaction of Ewing's sarcoma come under this heading (see Table 16–2).

One other interesting periosteal condition is hypertrophic pulmonary osteoarthropathy. The uniform thin but solid undulating new bone, often associated with bone pain, is a relatively infrequent roentgenographic finding in individuals suffering from benign and malignant thoracic tumors, chronic obstructive pulmonary disease, and chronic lung infec-

TABLE 16–2.—Roentgenographic Types of Periosteal Reactions

TYPES	EXAMPLES
Solid Periosteal Reaction	
Thin	Eosinophilic granuloma, osteoid osteoma
Thin undulating	Hypertrophic pulmonary osteoarthropathy
Dense undulating	Vascular
Dense elliptical	Osteoid osteoma
(with destruction)	Long-standing malignancy
Cloaking	Chronic infection
Interrupted Periosteal Reaction	
Perpendicular (spiculated or sunburst)	Osteosarcoma, Ewing's sarcoma, and infection
Lamellated (onion skin)	Osteosarcoma, Ewing's sarcoma, and infection
Amorphous	Malignant tumors
Codman's triangle	Malignant tumors, infection, and hemorrhage

Source: Edeiken, J., and Hodes, P. J. H.: *Roentgen Diagnosis of Diseases of Bone*. © 1967 Williams & Wilkins Co., Baltimore.

tions. The exact mechanism is uncertain, but it may be related to decreased arterial oxygen tension.

REGIONAL ANATOMICAL AND PATHOLOGIC ROENTGENOGRAPHY

Cervical Spine

ROENTGENOGRAPHIC EXAMINATION

The standard roentgenographic views of the cervical spine include anteroposterior, lateral, and both posterior oblique views as well as an open-mouth anteroposterior projection of the odontoid process and the first two cervical vertebral segments (Fig 16–2). The majority of cervical spine studies are performed for the evaluation of trauma. In the more severely injured individual, the most important views are a cross-table horizontal beam lateral image and an anteroposterior supine film. By keeping patient movement to a minimum, potentially fatal spinal cord injury is prevented.

On the lateral exposure, C7 and occasionally C6 will often be excluded, especially in heavy, short-necked individuals. In such instances it becomes necessary to depress the shoulders by gentle but firm downward traction of the arms.

If the cervicothoracic junction still has not been adequately visualized and severe injury to the neck has been excluded, a so-called swimmer's view may be obtained. The patient lies in a prone-oblique position with the higher tube-side arm above the head and the lower table-side arm beside his body. The x-ray tube is angled 15° to 20° toward the feet.

There are occasions when other special projections can be of assistance. Flexion and extension lateral views often will reveal minor degrees of subluxations resulting from damage to ligaments.

Dr. Don Weir of St. Louis University developed the "pillar view" for better evaluation of the lateral articulating masses, the superior and inferior articulating facets, and their intervening joints. Moreover, this view brings into focus the anterior and posterior margins of the lamina (Fig 16–3). The film is produced with the patient supine. Each side is done separately. The head is turned very slightly to one side, with the x-ray tube angled toward the feet 35° to 45° and centered over the middle to lower vertebrae. The opposite side is then examined in a similar manner.

ROENTGENOGRAPHIC ANATOMY

In order to properly evaluate the cervical spine, a thorough understanding of its roentgenographic anatomy is an absolute prerequisite. Each component of the individual vertebrae should be appraised separately on all views.

ODONTOID VIEW. – Of the seven cervical vertebrae, the first two are anatomically distinct. The odontoid represents a superior extension of the body of C2 and actually is the vestigial body of C1.

On the anteroposterior open-mouth film, the odontoid should be analyzed in terms of its position between the two lateral articulating masses of C1 (see Fig 16–2). The spaces between the lateral edges of the odontoid and the medial borders of the C1 articulating masses should be equal. However, minor degrees of rotation can produce spurious inequality of these interval distances. How can one determine this? The alignment of the densities of the spinous processes of C1 and C2 can be seen. If the C2 spinous process is to one side or the other, then rotation is present.

Also on viewing the odontoid film, the transverse processes and lateral borders of the articulating masses of C1 and C2 should not be overlooked. The horizontal joints between the atlantoaxial articulating masses should be symmetric (see Fig 16–2).

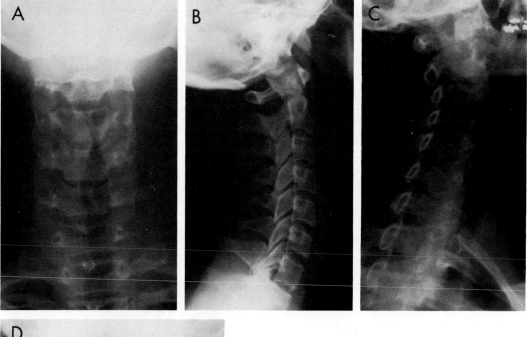

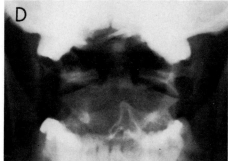

Fig 16–2.—Normal roentgenographic study of the cervical spine. **A,** anteroposterior view. **B,** lateral view. **C,** right oblique view. **D,** odontoid view.

Confusing artifacts superimposing the odontoid can be misleading and can result in misinterpretation of fractures of this structure. The inferior margin of the posterior arch of C1 can overlie the base of the odontoid, creating a "Mach" effect, a radiolucent line produced by the overlap of the edges of two bones. In a similar fashion, the space between the two incisor teeth may lay over the odontoid, yielding an artifactual vertical cleft (Fig 16–4).

ANTEROPOSTERIOR VIEW. — The straight anteroposterior film of the cervical spine demonstrates several specific structures. The vertical alignment of the spinous processes as well as the lateral margins of the articulating masses should be followed. The uncinate processes are the small triangular projections arising from the posterolateral margins of the vertebral bodies that by their apposition form the uncovertebral joints (also termed joints of Luschka). These establish the anterior boundaries of the intervertebral foramina. As synovial joints, they can be involved by degenerative osteoarthritis and produce the spurs that encroach on and narrow the foramina, resulting in impingement of the cervical nerve roots. In addition, being lined with

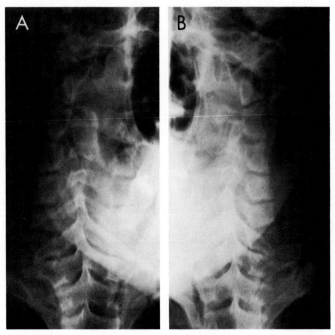

Fig 16–3. — Pillar views of the cervical spine. Right **(A)** and left **(B)** projections.

synovium, they are subject to the alteration of rheumatoid arthritis and rheumatoid spondylitis. The foramina, however, are best evaluated on the oblique films.

LATERAL VIEW. — Several important points must be remembered when viewing the lateral projection of the cervical spine (see Fig 16–2). Alignments of the anterior and posterior borders of the vertebral bodies, alignment of the lateral articulating masses, and alignment of the

spinolaminar line are studied. The latter is formed by the anterior margins of the spinous processes, which also describe the posterior surface of the spinal canal. The superior extension of this line is in direct alignment with the posterior margin of the foramen magnum.

The clivus at the base of the skull, which is a dense line continuous with the dorsum sella, is a helpful indicator for confirming normal craniovertebral alignment and should be included, at least in

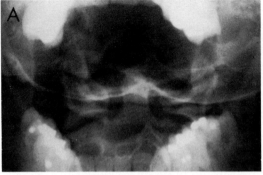

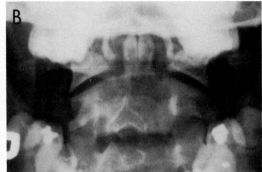

Fig 16–4. — Artifacts over the odontoid process simulating fractures.
A, anterior arch of C1. **B,** cleft of the incisor teeth.

part, on all lateral studies of the cervical spine. A line drawn along its margin will pass through the posterior one third of the odontoid.

The superior and inferior articulating facets ordinarily will be well visualized on the lateral film. The posterior borders of the lateral articulating masses should form a straight line (see Fig 16–2). If there is a slight offset, a facetal dislocation must be considered although slight rotation can give a similar appearance. The view should be repeated if there is any confusion and, if the problem persists, tomography should be considered.

Measurement of the space between the anterior border of the odontoid and the posterior margin of the anterior arch of C1 is mandatory. This is an indicator of a possible transverse ligament tear and should measure no more than 5 mm in children and 3 mm in adults in neutral, flexion, and extension positions.

Finally, evaluation of the lateral cervical spine film is incomplete without an analysis of the prevertebral soft tissues. There are minor differences in the measurement from physician to physician and from patient to patient, but the width of the soft tissues at the level of the inferior margin of the C3 body should not exceed 5 to 7 mm. Any increase in this measurement indicates swelling from hemorrhage or infection.

OBLIQUE VIEWS.—The intervertebral foramina and surrounding elements, including the pedicles and uncinate processes, are the most important components demonstrated on the oblique views. The foramina on the right side are visualized on the left posterior oblique projection and those on the left on the right posterior oblique film (see Fig 16–2).

TRAUMA

Recognition of an abnormal cervical spine should be a relatively simple task

TABLE 16–3.—CLASSIFICATION OF CERVICAL SPINE INJURIES ACCORDING TO THE MECHANISMS OF INJURY

Flexion
  Subluxation
  Bilateral interfacetal dislocation
  Simple wedge fracture
  Flexion teardrop fracture
  Clay-shoveler's fracture
Flexion-Rotation
  Unilateral interfacetal dislocation
Vertical Compression
  Bursting fractures
    Jefferson's C1
    Bursting fractures, other levels
Extension
  Posterior neural arch fracture
  Extension teardrop fracture
  "Hangman's" fracture

SOURCE: Harris, J. H., Jr., "Acute injuries of the cervical spine," Semin. Roentgenol. 13:53-68, 1978, by permission of Grune & Stratton, Inc.

---

once normal roentgenographic anatomy has been mastered. The primary objective, after a traumatic lesion has been identified, will be the establishment of whether or not the condition is stable. The stability of a fracture is best determined by grouping the type of injury according to the mechanisms of trauma, which are outlined in Table 16–3. From this classification, a statement of the instability of the injury can be made (Table 16–4).

FLEXION INJURIES.—There are a variety of flexion injuries, described below.

Subluxation.—The roentgenographic findings in this stable lesion may be minimal, often requiring flexion and extension lateral views for confirmation. The body and posterior elements remain intact, that is, show no fracture. However, there is major soft tissue involvement. The interspinous and posterior longitudinal ligaments as well as the interfacetal joint capsules are disrupted at the affected level. This allows the involved vertebral body to rotate anteriorly about its

TABLE 16–4.—CLASSIFICATION OF CERVICAL SPINE
INJURIES BASED ON STABILITY

Stable
    Subluxation
    Simple wedge fracture
    Unilateral interfacetal dislocation
    Bursting fracture, except Jefferson's fracture of C1
    Clay-shoveler's fracture
Unstable
    Bilateral interfacetal dislocation
    Flexion teardrop fracture
    Jefferson's bursting fracture of C1
    Hangman's fracture
    Extension teardrop fracture, unstable in extension but stable
      in flexion

SOURCE: Harris, J. H., Jr.: Acute injuries of the cervical spine,
Semin. Roentgenol. 13:53–68, 1978, by permission of Grune &
Stratton, Inc.

anterior and inferior corner, along with upward and forward displacement of its inferior articular facet on the lower adjacent vertebra's superior articular facet. The interspinous distance widens and the inferior intervertebral disc space narrows anteriorly and widens posteriorly. These alterations are accentuated on the flexion film (Fig 16–5). In young children under 8 years of age, with the head held in flexion, the second cervical vertebra will normally be displaced anteriorly over C3. This malalignment must not be mistaken for subluxation.

Bilateral Interfacetal Dislocation.—A more severe form of subluxation, a bilateral interfacetal dislocation represents a

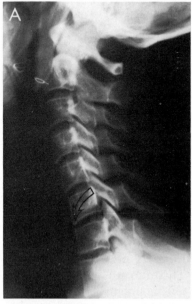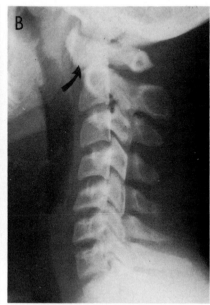

Fig 16–5.—Subluxation injuries of the cervical spine. **A,** mild subluxation of C6 on C7. **B,** atlantoaxial subluxation. Note increased width of space between the odontoid and the anterior arch of C1 in **B.**

true unstable situation. The inferior articular facets of the involved vertebra not only move up and forward but also over the superior articular facet of the distal vertebra, coming to rest within the intervertebral foramina. Oblique projections will be necessary to establish the diagnosis, but these have to be done with extreme caution.

Compression Fractures. — Forceful flexion of the neck can result in an uncomplicated, simple wedge-shaped compression fracture of one and sometimes two or three vertebral bodies. Because they are stable, extension and flexion films are permissible.

Flexion Teardrop Fracture. — Considered the most dangerous and unstable of all cervical spine injuries, flexion teardrop fractures are diagnosed on the cross-table lateral film only, with no indications or justification for acquiring further studies. The name of the lesion is derived from the fact there is a fracture through the inferior and anterior corner of the body, but the major component is comminution of the body. The posterior fragments become displaced backward into the spinal cord, with consequential acute and severe neurologic deficits. The posterior neural arch is also frequently fractured.

Clay-Shoveler's Fracture. — The name of this lesion is derived from the injury acquired by occupations in which heavy lifting is required. This injury consists of a fracture through the spinous process of either C6 or C7. There is no significant ligamentous damage, and therefore a stable condition exists. Since C7 is sometimes difficult to project on the lateral film, the fracture can be missed. A clue might be apparent on the frontal film, where an extraspinous process fragment is sometimes evident as the result of inferior displacement. An unfused apophysis of a spinous process must not be misinterpreted as a fracture (Fig 16–6).

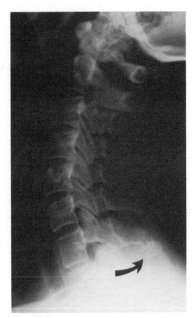

Fig 16–6. — Unfused apophysis of the spinous process of C7 simulating a fracture.

FLEXION-ROTATION INJURIES. — When the cervical spine is subjected to a rotational force in addition to flexion, a unilateral interfacetal dislocation may be observed (Fig 16–7). An inferior articular facet of one body is displaced over the adjacent superior articular facet of the next inferior vertebra on one side only. The dislocated facet is more or less locked in place, but due to associated ligament damage the lesion may be unstable; therefore, flexion and extension views are contraindicated. Oblique projections are most productive in identifying the displaced facet, but it may be suggested on the lateral film when the margins of the facets of a single vertebra do not superimpose on one another as the result of rotation. Additionally, a line drawn through the posterior borders of the bodies is offset at the level of the suspected injury.

EXTENSION INJURIES. — Various extension injuries are described as follows:

Posterior Neural Arch Fractures. — The neural arch of one vertebra may be com-

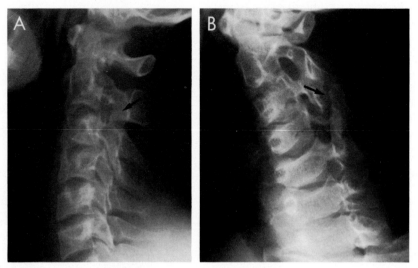

Fig 16–7. — Unilateral interfacetal dislocation. **A,** lateral view. **B,** oblique view.

pressed between the posterior elements of the two adjoining vertebrae during maximal forced extension. A unilateral or bilateral fracture may be sustained. If bilateral, the fragment can be displaced posteriorly yet there will be no encroachment on the neural canal; thus the situation is a stable one (Fig 16–8).

Extension Teardrop Fracture. — Similar to the flexion variety, an extension teardrop fracture demonstrates a triangular-shaped fragment at the anterior-inferior margin of the body, most often involving C2 although other levels are affected.

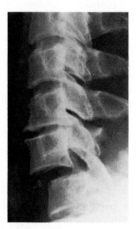

Fig 16–8. — Posterior neural arch fracture.

The injury, however, is not quite as severe as there is no posterior involvement. When the neck is held in flexion, there is stability of the spine, since the posterior ligament complex is intact. However, instability occurs during extension since the minor fragment remains attached to the anterior longitudinal ligament but not to the parent body.

Hangman's Fracture-Dislocation of C2. — This lesion consists of vertical disruption of both pedicles of C2 created by flexion forces against the extended vertebrae. The body of C2 is thrust forward over C3, with concomitant rupture of both the anterior and the posterior longitudinal ligaments giving rise to an unstable injury.

VERTICAL COMPRESSION FRACTURES. A considerable force directed through the vertical axis of the spine, such as a large object falling on top of the head, can produce the so-called bursting fractures of the cervical vertebrae. The least common type is the Jefferson fracture of C1. The anterior and posterior aspects of the ring are fractured on both sides, with bilateral lateral displacement of the fragments. This unstable injury can be apparent on the open-mouth anteroposterior film, but more reliably is distinguished on the lateral roentgenogram where the fractures are seen extending through the posterior arches.

Vertical compression or bursting fractures more frequently involve the middle and lower cervical vertebral segments. The longitudinally oriented pressures cause the intervertebral discs to impact against the end-plates of the bodies. Ordinarily there is no instability as the posterior elements remain intact. When viewed on the anteroposterior film, a vertical fracture line is identified within the involved body.

Thoracic and Lumbar Spine

ROENTGENOGRAPHIC EXAMINATION

The thoracic spine ordinarily is examined by means of anteroposterior and lateral films. However, due to the superimposition of the shoulders, the upper three to four vertebrae will be omitted from the lateral view and, if clinical symptoms point to this region, an oblique swimmer's projection should be obtained.

It is generally agreed that the above films will offer optimum information about the anatomy of the thoracic vertebrae. However, either or both oblique views of no more than 10° to 20° can be obtained, providing a different aspect of a questionable or subtle change in the vertebral bodies or articulating facets.

Routine roentgenographic examination of the lumbar spine must be composed of anteroposterior, lateral, and both oblique projections as well as a cone-down lateral film of the lumbosacral joint.

ROENTGENOGRAPHIC ANATOMY

ANTEROPOSTERIOR VIEW.—On the anteroposterior study, the 12 thoracic and five lumbar bodies will show a slight increase in size from top to bottom. The height, width, and alignment of the

bodies and their cortical margins and trabecular architecture and density need to be scrutinized carefully.

Subsequently, the round to oval pedicles need to be evaluated separately. They overlie the superolateral corner of each body and, like them, become progressively larger inferiorly. The density and sclerotic cortical margins should be noted for any alterations as they are involved in a number of pathologic processes.

The interpedicular distance, a line drawn between the inner boundaries of a vertebral body's pedicles, is an important observation throughout the spine. It affords an indirect evaluation of the size of the neural canal.

The transverse processes in the thoracic spine become smaller from superior to inferior, are oriented posterolaterally, and are located behind the intervertebral foramina. The normal articulations of the ribs should not be overlooked. In the lumbar spine the transverse processes are more laterally oriented and are much larger, the processes of the third vertebra usually being the largest.

On the anteroposterior projection, the spinous processes provide another guide for the evaluation of alignment. Rarely, they may be absent because of aplasia or due to malignant or infectious destruction.

Additionally, on the anteroposterior view, the paravertebral soft tissues should be studied. An increase in the width of the soft tissues will alert one to a possible fracture, neoplasm, or infection in the spine, the result of hematoma, infiltrating tumor cells, or bacterial extension, respectively. The psoas margins in the paralumbar region are fairly sensitive indicators to similar changes when they become obliterated. This abnormal change can also reflect lymphadenopathy or urinary lesions such as a perirenal abscess. In fact, when viewing the lumbar spine, one should always attempt to de-

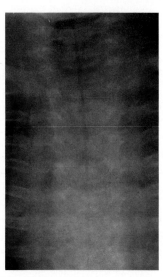

Fig 16–9.—Normal thoracic spine of an infant. Note vertical cleft of neural arch.

lineate the psoas and renal margins as well as search for urinary tract calculi as causes of back pain.

Lateral View.—One of the goals for studying the lateral views of the thoracolumbar spine is to ensure normal alignment of the anterior and posterior borders of the vertebral bodies. Furthermore, the cortical outlines and the internal structure of the bodies must be mentally recorded. Any narrowing of the intervertebral disc spaces can be established. In the thoracic spine, the intervertebral foramina can be seen on end but require oblique views for their proper visualization in the lumbar area.

The inferiorly directed spinous processes, as seen on the lateral film, may require a "hot" light to be adequately seen, but should not be neglected for reasons mentioned previously.

Oblique Views.—Important anatomical features are introduced on the oblique views of the lumbar spine. These details have been covered more extensively in chapter 7. On the left posterior oblique film (left side down against the film), the left half of the posterior neural arch elements, including the intervertebral foramina, are identified whereas the right half of these components are viewed on the opposite projection. In the cervical spine, the reverse condition exists.

DEVELOPMENTAL VARIATIONS AND CONGENITAL ABNORMALITIES

Confusing anatomical variations are seen in the developing and mature spine. In infancy the vertebral bodies are egg-shaped on lateral view. The upper and lower anterior corners are beveled until the apophyseal vertebral rings appear about each end-plate. They fuse with the body by the 15th year, but occasionally they remain ununited and, except for the presence of a complete sclerotic border, often are confused with a corner fracture.

On the anteroposterior film, a vertical radiolucent cleft is seen superimposing the vertebral bodies (Fig 16–9). This represents the normal uncalcified portion of the posterior neural arch and spinous process and is not to be confused with spina bifida. At approximately 3 to 5 years of age these will ossify and fuse. When they do fail to fuse completely, the cleft persists as a spina bifida occulta. This can occur anywhere in the spine, but is most common at L5. These are of no clinical importance.

True spina bifida is the result of a very wide defect in the posterior neural arch, usually involving multiple vertebrae and commonly found in the lumbar region. The widened spinal neural canal is evidenced by an increased interpedicular distance. These may be associated with a meningocele that produces a prominent posterior soft tissue density on the roentgenogram.

This wide gap of the dorsal arch and increased interpedicular width should also bring to mind the possibility of diastematomyelia, a condition in which the cord is divided by an intraspinal cartilaginous, fibrous, or bony spur. This has a predilection for the thoracolumbar junction. Syringomyelia can produce a similar appearance in the cervical spine where there is cystic dilation of the cord. The same type of appearance can also be seen with intraspinal tumors such as lipomas or dermoids.

Vascular channels may give rise to confusing appearances. Blood vessels perforate the anterior cortical borders of each body forming a radiolucent line termed the clefts of Hahn. A similar vascular defect that becomes more apparent in adulthood may exist along the posterior margin of the body.

Hypoplasia of the vertebrae, fusion or block vertebrae, and hemivertebrae constitute a few of the other spinal anomalies that may be encountered (Fig 16–10).

TRAUMA

The focus of attention will now be shifted to some of the traumatic lesions involving the thoracolumbar spine. The majority of injuries will disturb the muscular and ligamentous structures surrounding the spine. Just as in the cervical spine, the only visible roentgenographic findings may be scoliosis and/or straight-ening of the normal curvatures indicating muscle spasms.

When a fracture is present, the usual appearance is that of a wedge-shaped compression deformity, the result of hyperflexion forces. Avulsion-type corner fractures of the anterosuperior body result from extension forces. They appear as a very sharp, nonsclerotic fragment as opposed to an unfused apophysis.

Quite frequently, the dilemma of determining the age of a fracture presents itself. In long-standing compression fractures, degenerative changes with hypertrophic spurs arise along the articular margins and there may be an unpredictable degree of eburnation. Yet, at times, these changes are absent and the determination of age may be difficult if not impossible. Radioisotopic bone scans that utilize technetium Tc 99m phosphate compounds then become a valuable aid. Within two to five days of the injury, a recent collapse will show an increased uptake of the isotope, whereas older lesions will show no activity. However, the abnormal uptake may remain detectable for 18 to 24 months or longer, depending in part on the extent of the fracture and its location.

Biconcave deformities of the bodies, or

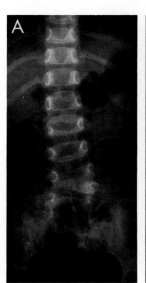 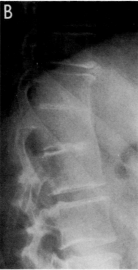

Fig 16–10.—Anomalies of the spine. **A,** hemivertebra of the lumbar spine. **B,** fusion or block vertebrae.

so-called fish vertebrae have a predisposition for the thoracic and lumbar location. They represent a chronic progressive form of compression characteristically seen in postmenopausal patients with osteoporosis. Vertebral body compression fractures with a history of minimal or no trauma should alert one to the possibility of a metastatic or primay malignant process.

Another important traumatic lesion, particularly of the lumbar spine, that can be easily ignored is the transverse process fracture (Fig 16–11). The importance of its recognition rests with the fact of frequently related renal injury. It is important not to mistakenly call the unfused apophysis of the transverse process a fracture.

A seldom-seen injury to the lumbar vertebrae is the Chance fracture. An extreme flexion force, often related to seatbelt injuries, causes a fracture through the spinous process, across the neural arch or lamina, and into the posterosuperior aspect of the vertebral body. An isolated fracture of the spinous process is uncommon in the thoracic and lumbar regions.

One more pitfall to watch for in the assessment of spinal trauma is the unfused ossification center of the articular facets. Their appearance can resemble a fracture (Fig 16–12). In evaluating the posterior elements, it is important to keep in mind the entities of spondylolysis and spondylolisthesis (chapter 7).

TUMORS

Except for metastatic neoplasms to the spine, tumors—both benign and primary malignant lesions—are very infrequent. The vertebrae are the most commonly affected portion of the skeleton for metastasis, accounting for approximately 40% of all secondary tumors of bone. A few of the common and not so common tumors will be discussed.

HEMANGIOMA.—Hemangiomas of the vertebral body may be the most common benign tumor, although few have been documented pathologically. Typically, their appearance is that of increased vertical trabeculations producing a somewhat striated pattern (Fig 16–13). They should not be confused with Paget's disease or osteoblastic metastasis, whose descriptions are forthcoming.

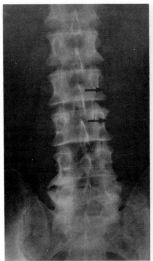
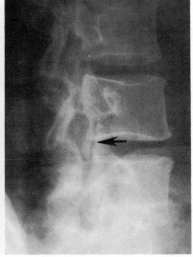

Fig 16–11 (left).—Transverse process fractures of the lumbar spine. Note lucent fracture lines *(arrows)* at bases of the processes of L3 and L4 on the left. Incidentally, the patient demonstrates lumbarization of the S1 segment.

Fig 16–12 (right).—Unfused apophysis of superior articular facet of L5.

ANEURYSMAL BONE CYST.—Of the benign tumors of the spine, aneurysmal bone cysts are possibly the next most frequent after hemangiomas. Of course, they are more commonly found in the extremities, especially the distal femur. In the spine they tend to involve the posterior elements as well as the body. Possessing a thin shell of peripheral bone, they are expansile and cystic in nature. Roentgenographically, a malignant appearance can be seen with a predominant cystic pattern. Unlike other tumors, benign and malignant alike, aneurysmal bone cysts have the unique capability of crossing over the cartilaginous disc space to involve adjacent vertebrae. A malignant chordoma also has this potential.

OSTEOID OSTEOMA.—A benign tumor that can produce significant and disabling pain is the osteoid osteoma. Most frequently found in the extremities, this tumor can involve the spine on rare occasions, and must be considered in the differential diagnosis of back pain. It is one of many causes of scoliosis. The lesion is almost always limited to the neural arch, a position that often prevents its detection on conventional roentgenographs. Tomography and isotopic bone scanning may be required for its recognition. It is composed of a small radiolucent nidus sometimes containing calcifications. A very dense reactive sclerosis surrounds the central nidus and often obscures it.

OSTEOBLASTOMA.—An osteoblastoma is a benign lesion that classically involves the spine, primarily the dorsal elements. Because of its varied histologic appearances, it has been described as a giant osteoid osteoma and certain cases may even mimic osteogenic sarcoma.

A wide variety of primary malignant tumors may involve the spine, of which only a few will be mentioned. Such tumors may be seen anywhere in the spine but have a preference for the sacrococcygeal region.

MULTIPLE MYELOMA.—The most common primary malignant tumor of bone is multiple myeloma. The classical picture of "punched-out" lesions, particularly evident in the skull, are characteristic but not that frequent. The usual presentation is diffuse demineralization. Multiple vertebral compression deformities form in a progressive nature.

SARCOMA.—Osteosarcoma, fibrosarcoma, and chondrosarcoma involve the spine only rarely and usually in the sacrum. These tumors may arise in an area of previous irradiation, Paget's disease, or fibrous dysplasia.

ROUND CELL TUMORS.—Ewing's sarcoma and reticulum cell sarcoma are rarely encountered in the vertebral column. They have more of a predilection for the appendicular skeleton, but must be included in the differential diagnosis of destructive lesions.

HODGKIN'S LYMPHOMA. — Hodgkin's disease can occasionally be seen within the bony spine and may present as an osteolytic or osteoblastic alteration or a combination of the two. More commonly, however, para-aortic lymph node involvement with lymphoma will produce erosive changes of the vertebral cortical margins.

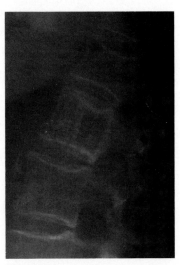

Fig 16–13.—Hemangioma of a vertebral body.

CHORDOMA AND SACROCOCCYGEAL TERATOMA. — There are two primary malignant tumors of the spine that are classified as developmental. A chordoma is an invasive lesion arising from remnants of the primitive notochord and therefore can presumably occur anywhere along the vertebral column, although there are no reported cases of its occurrence in the thoracic region. The sacrum is the most popular site, accounting for approximately 50% of cases. An intracranial chordoma located along the clivus represents about 30% of cases, and the remaining 20% originate in the cervical and lumbar areas. Roentgenographically, the tumor presents as an expansile, lytic process with moderate soft tissue extension. As noted previously, it may cross the disc space cartilage, an uncommon occurrence for any tumor but typical of infections. In one third of the tumors, calcifications are observed.

The second type of developmental primary malignant tumor is a sacrococcygeal teratoma. Sixty percent of these lesions, however, are benign but exhibit some degree of localized infiltration. They are found in infants within the pelvis around the parasacral region. Malformation of the spine can be an associated finding. They appear, roentgenographically, as variable-sized soft tissue masses, often with calcifications or ossifications within them. The rectosigmoid colon is extrinsically displaced forward. Destructive changes will be present to some extent within the sacrococcygeal bony structure.

INFECTION

For obvious reasons, infections involving the spine have decreased in frequency over the years. Nevertheless, this must be considered in the differential diagnosis of a painful back and abnormal roentgenograms.

Acute bacterial infections, or pyogenic spondylitis, can involve either the disc space, the vertebral body, or both. The former condition, termed pyogenic discitis, is more common in the younger population, apparently on the basis of a healthy vascularization of the cartilage and, therefore, easy access by blood-borne bacteria. This results in a closed space infection that can secondarily extend into the bodies.

On the other hand, infection of the vertebral body, particularly its anterior two thirds, is more commonly identified in the adult. Originating in the substance of the body, the infection may then secondarily involve the interspace by extension.

An important principle in pathophysiology should be reemphasized at this point. Cartilage serves as no barrier to the extension of infection and thereby is vulnerable to destruction. Conversely, the disc cartilage is very resistant to malignant cellular infiltration so that tumors tend to remain confined to the body.

In both pyogenic discitis and vertebral osteomyelitis, the earliest roentgenographic findings may be joint space narrowing. Depending on the aggressiveness of the offending bacteria and the time of institution of therapy, the surrounding bone will show varying degrees

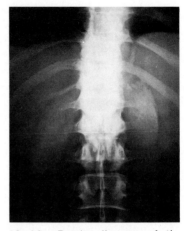

Fig 16–14. — Pott's disease of the spine. The chronic tuberculous process has resulted in calcified paravertebral psoas abscesses.

of demineralization brought on by hyperemia. The end-plates will then demonstrate progressive loss of continuity with irregular destruction and focal areas of subchondral reactive sclerosis. Extension into the posterior one third of the body, then into the dorsal appendages as well as into the adjoining vertebrae, may occur. The body may eventually collapse. Some degree of surrounding soft tissue swelling is invariably present and detectable on the roentgenograms.

Tuberculosis of the spine or Pott's disease is an extreme rarity among the abnormal spine studies of today. The vertebral column remains the most common skeletal site for this chronic infection. The midthoracic and thoracolumbar junctions constitute the most prevalent sites of involvement.

Because of its insidious and chronic nature, the spinal lesions are usually advanced when first examined roentgenographically, though this is not always the situation. An occasionally prominent feature is a large paravertebral soft tissue mass that constitutes the abscess. In the later phases, there may be extensive calcification within this mass. The bony structures will show a decrease in density and there will be narrowing of one or more of the disc spaces. The margins of the end-plates will manifest irregular destruction, and a mottled sclerotic and lytic appearance will extend into the bodies, which display varying degrees of compression (Fig 16–14).

PAGET'S DISEASE

One of the distinctive roentgenographic characteristics of spinal Paget's disease is that the disorder involves the entire vertebra—the body and all of the posterior elements, including the transverse and spinous processes (Fig 16–15). Generally, there is an increase in density produced by a thickened trabeculae. A picture-frame appearance can be imparted to the body, the result of a dense peripheral margin of thickened cortex. Furthermore, there is an actual increase in volume of the entire vertebra. This finding, along with total vertebral involvement, distinguishes Paget's disease from an osteoblastic metastasis.

The Shoulder

ROENTGENOGRAPHIC EXAMINATION

In the majority of cases, a complete and optimal roentgenographic study of the

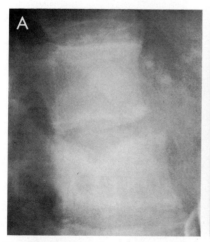 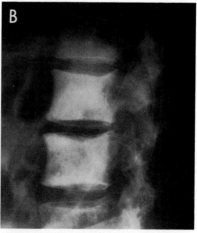

Fig 16–15.—Spinal Paget's disease and osteoblastic metastasis. **A,** Paget's disease demonstrates increased trabeculations, bone within bone appearance, and increased volume including the pedicles. **B,** osteoblastic metastasis.

shoulder girdle need only include up-right—standing or sitting—anteroposteri-or views with the humerus in internal and external rotation. These two projections will usually permit adequate evaluation of the bony structures constituting the shoulder.

On these roentgenograms the complete clavicle should be visualized as well as the entirety of the scapula and at least the proximal one third of the humerus. Special attention should be given to the alignments of the glenohumeral, acromio-clavicular, coracoclavicular, and sterno-clavicular joints. The tuberosities of the humeral head and its articular surface should be specifically scrutinized. The acromium and coracoid processes, in addition to the borders and flat surfaces of the scapula, require attention.

The standard examination, of course, may require modification as there are certain situations when special views must be obtained for better delineation of specific structures. In the acutely injured shoulder where immobilization of the shoulder is required, the humerus will ordinarily be held in internal rotation. In order to obtain roentgenograms of the humerus in external rotation without moving the arm, the patient can be positioned by rotating him 40° posteriorly with the affected side toward the film. Because of pain, this requires that the patient be sitting or standing.

Upright exposures are also beneficial in demonstrating fat-fluid levels. This occurs when a fracture has extended into the joint through the articular cortex that exists most often with fractures of the greater tuberosity. Such information is useful since articular cartilage damage is certain, and the patient should be informed that degenerative osteoarthritis in time is a possibility.

When there is suspicion of a fracture involving the shaft of the humerus below the neck, in addition to an anteroposteri-or view, a transthoracic lateral projection is necessary for evaluation of alignment (Fig 16–16). The glenohumeral relationship can also be accessed with proper exposure, but because of superimposed ribs, fractures above the neck are difficult to see. Instead, a transscapular study will be more helpful (Fig 16–17). This view

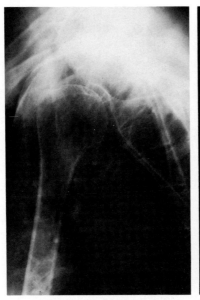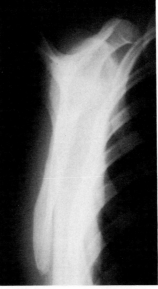

Fig 16–16 (left).—Transthoracic view of shoulder.
Fig 16–17 (right).—Transscapular view of shoulder.

is obtained by having the patient face the film at an angle of 45° with the affected side toward the film holder. The resultant picture forms a Y where the acromium, coracoid, and scapular body intersect. The humeral head will be superimposed on the Y. This is useful not only for fractures but also for posterior dislocations. This transscapular examination is always utilized when studying the scapula in addition to the routine anteroposterior roentgenogram.

Posterior shoulder dislocations are notorious for their ability to avoid detection on the standard anteroposterior views, and the tangential projection is an excellent means for detecting the abnormality. This is performed by angling the x-ray tube approximately 30°, so that the central ray passes tangentially across the glenoid articular surface. In this manner the glenohumeral relationship is much better defined than on the conventional straight anteroposterior view.

The axillary film also provides another perspective of the shoulder anatomy (Fig 16–18). The acromium, coracoid, glenohumeral joint, and humeral head are viewed in a different plane. By holding

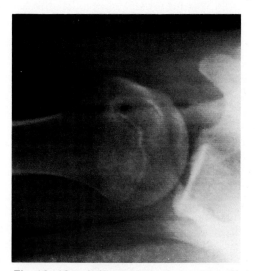

Fig 16–18. — Axillary view of shoulder. Note the glenohumeral relationship, the hook-like coracoid process, and the acromium behind the head of the humerus.

the film against the top of the shoulder, the picture is produced by abducting the arm and centering the x-ray tube through the axilla. It is helpful in determining the presence of a humeral head displacement, but it is not recommended when a dislocation has just been reduced since the required abduction may reluxate the joint.

The clavicle itself requires two projections in the anteroposterior plane in order to evaluate it properly. One film should be made perpendicular to the plane of the body, while the other exposure is made with a 15° to 20° cephalad angulation.

The acromioclavicular joints are best inspected with an anteroposterior film, tilting the x-ray tube 15° toward the head. Comparative films are necessary to determine the presence of a separation, and this should be performed with and without weight bearing.

ROENTGENOGRAPHIC ANATOMY AND DEVELOPMENTAL VARIATIONS

Needless to say, a considerable degree of confusion can be created by the ossification centers of the shoulder. The proximal humeral epiphysis does not become visible, as a rule, until the fourth to eighth month of life. There are two and occasionally three separate centers. By the 20th year, the proximal epiphysis fuses to the shaft of the humerus.

Before complete closure of the epiphyseal suture, the lucent line has a peculiar angulated appearance (Fig 16–19). Overlap of the suture line occurs no matter what projection is employed and consequently produces an image simulating a fracture.

A deceptive appearance of the proximal humeral shaft is the deltoid tuberosity, which, incidentally, receives the tendinous attachments of the deltoid muscle. The thickened cortex in this area may bring to mind the periosteal reaction of infection or tumor.

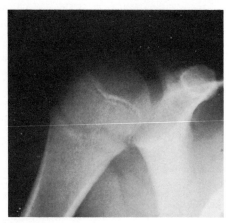

Fig 16–19. — Normal proximal humeral epiphysis in a child.

On a congenital basis, there may be complete absence of the clavicle or at least partial underdevelopment of its lateral end. This represents hereditary cleidocranial dysplasia, a disease that also affects the skull, pelvis, hips, and other skeletal regions.

The outer end of the clavicle appears less dense than the middle and sternal aspects, the result of a lesser thickness of overlying soft tissue. Soft tissues are also responsible for a discrete line density paralleling the superior border of the clavicle measuring no more than 4 mm in width and described as the "accompanying shadow." This shadow may be thickened in cases of subtle fractures.

The rhomboid fossa is a familiar anatomical variation of the clavicle and is found along the inferior border at its medial aspect as a notch-like depression. This represents the location of the insertion of the costoclavicular (rhomboid) ligament, which secures the first rib to the clavicle. Its irregular appearance has been misinterpreted as a destructive process.

TRAUMA

Of all the joints in the body, the shoulder is the most frequent site of dislocations. Over 97% are anterior in type and can be described as subglenoid or subcoracoid, depending on the location of the humeral head. Invariably this form of dislocation can be visualized by a single anteroposterior roentgenogram (Fig 16–20).

Whenever a dislocation occurs it is not unusual to have an associated fracture; this should be searched for on the film. With an anterior dislocation, a fracture of the greater tuberosity may exist; the les-

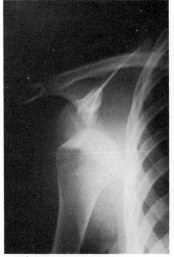 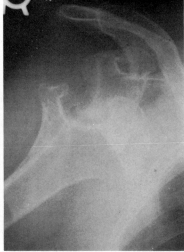

Fig 16–20 (left). — Anterior dislocation of the shoulder, subglenoid in type.
Fig 16–21 (right). — Hill-Sachs deformity in chronic recurring anterior shoulder dislocation.

ser tuberosity is vulnerable in posterior dislocations. The lower glenoid margin is also susceptible in either type of dislocation. An infraction of the articular cartilage without a visible fracture is also possible in dislocations and may require arthrography to demonstrate.

Not infrequently with intra-articular extension of a fracture in the absence of true dislocation, an intact joint capsule may become progressively distended with blood and, if enough blood accumulates, there will be inferior displacement of the humeral head away from the glenoid. This condition is termed pseudo-subluxation or "hanging shoulder."

With chronic recurring anterior dislocations, a defect becomes apparent along the superolateral aspect of the humeral head. This cortical infraction, present because of impaction against the anteroinferior rim of the glenoid, is commonly referred to as Hill-Sachs deformity. This abnormality is usually best demonstrated on an internally rotated anteroposterior view (Fig 16–21).

The less frequent posterior dislocation is much more difficult to visualize roentgenographically. The problem arises because the humeral head on the standard anteroposterior projections shows no apparent separation from the glenoid fossa when in fact it is separated. The posterolateral orientation of the glenoid articular surface accounts for this to some extent. Ordinarily, in the normal shoulder the head of the humerus overlaps about three fourths of the glenoid fossa. When it becomes posteriorly dislocated, due to lateral displacement of the head, this overlap is less but the change may be very subtle. This perplexing situation can usually be solved by employing the 30° tangential view, the axillary projection, or the transscapular film (Fig 16–22).

TUMOR

The proximal humerus is a relatively common location for a benign solitary cyst that may appear either as simple or as multiloculated (Fig 16–23). Such cysts are found within the metaphysis, exhibiting destruction of the medullary spongiosa with more or less expansion of the bone. Thinning of the cortex can attain paper thickness, and pathologic fractures are a very common event, even in the absence of significant trauma. When initially discovered the cysts extend to the epiphyseal line but do not involve the growth center itself. Followed serially until fusion of the epiphysis, the cyst appears to "migrate" toward the middle

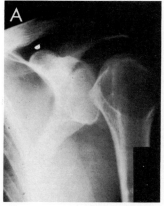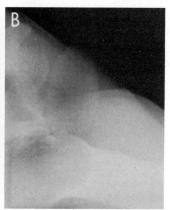

Fig 16–22. – Posterior shoulder dislocation. **A,** anteroposterior view showing some discrepancy in the glenohumeral joint. **B,** axillary view demonstrating posterior displacement of humeral head from the glenoid fossa (see Fig 16–18 for normal axillary film).

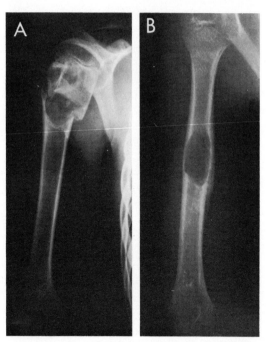

Fig 16–23.—Benign cysts of the humerus. **A,** multiloculated cyst in the metaphysis showing a fresh pathological fracture. **B,** simple solitary cyst in midshaft demonstrating healing fracture.

of the shaft as growth of the bone ends progresses.

Primary malignant tumors of the shoulder are a rarity and are often of the sarcomatous varity. Osteogenic sarcoma, as well as the round cell tumors, Ewing's sarcoma, and reticulum cell sarcoma, have already been described.

Secondary metastatic disease is much more prevalent than primary lesions, particularly of the proximal humerus. As with cysts, pathologic fractures frequently accompany these malignant changes.

ARTHRITIS

The roentgenographic alterations of osteoarthritis of the shoulder are similar to those seen in the knee and will be described under that heading. The process, however, more often has a posttraumatic relationship.

Rheumatoid arthritis of the shoulder, as in other joints, will demonstrate articular erosions without much bone production or osteophyte formation as is seen in osteoarthritis. But unique to this area, erosions of the lateral ends of the clavicles may be present. This pathologic change, nevertheless, is not specific for rheumatoid arthritis and may be seen in hyperparathyroidism and other less common diseases.

The Elbow

ROENTGENOGRAPHIC EXAMINATION

The standard examination of the elbow includes a straight anteroposterior film with the forearm fully extended and supinated, as well as a true lateral view with the joint flexed 90° and the forearm supinated. Not uncommonly, particularly with trauma, the patient is unable or unwilling to extend or flex the elbow. To delineate the distal humeral articulating surface when the elbow is held in flexion, the anteroposterior view can be obtained by orienting the central beam of the x-ray tube perpendicular to the distal humeral shaft. In the same way, the proximal radial and ulnar details and relationships can be observed by pointing the tube perpendicular to their shafts. Medial and lateral oblique exposures may become necessary to better analyze the radial head and shaft, the humeral condyles, or the coronoid process of the ulna.

ROENTGENOGRAPHIC ANATOMY

Before considering specific elbow lesions, pertinent roentgenographic anatomy of the elbow must be considered. Evaluating the different bony landmarks and their relationships can prove extremely useful.

In children a great deal of confusion arises because of the ossification sequence of the growth centers. The capitellum, trochlea, and the medial and lateral epicondyles compose the centers of the distal humerus. In addition, the elbow contains the olecranon apophysis and the radial head epiphysis (Fig 16 – 24).

The first of the distal humeral epiphyses to appear is the capitellum, which develops by the age of 2. At about age 6 the medial epicondylar center becomes visible. Next to become evident is the trochlea at age 10 and, finally, the lateral epicondyle appears near the 12th year of life.

The radial head epiphysis calcifies at about the same time as the medial epicondyle, in the vicinity of the sixth year. Before the age of 10 the olecranon ossification center is not visible.

The ossification centers normally fuse between the ages of 14 and 16, although union of the medial epicondyle may not occur until the 18th year.

Following their union, the medial and lateral epicondyles form the flared segment of the distal humerus. Between the condyles on both the ventral and dorsal surfaces are indentations identified as the coronoid and olecranon fossae, respectively, as they relate to the anatomical segments of the ulna. This area may be very thin and appear as a zone of rounded rarefaction on the anteroposterior film. In fact, an actual opening, termed the supratrochlear foramen, occasionally is present.

Contained within these recesses are the fat pads, fairly sensitive indicators of the presence of a distended joint capsule. In the normal elbow, providing a true lateral flexion film is obtained, the posterior fat pad is not visible. The anterior fat pad forms a slim triangular lucency adjacent to the anterior humeral cortex. With the presence of joint fluid, such as blood resulting from an intra-articular fracture, one or both of these fat pads will be elevated. The so-called fat-pad sign is not specific and may be seen in conditions other than trauma, such as pyarthrosis or rheumatoid arthritis. In cases of injury, a positive fat-pad sign should be searched for from the beginning and, if found, should initiate further investigation for an occult fracture, particularly of the radial head (Fig 16 – 25). Oblique views may be required and if necessary a repeated examination may be done in seven to ten days, at which time a fracture should be apparent. On occasion, no fracture will be found and the distended joint may be on the basis of a cartilage infrac-

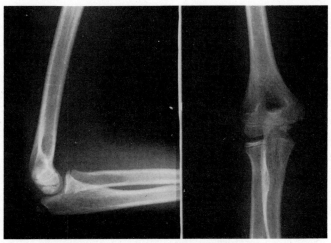

Fig 16–24. – Normal elbow of a 9-year-old child. **Left,** lateral view; **Right,** anteroposterior view.

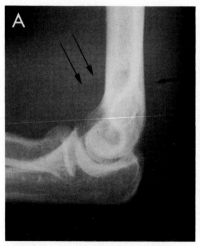

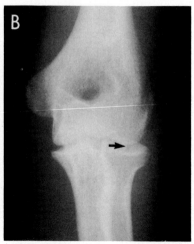

Fig 16–25. – Radial head fracture with a positive fat-pad sign. **A,** lateral view showing elevation of both anterior and posterior fat pads *(arrows).* **B,** fracture line through radial head *(arrow)* is well delineated on the anteroposterior projection.

tion or capsular tear. In adults an intra-articular fracture may be present in the absence of fat-pad elevation, but in children it is a more reliable indicator, being found in approximately 90% of elbow fractures (Rogers 1978).

Two other helpful relationships will be of assistance when evaluating normal elbow anatomy. The first is the anterior humeral line. On the lateral film, a line is drawn along the anterior margin of the humeral shaft and extended through the joint. If the capitellum is divided into equal thirds, this line normally passes through the middle one third. It is a simple and useful index in analyzing the normal 140° angle that the articular structures form with the shaft of the humerus. This easy maneuver often will alert one to a subtle transcondylar fracture in

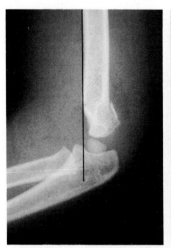

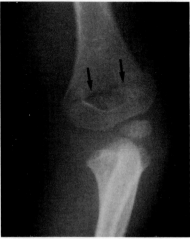

Fig 16–26. – Transcondylar fracture of the humerus. **Left,** lateral view revealing anterior and posterior fat-pad elevation. An obvious fracture is identified, but note how the anterior humeral line extends anterior to the capitellum. **Right,** Anteroposterior view clearly outlining the fracture *(arrows).*

children when the line will be seen extending through or anterior to the anterior third division of the capitellum (Fig 16–26).

The second practical indicator is the radiocapitellar line denoted by a line drawn through the longitudinal axis of the radius. This line will always pass through the capitellum, no matter what projection is being viewed. When the radial head is dislocated, this relationship no longer exists. Whenever there is a fracture of the ulnar shaft, this procedure should be utilized since the radial head often is dislocated in what constitutes a Monteggia fracture.

TRAUMA

Sixty percent of all elbow fractures in children are of the supracondylar type. The lateral epicondyle is involved about 15% of the time, and the medial epicondyle accounts for 10% of all fractures. The radial and olecranon ossification centers are infrequently traumatized.

In adults the radial head or neck mark the most common elbow area for fractures. Unlike the pediatric age group, adults seldom suffer fractures of the distal humerus.

A supracondylar fracture should more aptly be called a transcondylar fracture as it extends across the condyles and is seen through the coronoid and olecranon fossae (see Fig 16–26). The anterior humeral line will indicate posterior displacement of the distal fragment when the fracture is complete, which is seen in 75% of cases. The remainder, however, are incomplete, and visualizing the fracture line may be impossible. Almost always the posterior fat pad will be elevated.

When the lateral epicondylar epiphysis is traumatized it usually contains a fragment of metaphyseal bone. Because it serves for the attachment of forearm extensor tendons, the fragment becomes displaced posteriorly and inferiorly.

Little leaguer's elbow, discussed in chapter 5, describes the injury in which the medial epicondyle is separated. Ordinarily the avulsed center is best identified on the anteroposterior film, often lying adjacent to the capitellum. In rare instances the fragment may become displaced into the medial joint space, where it can simulate the trochlear ossification center before its actual appearance.

The coronoid process frequently is avulsed in posterior dislocations of the elbow being impacted against the trochlea. Whenever an elbow dislocation occurs, the radius and ulna are displaced lateral and posterior to the humerus in almost all instances. In children, when the radius and ulna are medial to the humerus, there is not a dislocation but rather a fracture through the entire distal humeral epiphysis. This is extremely important to recognize since treatment of the two are entirely different.

The Wrist and Hand

ROENTGENOGRAPHIC EXAMINATION

The routine roentgenographic study of the wrist consists of posteroanterior, oblique, and lateral projections. The oblique film is achieved by orienting the wrist at a 45° angle to the plane of the film with the ulnar side down.

There are several special wrist views that are necessary for the evaluation of specific anatomical features. One of the more frequently employed studies is that for the carpal navicular bone. A fracture of this bone may easily escape detection. When clinical symptoms point to a navicular injury yet the routine study appears normal, this view becomes mandatory. The palm is placed against the film holder with the thumb and index finger spread apart. The tube is angled 45° toward the elbow. This results in an elongated appearance of the navicular, but the distortion is minimal and it is projected free of superimposition from the other carpal bones (Fig 16–27). The midportion of the navicular where the majority of fractures occur is clearly outlined.

Roentgenographic examination of the phalanges and metacarpals is performed with posteroanterior and oblique films. When evaluating the fingers, the individual digits should also be examined with true lateral views.

ROENTGENOGRAPHIC ANATOMY, DEVELOPMENTAL VARIATIONS, AND PATHOLOGY OF THE INDIVIDUAL BONES

In this section on hand and wrist, anatomy, variations and abnormalities, especially of the individual carpal bones, will be considered together.

The carpus is composed of a proximal and distal row of four bones each. In order to remember their names, the infamous mnemonic of " . . . Tilly's pants . . . " still applies, but a picture sometimes is more than words can describe (Fig 16–28).

The proximal row is concave in alignment toward the hand, whereas the distal row is more or less convex in the same direction as seen on the anteroposterior film. The navicular, lunate, triquetral, and pisiform bones constitute the proximal column; the distal row is made up by the greater multangular (trapezium), lesser multangular (trapezoid), capitate, and hamate bones. For proper interpretation, each bone should be identified and scrutinized separately.

Throughout the skeleton, constitutional disease, such as congenital hypothyroidism (cretinism) and other endocrine and metabolic diseases, affect and alter the time of appearance and growth rate of ossification centers, but the wrist and hand provide one of the most sensitive indicators of growth retardation of bone age. A handbook for the normal growth and development of the hand and wrist is found in most radiology departments (Greulich and Pyle, 1959).

There are a few, infrequently de-

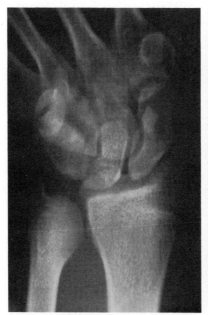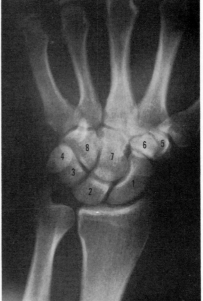

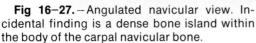

Fig 16–27.—Angulated navicular view. Incidental finding is a dense bone island within the body of the carpal navicular bone.

Fig 16–28.—Normal carpal bones: *1,* navicular; *2,* lunate; *3,* triquetrum; *4,* pisiform; *5,* greater multangular (trapezium); *6,* lesser multangular (trapezoid); *7,* capitate; and *8,* hamate.

scribed, congenital abnormalities affecting the carpus. Agenesis or hypoplasia of one or more of the bones may be found. Fusion anomalies or synostoses also are occasionally seen.

Anatomical variations occur with such frequency that some of the more common ones will be described to permit differentiation from pathologic conditions.

Accessory bones do appear about the carpal bones but are very infrequent. They are mentioned merely to make one aware of their existence, and they need to be recalled when considering the possibility of an avulsion fragment.

Small, well-defined, round to oval areas of increased density are often identified in any of the carpal bones, metacarpals and phalanges. They represent clinically insignificant bone islands (see Fig 16–27).

Tiny, rounded lucencies with well-delineated sclerotic margins coincide with vascular channels, but cyst-like areas are also frequently encountered within or along the cortical borders of any of the hand or wrist bones, especially the carpal bones. These may be the result of medullary fibrosis or hemorrhagic cysts. When related to the articular cortex, these cysts are the result of synovial herniation in osteoarthritis when the other classical signs of this disease are present. Erosive cysts at the juxta-articular margins are diagnostic of rheumatoid arthritis.

In the forthcoming discussion, all of the individual wrist and hand bones will be considered separately.

NAVICULAR. – The navicular bone becomes visible somewhat late, usually by the fifth to sixth year. This bone may be entirely absent (agenesis) or it may become assimilated (fused) with the radial epiphysis. A small hypoplastic navicular may result in a malformed radial-carpal joint. Quite often a tubercle arises from the distal and lateral corner of the bone. A partial division of the navicular resulting from incomplete fusion of two

ossification centers can simulate a fracture. This condition will require follow-up studies for the determination of healing, but the same may be found in the contralateral wrist.

LUNATE. – In the vicinity of the fourth to fifth year of life, the lunate bone becomes visible by ossification. Like the navicular, it may develop from two separate centers, which, if they fail to fuse, results in complete or partial fracture-like lines.

One of the most notable pathologic changes affecting the carpal lunate is Kienböck's aseptic necrosis. This form of osteochondritis has been described in more detail in chapter 6.

The carpal lunate is infrequently fractured, but is involved in one of the more important traumatic lesions of the wrist – dislocations. Three important types of wrist dislocations have been described. The first is a transnavicular perilunate dislocation (Fig 16–29). In this condition, there is a fracture at the midnavicular. The proximal pole fragment and the lunate maintain their normal relationship with the radial articulation, but the distal pole segment of the navicular bone and the remaining carpal bones become displaced posteriorly.

In a perilunate dislocation, the navicular is intact, and it along with the carpus becomes dorsally dislocated. The lunate remains in normal position.

The third type of carpal displacement is a pure lunate dislocation (Fig 16–30). The articular relationship between the lunate and the capitate is disrupted. The lunate rotates anteriorly, which is best appreciated on the lateral view. On the anteroposterior film, the lunate takes on a somewhat triangular appearance, which should alert one of this abnormality.

TRIQUETRUM. – The triquetrum or triangular bone, appearing between the second to third year, probably is the second most frequently fractured bone of the

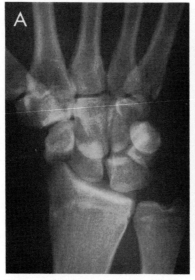
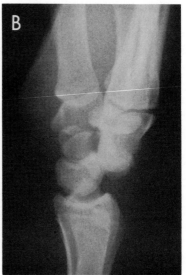

Fig 16–29.—Transnavicular perilunate dislocation. **A,** posteroanterior view. Note obvious displaced fracture of navicular and the overlap of the proximal pole fragment and the capitate, which should alert one to more than just a simple fracture. **B,** lateral view showing typical posterior displacement, particularly of the capitate, with the lunate, maintaining its normal position.

carpus. This usually consists of a posterior chip fracture, identified on the lateral roentgenogram, and is usually of no clinical importance.

PISIFORM.—The last and smallest bone of the carpus to ossify is the pisiform, usually in the ninth or tenth year of life. Because it often develops from multiple centers, its early appearance has often been misinterpreted as a fracture or aseptic necrosis. Traumatic lesions of the pisiform are almost nonexistent, although fractures and dislocations have been reported in the literature.

GREATER MULTANGULAR.—Progressing on to the distal row, the first bone to

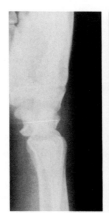
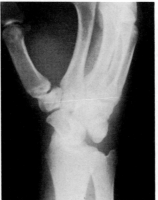
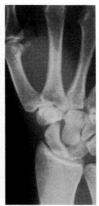

Fig 16–30.—Pure lunate dislocation. The lateral view *(left)* reveals the semilunar articular margin of the lunate faces forward. On the frontal view *(right)* note the abnormal relation of the lunate to the navicular, capitate, and triquetrum.

be considered is the greater multangular or trapezium. Appearing at approximately the fifth year, this carpal bone should be observed for its concave articulation with the base of the first metacarpal bone. A fusion between the two is not infrequent. In addition, it exhibits a tendency for fusion with the navicular. This bone, along with the lesser multangular, is somewhat difficult to evaluate because of the superimposition of the two.

Degenerative osteoarthritic alterations are very common at the first metacarpal-greater multangular joint. Joint narrowing, subarticular sclerosis, and spurring are characteristic findings of this process.

LESSER MULTANGULAR. — The lesser multangular or trapezoid makes its appearance sometime after the navicular visualizes. It is rarely involved in pathologic processes, including trauma. Synostosis between it and the adjoining capitate has been observed.

CAPITATE. — The first carpal bone to ossify and the largest of the eight is the capitate. Cyst-like lesions seem to predominate in the capitate bone. Its position appears to protect it from trauma.

HAMATE. — Finally, the last carpal bone to be visualized is the hamate. To the inexperienced observer the uncinate process or hamulus, the bony protuberance of the hamate extending toward the palm, will appear as a lucent lesion with a sclerotic border when seen en face in the anteroposterior projection. Because avulsion fractures of this hook-like process may happen, it is helpful to obtain an oblique view of the wrist with the posterior surface of the small finger resting against the film. This will project the hamulus free of overlapping bones.

DISTAL RADIUS AND ULNA. — When analyzing the wrist roentgenogram, the distal radius and ulna can hardly escape attention. We are all aware of what constitutes a Colles' fracture and its reverse,

a Smith fracture, but subtle impaction fractures of the distal radius may evade detection. A helpful rule to follow is to measure the anterior angle of the tilt of the distal articular margin of the radius, which normally measures 15° on the lateral view. The only indication of a fracture may be straightening or reversal of this tilt.

A transverse fracture of the radial styloid may be an isolated finding and constitutes the so-called chauffeur's fracture. A styloid fracture of the ulna usually accompanies another fracture, but it may be an isolated finding.

Dislocations of either or both the distal radius and ulna must not be overlooked, and this is easily accomplished if a true lateral roentgenogram is not performed. The displacement is invariably posterior.

METACARPALS AND PHALANGES. — When describing the individual fingers, the term "ray" is employed. Each of the five rays is composed of a metacarpal and its three associated phalanges, proximal, middle, and distal.

A number of congenital abnormalities exist at birth. Included are fusion of two or more of the digital rays, a condition referred to as syndactyly. Duplicative anomalies or polydactyly can involve any of the rays. Arachnodactyly of the fingers occurs in the generalized skeletal disorder of Marphan's syndrome, in which the digits are elongated and very thin.

When assessing the metacarpal bones, there are several important anatomical features to be considered (Fig 16–31). The epiphysis of the first metacarpal bone (the thumb) is located proximally, whereas the growth center occupies the distal aspect of the remaining four metacarpals. This property is consequential in terms of examinations made for assessing the presence of fractures in the growing patient. But, as is usual, there is always some variation to confuse the issue. On occasion one may see what appear to be

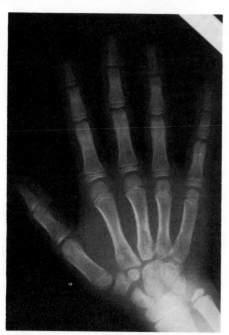

Fig 16–31.—Normal hand bones of a 9-year-old child. Note the position of the epiphyses of the metacarpal bones.

epiphyses involving the distal first metacarpal or the proximal second metacarpal and that are appropriately termed pseudoepiphyses.

Sesamoid bones about the hand and wrist deserve mention because of their frequency and occasional mistaken identity as fractures. They typically overlap the heads of the metacarpal bones. A fracture of a sesamoid is very rare, being more commonly found in the foot.

The appearance of the phalanges, particularly the terminal ones, is extremely variable, and the variants, for all practical purposes, should be considered normal. The ungual tuberosity or tuft of the distal phalanx can have many shapes and sizes, yet a number of disease processes may alter them considerably. Deformity and erosive changes of the tufts are seen in scleroderma, sarcoidosis, psoriasis, and leprosy.

Cyst-like or erosive changes in the tufts can be ascribed to glomus tumors that produce pressure erosion of bone and

are accompanied by severe pain. Enchondromas can involve any of the phalanges and are prone to pathologic fracture.

Of all the fractures involving the fingers, those of the tuft are probably the most common and may be avulsion types or comminuted. When analyzing the injured finger, the importance of obtaining a true lateral view, in addition to anteroposterior and oblique projections, cannot be stressed too much (Fig 16–32). This becomes particularly apparent in cases of volar plate injuries. A fragment of bone is avulsed from the palmer aspect at the base of the middle phalanx and involves the proximal interphalangeal joint. The result of hyperextension forces, the fragment may be obscured on all but the lateral film.

Rheumatoid arthritis produces distinctive transformations in the joints of the hand and wrist. The earlier roentgenographic finding may be periarticular soft tissue swelling. Later demineralization about the joint with slight widening of the joint space will be noted, the result of inflammatory hyperemia with intra-articular fluid and synovial thickening. This progresses to juxta-articular cortical erosions, which are related to synovial hypertrophy and panus formation. Eventually the joint space becomes narrowed and classical ulnar subluxations occur. Unlike degenerative osteoarthritis, there is no reactive spur production in rheumatoid arthritis.

Hyperparathyroidism produces a pathognomatic change in the hands. Typically, there is subperiosteal resorption along the radial aspect of the middle phalanges.

The Pelvis and Hips

ROENTGENOGRAPHIC EXAMINATION

The anteroposterior view is the only standard projection required for roentgenographic examination of the pelvis.

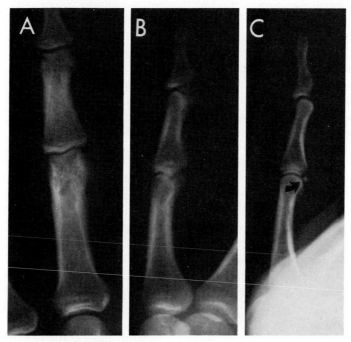

Fig 16–32. – Volar plate fracture of the finger. **A,** posteroanterior view. **B,** oblique view. **C,** lateral view. Note that the fragment is identified only on the lateral film.

This film should include the entirety of the bony pelvis, from iliac crests to the ischial tuberosities, which inherently encompasses the sacrococcyx and sacroiliac joints. Furthermore, both hips will be imaged on the film and this should include the femur to the subtrochanteric region (below the lesser trochanter) whenever possible.

There are special projections that will aid the analyses of certain pelvic segments and clarify suspected regions. Films performed in the anteroposterior direction with the x-ray tube angled 30° toward the head (cephalad) and 30° toward the feet (caudad) are practical under certain circumstances. These will give a different perspective of the sacroiliac joints, sacrococcyx, the iliac wings, and the anterior pelvic arch (the ischiopubic rami). Nondisplaced fractures of the rami may go undetected initially on the straight anteroposterior exposure but can be clearly delineated on these angled projections.

The anteroposterior views may suffice for complete preliminary pelvic assessment in cases of trauma. Minimal motion of the patient is the best policy to prevent possible compromise to already injured soft tissues, for example, blood vessels, and urinary bladder. However, oblique films can be helpful adjuncts on follow-up studies. The supine patient is first rotated 45° with the right hip down against the film (right posterior oblique) and then to the left 45° (left posterior oblique). Because of the outward orientation of the sacroiliac joints, the oblique films allow the viewer to look straight down the joints without confusing overlap of the free edges. Moreover, the ischiopubic rami and the margins of the obturator foramen will be visualized in a different manner. The posterior margin of the acetabulum can also lend itself to more direct inspection. Acetabular fractures, a topic that will be discussed later, require not only oblique roentgenograms but also lateral films for proper evaluation.

When the focus of attention is the hip, it is useful to include both sides on a single film for comparative reasons. The straight anteroposterior roentgenogram of the pelvis and hips is an appropriate examination but it is a must to view the hip from a lateral aspect when at all possible. This can be achieved in one of two ways: (1) a frog-leg position with the femur maximally rotated externally or (2) a horizontally directed roentgenogram with the tube placed along the inner aspect of the thigh and directed through the hip to a grid film placed alongside the hip. This latter method is generally the desired technique in cases of fracture as the patient usually will not tolerate rotation of the leg and hip, and little or no motion of the injured part is preferred.

ROENTGENOGRAPHIC ANATOMY AND DEVELOPMENTAL VARIATIONS

The pelvis is formed by two innominate bones each consisting of an ilium, an ischium, and the pubis, which are distinct entities in youth but fuse to form a singular solid structure in the adult. The sacrum serves as a posterior bridge between the two by way of the essentially nonmobile sacroiliac joints.

The epiphyses and apophyses of the pelvis and hips ordinarily do not unite until the second decade of life. The apophyses of the iliac crest normally make their appearance by the 12th to 15th year and fuse by age 21 to 25. They are separated from the body of the ilium by no more than 2 to 3 mm, often have an irregular, rippled appearance, and may show segmentation into two or more parts.

Small centers of ossification arise from the anterior inferior iliac spines by the 13th year and fuse two to three years later. Athletes are prone to avulsion of these centers and this should be looked for when there is localized pain in a sports-related injury. Oblique films are most useful in such situations, and a view of the opposite side is almost always needed to make the diagnosis.

The cheerleader's "splits" can create a similar avulsion of the ischial tuberosity apophysis on one or both sides (Fig 16–33). The time of appearance and fusion of these ossification centers parallels those of the iliac crest.

Until the eighth year of life, a radiolucent cartilage separates the ischium and pubis along the inferior ramus (Fig 16–34). This area of normal development is frequently misjudged as a fracture. During the process of union this region appears more dense and expanded, giving the impression of callus formation or tumor. The bilateral appearances are often asymmetric.

The triradiate cartilage forms a Y-shaped configuration at the acetabulum and constitutes the junctures of the pubis, ischium, and ilium (see Fig 16–34). This will become completely filled in with bone at about the time of puberty.

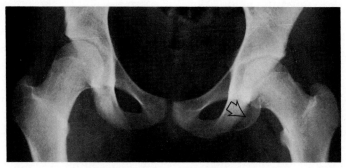

Fig 16–33.—Avulsion fracture *(arrow)* of the ischial tuberosity on the left side.

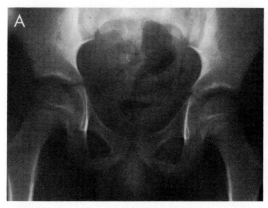

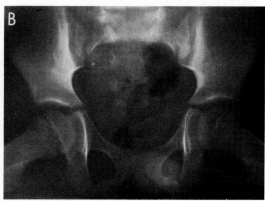

Fig 16–34.—Normal pelvis and hips of a 10-year-old child. **A,** anteroposterior view with hips in neutral position. **B,** anteroposterior view with hips in frog-leg lateral position. Note the triradiate cartilage and the bulbous appearance of the ischiopubic synchondroses of the inferior rami.

There have been many occasions when this, too, has been called a pelvic fracture.

In evaluating the symphysis pubis, it is more important for the inferior margins to align, whereas the superior borders are frequently and normally offset. Ordinarily, the width of the symphysis pubis joint measures no more than 8 mm in adults and 10 mm in children. Widening of the joint is characteristic of late pregnancy.

The posterior margin of the acetabulum, somewhat obscured by the femoral head and requiring an oblique view to see adequately, may arise from a separate ossification center and easily simulate a fracture because of its linear appearance. This variation is often a bilateral finding.

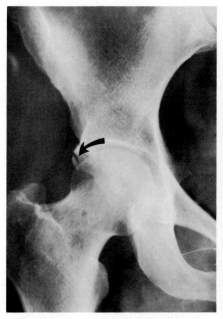

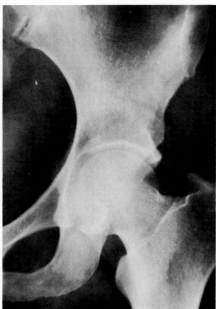

Fig 16–35.—Os acetabuli. The right side demonstrates this normal variant. None is seen on the left.

A variable-sized ununited center, the os acetabuli, may persist throughout life and is located along the superolateral margin of the acetabulum (Fig 16–35).

Proceeding now to the anatomy of the hip, the developmental features are of utmost importance. The femoral capital epiphysis appears during the first year. Synostosis of the head with the femoral neck is completed by the 18th year, but a cartilaginous fissure may persist. A central indentation along the articular margin of the femoral head corresponds to the fovea centralis in which the ligamentum teres is embedded.

The greater trochanter apophysis becomes visible by the fifth year and unites at the same time as the femoral capital epiphysis, namely, 18 years. The line of fusion may also persist for a long time and result in confusion.

In addition to the bones themselves, there are certain soft tissue densities about the hips and pelvis that demand attention. The shadows of the obturator internus, the iliopsoas, and gluteus medius muscles are ordinarily outlined by radiolucent adipose tissue. Because of their close approximation to the joint capsule, blood or pus that will distend the joint will be reflected on the roentgenogram by displacement of these fat stripes.

TRAUMA

A rather significant degree of correlation exists between the presence of an extracapsular subtrochanteric hip fracture and a pathologic process. In other words, do not take for granted that such a fracture is related purely to trauma, since this is a favorable site for metastasis.

Hip dislocations have been dealt with in chapter 9. From a radiologist's point of view, it is useful to comment on some of the roentgenographic changes seen in this type of injury. First of all, hip dislocations are classified as anterior, posteri-or, and central. In the most common posterior form of dislocation, the injury may not always be readily apparent on the anteroposterior film. There may be a slight difference in the size of the femoral heads as a result of slight rotation of the displaced hip. Shenton's line may be askew. This is a continuous, smooth line formed along the sweep of the inner margin of the femoral neck and it normally follows the inferior boundary of the arched contour of the superior ischiopubic ramus. Any disruption of this line would indicate a dislocation. The posterior lip of the acetabulum may be fractured but, as previously noted, a persistent unfused apophysis is sometimes located here.

When an anterior dislocation is present, the femoral head may lie medial and below the acetabulum, sometimes superimposed on the obturator foramen. However, the head infrequently may overlie the acetabular roof, simulating a posterior dislocation. This will require a horizontal groin lateral roentgenogram for differentiation.

When either a posterior or an anterior dislocation has been reduced, postreduction roentgenograms should be inspected for associated fractures. Also, the width of the hip joint space requires measurement. A difference of more than 2 mm should make one suspect the possibility of interposed tissue, such as a portion of the torn capsule, which will necessitate surgical removal. Short of surgical exploration, the diagnosis may need tomography or even hip arthrography with radiopaque material.

A central dislocation of the hip is always associated with an acetabular fracture; hence the condition is termed a central fracture-dislocation (Fig 16–36). A central acetabular fracture, however, may exist without a dislocated hip. There are four basic types of acetabular fractures, but the central form constitutes the most common.

As seen in Figure 16–37, the central

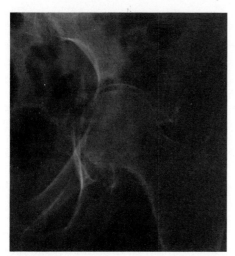

Fig 16–36.–Central fracture dislocation of the hip.

acetabular fracture may be transverse or oblique. The transverse type extends from the anterior acetabular margin backward through the ischial spine, whereas the oblique form is directed more superiorly to the greater sacrosciatic notch. Both

actually divide the innominate bone into superior and inferior segments.

The second variety of acetabular fracture, as discussed previously, involves the posterior rim. This most often is produced by a posteriorly dislocated hip.

Two other categories of acetabular fractures are depicted in the schematic drawing of Figure 16–37: anterior (iliopubic) and posterior (ilioischial) column fractures. Oblique films will be required for their proper interpretation.

In addition to acetabular fractures, the remainder of the pelvis can be fractured in various ways. It is best to classify these as either stable or unstable.

Stable fractures can be categorized into avulsions, ischiopubic rami fractures, iliac wing fractures, and fractures of the sacrococcyx. Avulsions of the anterior superior and inferior iliac spines as well as the ischial tuberosities have already been commented on.

The most frequent pelvic fractures are those involving the ischiopubic rami.

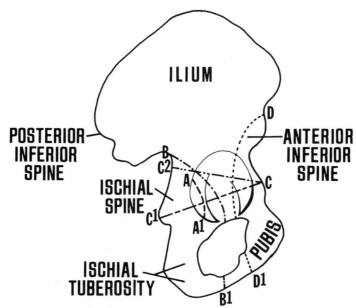

Fig 16–37.–Types of acetabular fractures. This drawing of a lateral view of the pelvis describes the basic fractures that can involve the acetabulum: A-A^1 = posterior rim fracture; B-B^1 = posterior column fracture (ilioischial); C-C^1 = central transverse fracture; C-C^2 = central oblique fracture; and D-D^1 = anterior column fracture (iliopubic). (From Thaggard, A., Harle, T. S., and Carlson, V.: Fractures and dislocations of bony pelvis, Semin. Roentgenol. 13:117-133, 1978, by permission of Grune & Stratton, Inc.)

Occasionally, these may be stress-type infractions. Their visualization may call for cephalic and caudal tilt films.

A fracture of the iliac wing often results from a direct lateral blow to the pelvis. These are best depicted with an oblique roentgenogram.

A variety of fractures and/or dislocations result in unstable conditions of the pelvis. Among the more common types that might be encountered is the straddle fracture (Fig 16–38, A). This situation exists when there are vertical fractures involving the superior and inferior ischiopubic rami on both sides. Less frequently, the fractures are unilateral but with separation of the symphysis pubis. Approximately 30% of such injuries will have associated urethral or bladder trauma.

More serious forms of unstable fractures are classified as double vertical fracture-dislocations (see Fig 16–38). There are three such types, and all have in common a double component involving the pelvic ring, anterior and posterior to the acetabulum.

When there is unilateral vertical fractures of the ischiopubic rami or a dislocation of the symphysis pubis in combination with a fracture about the ipsilateral sacroiliac joint or a dislocation of that joint, the condition is termed Malgaigne's fracture (Fig 16–38, B and C). The hemipelvis on the involved side may become displaced up or down, creating a true unstable situation.

A "sprung pelvis" is another form of an unstable double vertical injury. Here, there is separation of one or both sacroiliac joints and a disjunction of the symphysis pubis (Fig 16–38, D). Careful inspection of the sacroiliac joints should be made in any case showing displacement of the pubis.

The third type of double vertical pelvic injury is the so-called bucket-handle fracture (Fig 16–38, E). There will be fractures through the upper and lower rami of the anterior pelvic ring. The opposite or contralateral sacroiliac joint will be separated or will demonstrate a juxta-articular fracture.

TUMOR

Our attention is now directed to neoplastic disease of the pelvis. Primary tumors are seldom seen and usually present no diagnostic dilemmas. Most of these are similar to those described in the discussion of the spine.

On the other hand, metastatic disease is quite common in the pelvis, constituting approximately 12% of all bone metastatic sites. Difficulty in distinguishing minimal involvement may be related to confusing overlying intestinal gas and fecal material. Here is where the sensitivity of nuclear bone scanning will help to solve these difficult situations.

Not infrequently a pelvic roentgenogram will be seen showing a marked increase in density. The majority of these cases will represent either diffuse osteoblastic metastasis or Paget's disease. The differentiation, as already observed, can often be made utilizing basic characteristics of each (Fig 16–39). Notably, Paget's disease will disclose increased volume of bone and a greatly thickened trabecular pattern. Moreover, it may be confined to one side of the pelvis, a less likely occurrence in metastasis. In a small percentage of individuals (less than 1%), Paget's disease may transform to osteogenic sarcoma.

INFECTION

Infections involving the hips and pelvis, such as acute pyogenic arthritis and tuberculous osteomyelitis, are extremely rare today. Secondary seeding of infection, either directly from pelvis inflammation or through the bloodstream, can take place, resulting in either an infected joint or osteomyelitis.

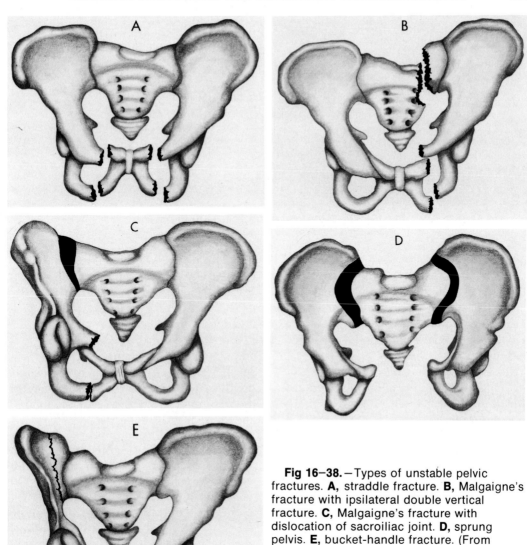

Fig 16–38.—Types of unstable pelvic fractures. **A,** straddle fracture. **B,** Malgaigne's fracture with ipsilateral double vertical fracture. **C,** Malgaigne's fracture with dislocation of sacroiliac joint. **D,** sprung pelvis. **E,** bucket-handle fracture. (From Dunn, A. W., and Morris, H. D.: Bone Joint Surg. 50:1639–1648, 1968.)

The Knee

ROENTGENOGRAPHIC EXAMINATION

The basic minimum examination of the knee consists of supine anteroposterior and flexed lateral views. The latter film should be obtained with the knee bent at least 45°, although this may be impossible in an acutely injured, fluid-filled joint or in a severely osteoarthritic knee.

Certain situations will call for other views. Internal and external oblique films may help visualize otherwise non-visible subtle fractures of the tibial plateaus or femoral condyles. These features, as well as the intercondylar space and the tibial spine (intercondylar crest), can also be evaluated with a tunnel film. The "sunrise" or tangential projection

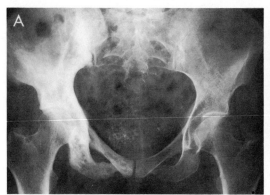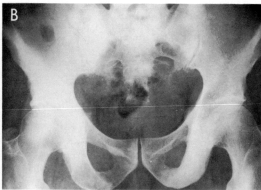

Fig 16–39.—Increased bone density in the pelvis.
A, Paget's disease. **B,** osteoblastic metastasis.

affords another perspective of the patella and the femoropatellar joint. A fat-blood level may be detected on an across-the-table horizontal beam roentgenogram, indicating an intra-articular fracture in which marrow fat and blood have been extruded into the joint.

Stress films, including valgus and varus manual forces, can bring out ligamentous injuries or laxity. Standing anteroposterior weight-bearing studies give information related to subtle joint space narrowing in degenerative osteoarthritis. Occasionally, tomography will elucidate abnormalities not identifiable on the standard films. With the advent of better fluoroscopic equipment, intra-articular changes of the invisible cartilaginous menisci, articular cartilage, and ligaments can be successfully evaluated by means of double air-contrast arthrography.

ROENTGENOGRAPHIC ANATOMY AND DEVELOPMENTAL VARIATIONS

The distal femoral epiphysis normally appears in the ninth month of gestation and therefore is utilized in determining fetal maturity. At birth it measures approximately 5 mm. The distal femoral epiphysis normally fuses at age 20. As in other areas of the skeleton, the epiphyseal line may persist as a faint track.

The intercondylar fossa, best evaluated on the tunnel film, forms a smooth arch. It serves primarily as a compartment for the proximal origins of the anterior and posterior cruciate ligaments.

The joint space, divided into medial and lateral compartments, normally measures 3 to 5 mm in height. It represents the thickness of the articular cartilages of the femur and tibia as well as the medial and lateral semilunar cartilages.

The proximal tibial epiphysis becomes visible by ossification in the last two months of fetal life. Like the femoral epiphysis it fuses to the shaft by the 20th year. Between the ages of 7 and 15, the tongue-shaped anterior and inferior extension of the epiphysis is visible, forming the anterior tibial tuberosity or spine (Fig 16–40, *A*). The tuberosity is an extremely variable structure, developing in an irregular fashion and often having a fragmented appearance. This should not be confused with a fracture or Osgood-Schlatter disease. Its features on the anteroposterior view can be particularly bewildering (Fig 16–40, *B*). On the frontal view, a radiolucent cleft often appears over the proximal tibial shaft.

The patella is considered a large sesamoid bone embedded in the quadriceps tendon. It should always be examined with a tangential film in addition to the lateral and frontal roentgenograms. On

characteristic layered periosteal thickening resembling an "onion skin." A variable patchy dissolution without significant expansion is imparted to the osseous architecture. Unfortunately, the symptoms of fever and pain and the sarcoma's roentgenographic manifestations can resemble those of osteomyelitis in the child and adolescent, and indeed the distinction may be extremely difficult to make.

ARTHRITIS

Osteoarthritis is a familiar affliction of the knee (Fig 16–45). Degenerative wear and tear produces the changes with progressing age, but secondary posttraumatic arthrosis is also a leading offender. Minimal joint space narrowing will be one of the earliest roentgenographic changes reflecting wearing and thinning of the articular cartilage. Standing weight-bearing films might be required to demonstrate this finding. The decreased height of the joint space may be accompanied by increasing sclerosis of the subarticular region of the tibia, quite often the medial condyle. The femoropatellar joint will undergo similar alterations of narrowing and associated sclerosis of the articular surface of the patella. Eventually the process leads to bony spurs arising from the articular margins of the femur, tibia, and patella. These osteophytes may become significantly large so that function is impaired.

Subchondral cysts, which are not always evident, are a unique feature of osteoarthritis even in joints other than the knee. They are well-defined round to oval lucencies, one or more in number, and measure anywhere from a few millimeters to 3 to 4 cm. One proposed theory for their evolution states that, because they are lined with synovium, they represent protrusions of the membrane through a defect in the articular cartilage. A small channel forms a direct communication between the cysts and the joint space, and this has been proved on pathologic dissections. A change in the intraarticular fluid and pressure dynamics of the disorganized joint is thought to be the mechanism for their formation.

The actual size of the intercondylar fossa, as seen on the tunnel view, may enlarge somewhat in osteoarthritis. This feature, however, is more pronounced in rheumatoid arthritis and the arthrosis of hemophilia with repeated intra-articular hemorrhages.

OSTEOCHONDRITIS

There are several disease entities classified as osteochondritis or aseptic necrosis involving the knee. The abnormalities of osteochondritis dissecans have already been described (chapter 10). Osgood-Schlatter disease is another form involving the anterior tibial tubercle. As mentioned previously, there is a significant variation in the roentgenographic appearance of the normal tuberosity, and the diagnosis is primarily a clinical one. Even though there may be sclerosis and/or fragmentation, this does not necessarily constitute Osgood-Schlatter disease. The only roentgenographic abnormality, almost universally present in the acute phase, is overlying soft tissue swelling. The principal purpose for obtaining the films is to exclude some other lesion, such as tumor or infection.

One other type of osteochondritis that might be encountered in the knee is Blount's disease or tibia vara. For some unknown reason, possibly stress, a localized growth disturbance occurs along the medial-posterior aspect of the tibial metaphysis. The changes may appear between the ages of 1 through 12 and culminate in outward bowing of one or both legs.

Roentgenographically, the medial tibial metaphysis is widened, forming a broad spur that extends both medially and posteriorly. The medial surface of the tibial epiphysis becomes flattened, producing a slope or concavity where this growth center is normally convex.

Without correction, the fully developed knee may exhibit a persistent downward slope of the medial tibial articular surface. The medial femoral condyle hypertrophies to compensate for the tibial deformity.

The Ankle and Foot

ROENTGENOGRAPHIC EXAMINATION

Three views are mandatory for proper evaluation of the ankle, and three projections are necessary for the foot examination. As elsewhere in the skeleton, modified and special films can clarify suspicious areas.

For the ankle, the three films include anteroposterior, lateral, and oblique projections (Fig 16–46). The oblique study, or mortise view, is obtained by rotating the foot internally 10° to 15°. Even though the calcaneus, tarsal bones, and bases of the metatarsal bones are not considered anatomically a part of the ankle, they should be included since associated or isolated injuries to these structures may be found when symptoms point only to the ankle. A good example of this is a fracture of the base of the fifth metatarsal bone.

An external oblique view might be requested when there is still a question of an abnormality in the absence of findings on the three standard x-ray films. A subtle fracture of either malleoli may be brought out in this way.

The standard roentgenographic study of the foot should include anteroposterior, internally rotated oblique, and lateral projections. Because of superimposition, the metatarsal and phalangeal bones cannot be evaluated to any extent on the lateral film, but the talus, calcaneus, and tarsal bones are relatively clearly outlined. Additionally, the talocalcaneal, talonavicular, and calcaneocuboid joints are well depicted. On the anteroposterior film, the cuboid and lateral cuneiform bones are superimposed and the bases of the metatarsals tend to be obscured by overlap. These bones are projected into profile with the internal oblique film. An externally rotated oblique view will delineate the first metatarsal and medial cuneiform bones.

The toes should be examined with an-

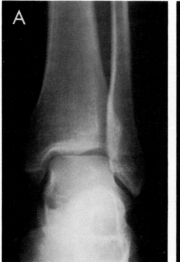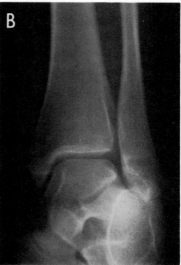

Fig 16–46. – Normal ankle films. **A,** anteroposterior view; **B,** oblique (mortise) view (see Fig 16–47 for lateral view details).

teroposterior and internal and external oblique films. An individual toe of concern requires a lateral view. This may be performed by having the patient hold the toe in extension with a pencil while the other toes are held in flexion, a maneuver that also is utilized for finger roentgenograms.

The heel is best demonstrated with lateral and axial (tangential) films. However, as will be pointed out later, oblique exposures sometimes aid in the study of this bone.

ROENTGENOGRAPHIC ANATOMY, VARIANTS AND PATHOLOGY

ANKLE.—The ankle mortise is formed by the distal fibula (lateral malleolus), styloid process of the tibia (medial malleolus), the horizontal articular plate of the tibia (plafond), and the dome-shaped articular surface of the talus (tenon) (see Fig 16–46).

On the lateral view, the width of the joint space between the tibia and talus narrows from anterior to posterior in the normal subject. Because of this, most ankle dislocations are anterior, except where there is a disruptive fracture of the mortise.

As has been mentioned previously with other growth centers, a linear sclerotic zone of bone condensation or a lucent line of incomplete union may persist in the distal tibia where the epiphyseal line existed. Additionally, just as in the distal radius or femur, a variable number of regular transverse bands of increased bone density may be observed in the tibial metaphysis. These so-called growth lines are normal; they tend to disappear with age and should not be confused with a pathologic process, such as the lines of lead poisoning.

Not infrequently, the tip of the medial or the lateral malleoli arises from separate ossification centers that fail to fuse. The resultant os subtibiale and os subfibulare can be variable in size, but, like all accessory bones, they have a well-defined thin cortical margin throughout their circumference. This will differentiate them from recent fractures.

Because of the high frequency of accessory bones in the ankle and foot, comparative views are recommended since the findings are usually but not always bilateral. If the distinction between fracture and accessory ossicle is difficult, one should consider one of several textbooks dealing with normal variants (Birkner, 1978; Keats, 1974; Kohler and Zimmer, 1968).

One of the best-known accessory skeletal elements of the ankle in addition to the os subtibiale and os subfibiale is the os trigonum (Fig 16–47). Situated behind the talus near the posterior aspect of the talocalcaneal joint, it is best viewed on the lateral roentgenogram. Its shape and size are variable and it may measure a centimeter or more. Despite its frequency, it still is commonly misinterpreted as a fracture.

Rarely, the os trigonum may be mimicked by a fracture of the posterior tubercle of the talus. This may occur when the posterior talar process becomes wedged between the posterior articular rim of the tibia and the calcaneus with severe forced plantar flexion.

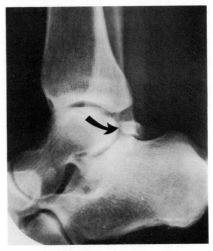

Fig 16–47.—Os trigonum.

On the anteroposterior projection of the ankle, the Achilles tendon is seen as a thick band of slightly increased density behind the tibia. The resultant shadow at times can create a bewildering roentgenogram. On the mortise film, one may see a horizontal V-shaped lucency through the medial margin of the talus. This corresponds to the inner margin of the talocalcaneal joint.

Overlap of the cortical margins of the fibula and tibia occurs in most views of the ankle, except a correctly positioned mortise film. This results in an apparent radiolucent defect termed a "Mach" effect and often leads to fracture misinterpretation.

On the lateral view of the ankle, distention of the joint capsule with blood can be discerned in either or both the anterior or posterior soft tissue compartments. Such a finding is often indicative of a fracture of the distal tibia or talus but not the lateral malleolus, since the synovial membrane of the capsule invests only the talus and tibia but not the distal fibula.

Benign cortical defects are a relatively frequent finding in the distal tibia in children and are just as common in the femur and tibia about the knee. Their characteristics have been described under the section on the knee. They are easily distinguishable on roentgenograms from more serious lesions.

The distal tibia is a favorite site for the development of Brodie's abscess. This lesion results from a sharply localized pyogenic infection of low virulence. This isolated form of osteomyelitis, seen primarily in children, quite often involves the metaphysis. Its intramedullary location is usually eccentric. It is seen on roentgenogram as a central irregular lucency surrounded by a thick capsule of sclerotic bone.

FOOT. — Overlap of the individual bony elements of the foot tends to make evaluation of the roentgenographic anatomy somewhat difficult. Anatomically, the bones of the foot include the phalanges, metatarsals, cuboid, the three cuneiforms, navicular, and the calcaneus, as well as the talus, although the latter is also considered a component of the ankle.

Of the tarsal bones, the talus is second only to the calcaneus as the most frequent bone to be fractured. The majority of these injuries are chip and avulsion types. They may occur along the anteroposterior surface of the neck and, therefore, a lateral film is required. Such fractures have also been described along the medial, lateral, and posterior processes. A fragment of the posterior eminence may simulate the os trigonum. Less commonly, the talus is fractured through the neck.

The talus is more susceptible to dislocation than the other tarsal bones because it is the only bone in the lower extremity not having direct muscle attachments. Furthermore, due to its tenuous vascular supply, posttraumatic aseptic necrosis of the talus may eventually take place.

The calcaneus anatomically consists of a body and a large posterior tuberosity. The sustentaculum tali forms a platform

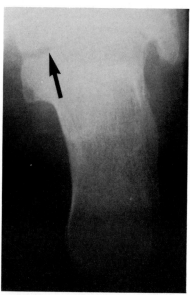

Fig 16–48.—Axial view of os calcis. Note sustentaculum tali *(arrow)*.

of bone along the inner superior surface of the body providing support to the anterior portion of the talus. The posterior facet, behind the sustentaculum tali, is that portion of the talocalcaneal (subtalar) joint that slopes downward, as seen on the lateral roentgenogram, and into which the lateral triangular process of the talus projects (Fig 16–48).

In order to properly evaluate the heel, especially in cases of trauma, in addition to the lateral film a tangential (axial) projection (Fig 16–49) as well as both oblique views are required. To obtain the axial exposure, the patient is seated on the table with his heel against the film. A towel or long piece of gauze is placed around the ball and toes of the foot and the individual is instructed to flex the foot by pulling on the cloth. The tube is angled 40° toward the head and centered over the heel. Multiple axial films from angles of 20° to 40° may be necessary to properly demonstrate the location and extent of a fracture.

The lateral convex and medial concave surfaces of the calcaneus should be well delineated on the axial view. If the film is accurately exposed, the sustentaculum tali along the medial aspect will also be identified.

When viewing the os calcis on the lat-

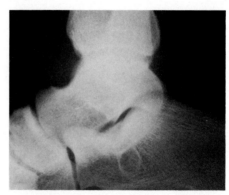

Fig 16–50.—Normal lucency within the os calcis simulating a cyst.

eral examination, it is mandatory that Boehler's angle be measured. This is formed by the intersection of (1) a line drawn from the dome of the os calcis at the talocalcaneal joint to the anterior process of this same bone, and (2) a line extending from the posterior tubercle to the dome of the calcaneus (see Fig 16–49). Normally this measures 20° to 40°. With compression fractures, this angle will be reduced. Subtle compression fractures may be overlooked without measuring this angle.

A somewhat rounded to triangular area of lucency that is relatively well circumscribed occasionally will be observed in the body of the calcaneus on the lateral roentgenogram (Fig 16–50). This finding can create interpretive difficulties since it simulates a cyst. This has been proved anatomically to represent a normal area of thinned, deficient trabeculae. This is usually an incidental finding and can be very disturbing when seen.

When considering the tarsal navicular bone roentgenographically, there are several lesions that deserve discussion because of their relatively common occurrence. Traumatic injuries of the tarsal navicular are uncommon. Avulsion fractures along the dorsal surface may be found near the talonavicular joint and require differentiation from an os supranaviculare. The medial tuberosity that serves for the insertion of the posterior

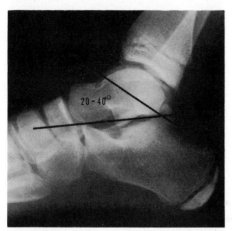

Fig 16–49.—Lateral film of ankle demonstrating Boehler's angle. Normal measurement is 20° to 40°.

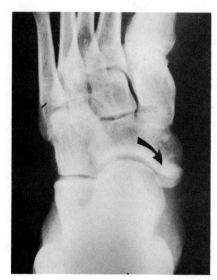

Fig 16–51. — Os tibiale externum *(arrow).*

tibial tendon may be subjected to forces resulting in fracture. Importantly, such a fracture may be associated with a fracture of the cuboid bone often with dorsal subluxation of the navicular. An accessory bone, the os tibiale externum, located behind the tuberosity, is more frequent than tuberosity fractures and may be confused with one (Fig 16–51).

Of all the tarsal bones, the cuboid initially has the most striking features due to its multifragmented appearance. After a short interval, the fragments become united into one solid structure.

Rarely encountered, cuboid anomalies are synostoses to the calcaneus, talus, navicular, or metatarsals. Accessory bones closely related to the cuboid are the relatively common os peroneum and less frequent os vesalianum. Their distinction from avulsion fractures is not always simple.

It is a rare occasion for the cuboid to exhibit an isolated fracture. Ordinarily, there are associated tarsal injuries, usually the tuberosity of the navicular or anterior process of the calcaneus.

The three cuneiform bones are anatomically labeled and numbered as follows: (1) medial or internal, (2) middle, and (3)

lateral or external. Like the navicular and cuboid bones, the internal cuneiform may demonstrate multicentric ossification. A not so infrequent finding is division of the first cuneiform into dorsal and plantar segments, representing a true bipartite condition. Isolated fractures of any of the three cuneiforms is definitely an uncommon situation.

With the correct roentgenographic projection on the internal oblique film, the joint space between the first and second cuneiform bones can appear quite wide and might lead one to a false impression of a separation. The middle and external cuneiforms often elude appropriate inspection due to their inconspicuous positions within the framework of the bony arch.

In the growing foot, the epiphyseal centers of the metatarsal bones are essentially similar in location to those of the hand. They appear in the third year, and normally fuse about 15 years of age. Each of the metatarsals contains one epiphysis, but the fifth metatarsal also possesses an apophysis at its proximal end. The epiph-

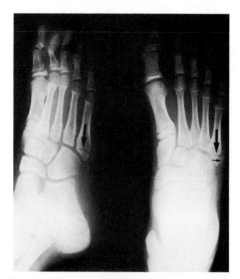

Fig 16–52. — Transverse fracture *(large arrows)* through the base of the fifth metatarsal bone. Note the normal shell-like apophysis *(small arrow)* that will increase in size before fusion.

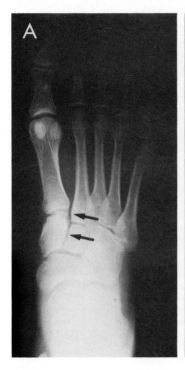
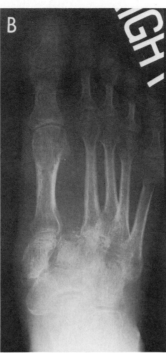

Fig 16–53. — **A,** normal alignment of the second metatarsal and middle cuneiform bones *(arrows).* **B,** lateral dislocation of the three middle metatarsal bones.

yses of the second through fifth metatarsals are distal, whereas that of the great toe is proximal. On rare instances, one may encounter pseudoepiphyses at the bases of the lateral four metatarsals, particularly the third and also the head or distal aspect of the first metatarsal. Occasionally, a cleft divides the epiphysis of the great toe metatarsal bone and should not be misconstrued as a fracture.

Several interpretive challenges are presented by the appearance of the base of the fifth metatarsal bone. The longitudinally oriented shell-like apophysis can be roentgenographically dissimilar in the feet of the same individual, varying in size and shape. Furthermore, it may persist unfused throughout life, but this is an uncommon event. Ordinarily the distinction between the apophysis and a fracture is relatively simple since the growth line is oriented to the axis of the shaft, whereas a fracture is transverse in almost all instances (Fig 16–52). An accessory bone, the os vesalianum, alluded to previously, is located near the junction of the

proximal metatarsal tuberosity and the cuboid. This fact should be remembered when evaluating trauma to this area.

A moderate degree of overlap of the bases of the metatarsal bones is noted to a greater or lesser degree on all views, but more so on the anteroposterior projections. Keeping the "Mach" effect in mind, this can and has led to the diagnosis of many erroneous fractures. The internal oblique film tends to reduce this problem to some extent.

When viewing the foot, the tarsometatarsal joints form a somewhat curvilinear line convex toward the toes. This is disrupted only by the recessed base of the second metatarsal bone resulting from a relatively short middle cuneiform. The base of this metatarsal is therefore wedged between the first and third cuneiform bones. Furthermore, the medial margins of the base of the second metatarsal and the middle cuneiform are always in line (Fig 16–53).

In the proximal space between the bases of the first and second metatarsal bones may be found the os intermetatarseum. It is located along the dorsal surface and, like most accessory ossicles, can assume variable sizes and shapes. Radioopacities in the form of arteriosclerotic vascular plaques can also be seen in this same interdigital space. Both of these can simulate avulsion fractures.

There is one traumatic lesion involving the metatarsal area that deserves special attention but, fortunately, is infrequent. The Lisfranc fracture-dislocation involves the tarsometatarsal junction and consists essentially of dorsal displacement of the metatarsal bases. Two basic forms exist: homolateral and divergent. In the homolateral type, the lateral four metatarsals are dislocated posteriorly and laterally, often with associated fractures at the bases. The divergent type exists when the first metatarsal is displaced medially and the others are dislocated laterally. The disfigurations may be subtle, and use of the normal straight alignment of the second metatarsal and middle cuneiform bones should be utilized.

BIBLIOGRAPHY

Aegerter, E.: Diagnostic radiology and the pathology of bone disease, Radiol. Clin. North Am. 8:215, 1970.

Beabout, J. W., McLeod, R. A., and Dahlin, D. C.: Benign tumors of the spine, Semin. Roentgenol. 5:419, 1970.

Birkner, R.: *Normal Radiologic Patterns and Variances of the Human Skeleton* (Baltimore: Urban and Schwarzenberg, 1978).

Brodeur, A. E.: *Radiologic Diagnosis in Infants and Children* (St. Louis: C. V. Mosby Co., 1965).

Caffey, J.: *Pediatric X-ray Diagnosis*, Vol. 2 (6th ed.; Chicago: Year Book Medical Publishers, Inc., 1973).

Christenson, P. C.: The radiological study of the normal spine: Cervical, thoracic, lumbar and sacral, Radiol. Clin. North Am. 15: 133, 1977.

Dahlin, D. C.: *Bone Tumors: General Aspects and Data on 3,987 Cases* (2d ed.; Springfield, Ill.: Charles C Thomas Publisher, 1967).

Dunn, A. W., and Morris, H. D.: Fractures and dislocations of the pelvis, J. Bone Joint Surg. 50:1639, 1968.

Edeiken, J., and Cotler, J. M.: Ankle trauma, Semin. Roentgenol. 13:145, 1978.

Edeiken, J., and Hodes, P. J.: *Roentgen Diagnosis of Diseases of Bone* (Baltimore: Williams & Wilkins Co., 1967).

Epstein, B. S.: *Atlas of Tumor Radiology: The Vertebral Column* (Chicago: Year Book Medical Publishers, Inc., 1974).

Forrester, D. M., Brown, J. C., and Nesson, J. W.: *The Radiology of Joint Disease* (2d ed.; Philadelphia: W. B. Saunders Co., 1978).

Foster, S. C., and Foster, R. R.: Lisfranc's tarsometatarsal fracture dislocation, Radiology 120:79, 1976.

Freedman, G. S.: Radionuclide imaging of the injured patient, Radiol. Clin. North Am. 11: 472, 1973.

Freiberger, R. H.: *Bone Disease Syllabus*, Set 9, American College of Radiology Self-evaluation and Continuing Education Program (Baltimore: Waverly Press, Inc., 1976).

Goldman, A. B., and Freiberger, R. H.: Localized infectious and neuropathic diseases of the spine, Semin. Roentgenol. 14:19, 1979.

Greenfield, G. B.: *Radiology of Bone Diseases* (2d ed.; Philadelphia: J. B. Lippincott Co., 1975).

Greulich, W. W., and Pyle, S. I.: *Radiographic Atlas of Skeletal Development of the Hand and Wrist* (Stanford, Calif.: Oxford University Press, 1959).

Harris, J. H., Jr.: Acute injuries of the spine, Semin. Roentgenol. 13:53, 1978.

Harris, J. H., and Edeiken, J.: Acute cervical spine trauma, Radiol. Sci. Update Series, No. 17, 1976.

Harris, J. H., and Harris, W. H.: *The Radiology of Emergency Medicine* (Baltimore: Williams & Wilkins Co., 1975).

Hill, H. A., and Sachs, M.D.: The grooved defect of the humeral head: A frequently unrecognized complication of dislocations of the shoulder joint, Radiology 35:690, 1940.

Jacobson, H. G.: *Bone Disease Syllabus: Disorders of the Skeleton*, Set 2, American College of Radiology Professional Self-evaluation and Continuing Education Program (Baltimore: Waverly Press, Inc., 1972).

Kaye, J. J.: Fractures and dislocations of the hand and wrist, Semin. Roentgenol. 13:109, 1978.

Keats, T. E.: *An Atlas of Normal Roentgen Variants That May Simulate Disease* (Chicago: Year Book Medical Publishers, Inc., 1974).

Kohler, A., and Zimmer, E. A.: *Borderlands of the Normal and Early Pathologic in Skeletal*

Roentgenology (3d Am. ed.; New York: Grune & Stratton, Inc., 1968).

Lichtenstein, L.: Bone Tumors (4th ed.; St. Louis: C. V. Mosby Co., 1972).

Lodwick, G. S.: *Atlas of Tumor Radiology: The Bones and Joints* (Chicago: Year Book Medical Publishers, Inc., 1971).

Meschan, I.: *Roentgen Signs in Clinical Practice*, Vol. 1 (Philadelphia: W. B. Saunders Co., 1966).

Mounts, R. J., and Schloss, C. D.: Injuries to the bony pelvis and hip, Radiol. Clin. North Am. 4:307, 1966.

Murray, R. O., and Jacobson, H. G.: *The Radiology of Skeletal Disorders* (Baltimore: Williams & Wilkins Co., 1971).

Nelson, S. W.: Some important diagnostic and technical fundamentals in the radiology of trauma, with particular emphasis on skeletal trauma, Radiol. Clin. North Am. 4:241, 1966.

Paul, L. W., and Juhl, J. H.: *Essentials of Roentgen Diagnosis of the Skeletal System* (New York: Harper & Row, 1967).

Pavlov, H., and Freiberger, R. H.: Fractures and dislocations about the shoulder, Semin. Roentgenol. 13:85, 1978.

Pyle, S. I., and Hoerr, N. L.: *Radiographic Atlas of Skeletal Development of the Knee* (Springfield, Ill.: Charles C Thomas Publisher, 1955).

Rogers, L. F.: Fractures and dislocations of the elbow, Semin. Roentgenol. 13:97, 1978.

Rogers, L. F., and Campbell, R. E.: Fractures and dislocations of the foot, Semin. Roentgenol. 13:157, 1978.

Rogers, L. F., and Lowell, J. D.: Occult central fractures of the acetabulum, A. J. R. 124:96, 1975.

Sherman, R. S.: General principles of the radiologic diagnosis of bone disorders, Radiol. Clin. North Am. 8:173, 1970.

Sherman, R. S.: The nature of radiologic diagnosis in diseases of bone, Radiol. Clin. North Am. 8:227, 1970.

Siberstein, E. B., Saenger, E., and Tofe, A. J.: Imaging of bone metastasis with Tc-99m EHDP and skeletal radiography, Radiology 107:551, 1973.

Smith, G. R., and Loop, J. W.: Radiologic classification of posterior dislocations of the hip: Refinements and pitfalls, Radiology 119:569, 1976.

Subbarao, K., and Jacobson, H. G.: Fractures and dislocations around the adult knee, Semin. Roentgenol. 13:135, 1978.

Subbarao, K., and Jacobson, H. G.: Primary malignant neoplasms of the spine, Semin. Roentgenol. 14:44, 1979.

Thaggard, A., Harle, T. S., and Carlson, V.: Fractures and dislocations of the bony pelvis and hip, Semin. Roentgenol. 13:117, 1978.

Vix, V. A., and Ryu, C. Y.: The adult symphysis pubis: Normal and abnormal, A. J. R. 112:517, 1971.

Wilkinson, R. H., and Kirkpatrick, J. A.: Pediatric skeletal trauma, Curr. Probl. Diagn. Radiol. 6:3, 1976.

Wilkinson, R. H., and Strand, R. D.: Congenital anomalies and normal variants of the spine, Semin. Roentgenol. 14:7, 1979.

Wiot, J. F., and Dorst, J. P.: Less common fractures and dislocations of the wrist, Radiol. Clin. North Am. 4:261, 1966.

Zatzkin, H. R.: Trauma to the foot, Semin. Roentgenol. 5:419, 1970.

17 / Maxillofacial Fractures

JOHN J. HEIECK, M.D.

INCREASING VIOLENCE in today's society combined with the development of local hospital emergency rooms as trauma centers have placed many emergency and primary care physicians in a position of initial responsibility for the isolated or multicomplex injured patient. Usually these physicians are able to recognize potential thoracic or abdominal injuries more easily than the maxillofacial defects. Their ability to identify maxillofacial injuries, of course, is necessary for the complete evaluation of the condition of any trauma patient. Although not lethal per se, undiagnosed facial fractures may have potential lethal complications or may produce contour deformities or functional disabilities.

The surgical literature lists many causes for maxillofacial injuries. The automobile accident, however, is the most frequent cause overall. Other causes include motorcycle accidents, fistfights, sports, falls, bicycle accidents, and convulsive disorders. Identification of the cause is important since one third of patients with maxillofacial injury caused by motor vehicle accidents will have associated life-threatening cranial, pulmonary, or intra-abdominal injuries. About one third will also be accompanied by nonlethal injuries, such as extremity fractures or eye loss. On the other hand, patients with maxillofacial injuries secondary to low-velocity causes (assaults or falls) have a markedly decreased incidence of associated injury: life-threatening (4%) and nonlethal (10%).

ASSOCIATED INJURIES

The primary physician's initial introduction to the maxillofacial injured patient may be as an isolated injury or as part of a multisystem involvement. However, the principles of treatment are similar in either case. Establishment of a patent airway should be the most immediate concern. Control of hemorrhage from open wounds or bleeding orifices by pressure dressing or packing should be attended to next. If shock does exist, treatment should include rapid infusion of intravenous lactated Ringer's solution followed by blood administration as soon as possible. Investigation of possible cranial, thoracic, or intra-abdominal injuries should be completed before identifying the maxillofacial abnormalities.

Airway obstruction with subsequent hypoxemia can easily develop in the patient with a maxillofacial fracture. Blood clots, broken teeth or dentures, and foreign bodies, such as dirt or glass, can physically obstruct the airway. The posterior displacement of the tongue secondary to the patient's position or to a mandibular fracture may occlude the airway. Other potential causes include glossopharyngeal edema and expanding hematoma. In all situations, a patent airway must take immediate priority. Sweeping debris from the oropharynx and mouth by using one's finger may be a life-saving technique. Suction, if available, will be helpful. Simple traction on a posteriorly displaced tongue by suture or towel clip may alleviate obstruction. If these methods fail, oral intubation must be instituted. If facial edema, facial fractures, or cervical spine fractures prevent oral or nasal intubation, a cricothyroidotomy can be performed through the membrane between the thyroid and cricoid cartilages. This is a bloodless field and the procedure can easily be done in the emergency room with only a scalpel. Later, an elective lower tracheotomy can be performed under controlled circumstances in the operating room. A low tracheotomy performed in the emergency room may be very hazardous and should be avoided.

Hemorrhage from open wounds can be controlled most easily by pressure dressings consisting of layers of Kerlix and Ace bandages. Occasionally, an active bleeder in a facial wound can be easily clamped and ligated. However, blind clamping of possible bleeding sites is condemned due to the high incidence of iatrogenic complications, such as facial nerve dysfunction. Nasal hemorrhage may require packing. Shock occurs very seldom from an isolated maxillofacial injury and is most commonly due to a thoracic or abdominal injury.

All patients should be considered candidates for cervical spine fractures, which occur in 4% to 7% of maxillofacial injuries. The initial examiner should palpate the neck for tenderness over the cervical spines and evaluate the grip strength and motion in all extremities. Before other roentgenograms are taken, a cross-table lateral view of the cervical spine with all seven vertebrae visible should be examined for fracture or dislocation.

Other associated injuries in the maxillofacial patient may involve one or more other systems. Subdural, epidural, or intracerebral hematoma may be present in a comatose or semilucid patient, indicating the need for skull roentgenograms and computerized axial tomographic scan. Possible chest injuries include rib fractures, pneumothorax or hemothorax, flail chest, aortic rupture, and pulmonary or cardiac contusion. Chest films and arterial gas studies may be indicated. Intra-abdominal injuries, of course, would include a ruptured spleen, transected liver, major vessel injuries, and/or perforated intestine. A pregnant woman may suffer an abortion as a result of the accident. Single or multiple extremity fractures may also be present.

All life-threatening associated injuries must receive first priority in the treatment of the multi-injured patient. After repair and/or stabilization of the associated injuries has been accomplished, reduction of the maxillofacial fractures may be performed.

EXAMINATION AND DIAGNOSIS

An accurate history should be obtained whenever possible from the patient and/or witnesses at the scene of the accident. The type of accident, the patient's position in the car, the use of safety belts, the mode of impact, and the patient's condition at the time of injury are all important considerations in the initial assessment. Since alcohol is involved in 50% of automobile accidents, a blood alcohol sample should be drawn. Ingestion of other drugs should be ruled out. A review of the patient's past history should include other illnesses, previous surgery, allergies, and all current medications.

A diagnosis of facial bone injury can be established by three methods: observation, palpation, and radiologic evaluation. Moderate to severe facial edema may mask bony irregularities and asymmetries (Fig 17–1). However, after resolution of the edema, facial asymmetry is suggestive of an underlying fracture. Light manual palpation is important in making the initial diagnosis. A systematic approach should be used routinely in examining all potential facial fracture

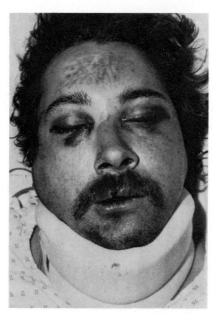

Fig 17–1.—This 32-year-old man suffered a Le Fort III maxillary fracture, nasal fractures, a displaced mandibular fracture, and an undisplaced fracture of the seventh cervical vertebra. The nasal deformity is easily recognized, but the remaining deformities are masked by facial edema.

patients. One should palpate the boundaries of the orbit, the projection of the malar eminences and zygomatic arches, the maxillary and mandibular arches, and the nasal bones. During palpation, one should assess possible asymmetry by noting any depressions or step deformities, as well as observing tenderness in areas of potential fracture. Evaluation of the function of the extraocular muscles may demonstrate superior gaze impairment with subsequent diplopia. Orbital ridge or floor fractures will commonly result in infraorbital nerve numbness of the cheek and of the maxillary gingiva on the side of the fracture. Crepitus to light touch suggests fracture extension through the nasal airways or paranasal sinuses. Rhinorrhea confirms the involvement of the fracture through the cribiform plate. The presence of trismus may indicate a hematoma or contusion in the muscles of mastication or could suggest either zygomatic arch or mandibular fractures. However, most important is the evaluation of dental occlusion.

Radiologically, the Waters' view is the single, most informative roentgenogram to obtain in evaluation of the maxillofacial patient (Fig 17–2). This study visualizes the floors and rims of the orbits, the walls of the sinuses, the zygomatic bones, the zygomatic arches, and the nasal septum with minimal interference of other bony structures. Opacity of a sinus suggests hemorrhage as a result of an orbital ridge and/or floor fracture. However, this view requires the cooperation of the patient and a normal cervical spine since the patient must be in the prone position during the examination. If the patient is comatose, uncooperative, or suspected of having a cervical fracture, a reverse Waters' view with the patient in the supine position is a satisfactory substitute since it gives almost the same detail of information. Other films worth consideration in the emergency room are the submental vertex view of the zygomatic arches, posteroanterior and lateral oblique views of the mandible, and the Towne's projection. More sophisticated and detailed studies can be obtained later during the hospitalization and after the facial edema has resolved.

MANDIBULAR FRACTURES

Although it is the thickest and heaviest of the facial bones, the mandible is the most commonly fractured, if one excludes nasal bone fractures. Mandibular fractures may occur as isolated injuries or as components of complex maxillary and mandibular fractures.

The most frequent cause of mandibular fractures are acts of violence that encompass simple falls, assaults, or motor vehicle accidents. Occasionally, systemic diseases such as hyperparathyroidism and osteomalacia may predispose to mandibular fractures. Infrequently, benign or malignant tumors, cysts, or osteo-

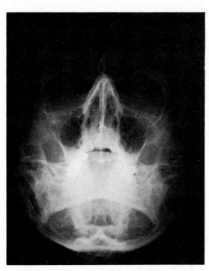

Fig 17–2.—The Waters' view is the best single roentgenographic study of the facial bones. It most clearly visualizes the rims of the orbits, the zygomatic bones and arches, and the maxilla. Note the clarity of the maxillary sinuses.

myelitis may precipitate such fractures.

Factors influencing the severity of the displacement of the fracture segments are multiple and interrelated. The direction and intensity of the force of injury will cause different fractures. High-velocity injuries cause a fracture at the site of impact, whereas a slow, less violent force not only causes a fracture at the impact site but also may fracture the opposite condylar neck. A blow to the area of the symphysis may cause fractures of both condylar necks. Second, the site of the fracture may influence the amount of displacement of the segments depending on the direction of the fracture line and the direction of the different muscle movements in the area. A fracture line that runs downward and forward from the molar area has less displacement than a line that runs downward and backward. The muscle groups that operate the mandible include the anterior (depressor-retractor) group and the posterior (elevator) group. The anterior muscle group will displace fragments in a downward, pos-terior, and medial direction, whereas the posterior group displaces fragments in an upward, forward, and medial direction. Consequently, a fracture through the angle of the mandible in a downward and backward direction will have a far greater displacement due to the distracting forces of the posterior muscle group. If the fracture line, however, was in a downward and forward direction, the muscle pull of the posterior group would tend to keep the fracture segments in an anatomical position. Third, the presence or absence of teeth will influence displacement of the fractures. Teeth on the proximal segment may decrease the displacement of the fractures by meeting the corresponding teeth of the maxilla. Finally, the presence and extent of soft tissue wounds will result in a larger displacement with larger defects.

Clinically, the patient may present with varying degrees of malocclusion. He may simply admit "my teeth don't feel right," or physical examination may demonstrate gross malocclusion. Anesthesia of the lower lip is common in fractures of the body of the mandible. Edema and ecchymosis may mask mandibular asymmetry. On examination, tenderness to palpation over the fracture site and pain with movement will be observed. Crepitation may be seen with motion. However, the principal physical abnormality will be malocclusion.

Although the clinical examination most frequently establishes the diagnosis of mandibular fractures, roentgenographic studies more clearly define the direction of the fracture line, the relationship of the teeth to the fracture, and the degree of displacement. Posteroanterior and oblique lateral views of the mandible will demonstrate fractures of the body and the angle without difficulty (Figs 17–3 and 17–4). If available, a Panorex view of the mandible is an excellent study and will show fractures at any site. However, fractures of the temporomandibular joint

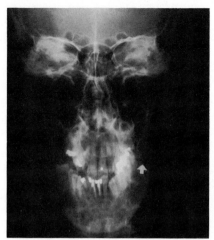

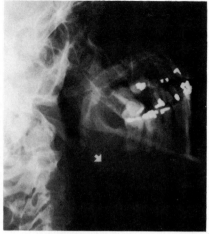

Fig 17–3.—A fracture through the left angle of the mandible is evident in this posteroanterior view of the mandible.

Fig 17–4.—Lateral view of the fracture shown in Figure 17–3.

and condylar area are sometimes difficult to demonstrate on routine mandibular roentgenograms and may require tomograms for the final diagnosis (Fig 17–5).

The most frequent fracture of the mandible is in the neck of the condyle. According to Dingman and Natvig (1964), 36% of all fractures occur in the condylar process. This site is closely followed by

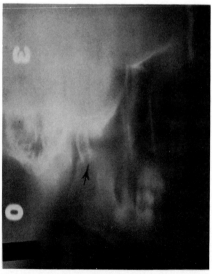

Fig 17–5.—Tomograms of the condylar process are often required to establish a fracture of the condylar neck *(arrow)*.

the angle of the mandible (20%), the body (21%), and the area of the symphysis (14%). Other sites are much less frequently involved.

The principles of treatment for mandibular fracture include early anatomical reduction of the fracture, immobilization, and control of infection. An isolated mandibular fracture should be reduced at the time of injury. However, if other life-threatening injuries are present, treatment of the mandibular injury may be postponed for seven to ten days. All mandibular fractures are considered compound if the slightest displacement is present and, consequently, preoperative and postoperative antibiotics are recommended. Immobilization will require at least the application of arch bars and intermaxillary fixation with rubber bands for a minimum of five weeks.

Specific treatment for each mandibular fracture will vary with the site of the fracture, the degree of displacement, and the presence or absence of teeth. Whenever possible, closed reduction of the mandibular fracture with application of arch bars and intermaxillary fixation is the treatment of choice. Fractures in the region of the symphysis or at the angle of the mandible often require open reduction and internal fixation supplemented with application of arch bars and intermaxillary fixation. Fractures in the body of the mandible, with teeth absent on the proximal side or with no teeth present on either side of the fracture, will require open reduction and internal fixation.

The edentulous patient presents a different problem. If dentures are intact, arch bars can be applied to the dentures. The upper denture is suspended from the zygomatic arches. The mandibular fracture is reduced and held in place by the lower denture secured by circumferential wires around the mandible. Intermaxillary fixation completes the procedure. However, if the dentures are not intact or if the lower denture will not maintain the anatomical reduction, open reduction and internal fixation will be required.

Postoperatively, the immobilization will be needed at least five weeks for a solid union to develop, even though roentgenograms will not demonstrate healing at that time. The use of the Water-Pik is highly recommended to maintain good oral hygiene during the period of immobilization. Nutrition is maintained very simply be blenderizing a regular diet. The patient should be seen weekly to check the dental occlusion and to replace broken rubber bands to maintain immobilization. Dental wax may be applied to irritating wires. At the end of five weeks, the rubber bands are removed and the patient is allowed to eat for a week. If the patient experiences no pain with oral ingestion, the arch bars are removed with the patient under intravenous sedation. However, if pain or movement at the fracture site can be elicited with eating, the rubber bands are reapplied for another seven to ten days of immobilization.

Occasionally, after removing the arch bars, the patient experiences a transient period of trismus due to the prolonged contraction of the muscles of mastication during the period of immobilization. By sliding tongue blades between his teeth, the patient should be able to forcibly open his mouth over a period of time and, consequently, regain the proper use of his mandible.

Early complications of mandibular fracture may include infection, avascular necrosis, osteitis, and osteomyelitis. Predisposing factors to infection are poor oral hygiene, multiple caries, or a compound fracture. Diabetic patients are more susceptible to infections. Acute infection will be manifested as an abscess and would be reflected by pain, swelling, and erythema in the area of the abscess. Incision, drainage, and systemic antibiotics constitute the treatment of choice. Chronic infections, such as osteitis and osteomyelitis, usually occur when a comminuted fracture with an avascular bone segment has occurred. Pain and roentgenographic changes suggestive of osteomyelitis usually are evident.

FRACTURES OF THE MAXILLA

Fractures of the maxilla or midface have increased in frequency correspondingly with the increased use of high-speed vehicles. Displacement of the fracture is directly related to the force of the injury and not to the effects of muscle contraction.

Maxillary fractures can be divided into two groups: vertical and horizontal. Vertical fractures will split the palate on either side of the septum. However, the three classical fractures of the maxilla are those horizontal defects described by Le Fort. The Le Fort I (transverse) fracture is a horizontal fracture immediately above the level of the teeth. The Le Fort II fracture has the configuration of a pyramid, with the apex being the nasal bridge. It extends through the nasal bones, the frontal processes of the maxilla, the lacrimal bones, the inferior rim and floor of

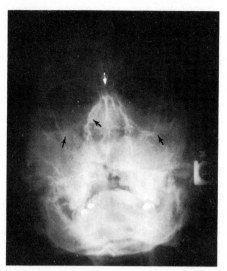

Fig 17–6.—A Waters' view visualizes Le Fort II fractures with involvement of the infraorbital rims, nasal bridge, and the right naso-orbital complex. The opacity of the maxillary sinuses is due to the presence of blood.

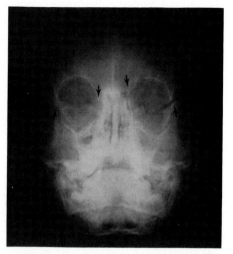

Fig 17–7.—A Le Fort III craniofacial separation is evident in a Waters' view of an 8-year-old patient. The opacity of the left maxillary sinus is more severe than the right.

both orbits, and the maxillozygomatic suture line (Fig 17–6). From this last point, the fracture continues posteriorly through the lateral wall of the maxilla, the pterygoid plates, and into the pterygoid maxillary fossa. The Le Fort III fracture separates the craniofacial complex and extends through the zygomaticofrontal, maxillofrontal, and nasofrontal suture lines, the floors of the orbit, and the ethmoid and sphenoid bones (Fig 17–7).

Clinically, the patient may complain of the inability to "match" his teeth properly. Infraorbital nerve numbness may be present. In Le Fort II or III fractures, nasal hemorrhage is usually evident. On physical examination, facial deformities may be masked by edema and ecchymosis. Bimanual palpation along the orbital ridges may detect step-like deformities or separations and tenderness. Forward movement of the maxilla will be elicited with all three Le Fort fractures; in the Le Fort III fracture, the entire midthird of the face may move. However, occasionally these fractures may be impacted and

no movement will be evident. Malocclusion can be an initial sign and should suggest a maxillary fracture if the mandible is intact. Extraocular muscle dysfunction may be manifested by diplopia with superior gaze.

With extension of the maxillary fractures into the cribiform plate, rhinorrhea mixed with blood will be detected as a result of the dura defect. The patient may admit to a salty taste in the back of his mouth. If sugar is demonstrated in the rhinorrhea, the presence of CSF has been confirmed and a tear in the dura has occurred. Consequently, the patient's nose should not be packed despite the possible presence of depressed nasal fractures, and the patient should be instructed not to blow his nose. Prophylactic antibiotics that cross the blood-brain barrier should be instituted to decrease the possibility of the development of a retrograde infection. When meningitis has occurred in this type of injury, the most common organism isolated has been *Pneumococcus*, sensitive to penicillin.

Roentgenographically, the Waters' view is the most reliable in demonstrating maxillary fractures. After resolution of the facial edema, tomograms of the facial bones will detail more accurately the full extent of the fractures. For vertical or alveolar fractures, occlusal views are more suitable.

Initially, the airway may be compromised by the posterior displacement of the maxillary fractures or by the combination with mandibular fractures. An endotracheal tube is the preferred treatment, although a cricothyroidotomy occasionally may be necessary.

After adequate resolution of facial edema, open reduction and internal fixation of the maxillary fractures will be required in order to establish the proper dental occlusion and to maintain an adequate midface projection. Definitive treatment includes stabilizing the maxillary segments by interosseous fixation, applying arch bars and intermaxillary fixation, and dropping suspension wires from either the zygomatic arches (Le Fort II fractures) or the frontal bone (Le Fort III fractures) to the arch bars. The orbital floors are explored bilaterally and large defects are reconstructed with either synthetic implants or bone grafts. Very infrequently is a tracheotomy required in the isolated midface fracture. However, maxillary fractures combined with pulmonary or thoracic injuries may require a tracheotomy to insure proper ventilation and adequate pulmonary toilet postoperatively.

In the edentulous patient with minimal displacement of the midface, correction of the anatomical defect may be maintained by adjustment with new dentures. However, any significant displacement will require open reduction and internal fixation, as previously described, using the intact dentures or dental splints to maintain the intermaxillary fixation.

Occasionally, the patient with extensive maxillary fractures will also suffer a severe head injury with resultant coma. After the stabilization of the neurologic status and with the approval of the neuro-surgeon, correction of the maxillary fractures is recommended. If treated within three weeks of injury, adequate reduction and fixation of the fracture can be accomplished. Otherwise, months may elapse before some degree of consciousness occurs, and surgical intervention then will be markedly more difficult, will probably require osteotomies with bone grafting, and will have less satisfying postoperative results.

Usually, the presence of rhinorrhea will spontaneously cease about five days after injury. Alternatively, the CSF leak will cease with adequate reduction of the maxillary fractures. If rhinorrhea continues three weeks after reduction, a craniotomy will be required to close the dura defect.

Postoperative treatment for the maxillary fracture patients is basically the same as described for mandibular fractures. Even in patients without rhinorrhea, preoperative and postoperative antibiotics are advocated as precaution against infection secondary to sinusitis. Oral hygiene is maintained by the use of the Water-Pik and adequate mouthwashes. A blenderized diet should be outlined prior to discharge. Weekly visits to the office are needed to insure the maintenance of proper dental occlusion. Rubber bands are replaced as necessary. At the end of the fifth week, the rubber bands are removed and the mobility of the maxilla is tested clinically. If the maxilla is immobile, the patient is allowed to eat for a week. If he experiences little pain during the sixth week, the arch bars and suspension wires are removed with the patient under intravenous sedation.

Late complications of maxillary fractures include nasal obstruction, chronic sinusitis, and lacrimal duct dysfunction. Anesthesia or hypoesthesia of the infraorbital nerve may persist. Malunion of the fracture may occur and, if unrecognized until four months after reduction, will require planned osteotomies with bone grafting for correction. If recognized within four months of the initial reduction, the malunion may be corrected by a second attempt at open reduction and internal fixation.

FRACTURES OF THE ZYGOMA

The zygoma or malar bone forms the prominence of the cheek and, consequently, is frequently injured. The usual cause of a zygoma fracture is the low-intensity, less violent type of injury: fistfights, falls, collisions.

The zygoma articulates with the maxilla, frontal, and temporal bones. Injury to it may cause a separation at the suture lines in an isolated injury or may be combined with fractures of the middle third of the face. If displaced, the zygoma will be depressed in the direction of the traumatic force, which most commonly is in the posterior, downward, and medial direction. Although six different groups of malar fractures have been described, fractures of the zygoma basically are either an isolated zygomatic arch fracture (Fig 17–8) or the "tripod" fracture (Fig 17–9).

Clinically, the patient may complain of pain in the area of the zygomatic arch when attempting to open his mouth. Infraorbital nerve anesthesia may be present in both the ipsilateral cheek and the maxillary gingiva (gingival numbness suggests orbital floor and rim fractures). The patient may also admit to diplopia with upward gaze.

On initial examination, the anatomical abnormalities may be masked by significant edema. Ecchymosis may involve the conjunctiva and sclera, as well as the eyelids. Bimanual palpation of both the orbital rims and the zygomatic arches should be done simultaneously and may elicit tenderness at the fracture site. After resolution of the edema, one may be able to identify depression over the zygomatic arch, step-off deformities of the orbital rim, flattening of the malar eminence, or

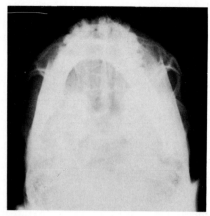

Fig 17–8. — A markedly depressed zygomatic arch fracture is demonstrated by a submental-vertex view.

inferior displacement of the lateral canthus. Oral excursion may be limited to less than 2 cm. (Limitation of oral excursion can occur if the zygomatic arch is depressed 1 cm and impedes the movement of the coronoid process of the mandible.) Diplopia with superior gaze may be present if the inferior rectus muscle is trapped by an orbital floor fracture.

The best roentgenographic studies obtainable from the emergency room are the Waters' view of the facial bones and the submental-vertex view of the zygomatic arches. Opacity in the maxillary sinus in a tripod fracture is readily visible on a Waters' view. After resolution of the edema, tomograms of the orbits can be obtained to further delineate the extent of the fractures.

Actual treatment depends on the type of fracture, the degree of fragmentation, and the direction and degree of displacement of the fracture sites. Resolution of the facial edema is necessary to assess the malar deformity and to insure good symmetry with the opposite malar prominence during reduction. A nondisplaced tripod malar or zygomatic arch fracture does not need surgical intervention. Antibiotics are prescribed for tripod fractures since the maxillary sinus is usually violated, creating a compound fracture.

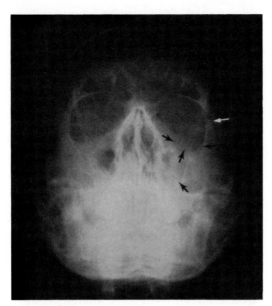

Fig 17–9.—A comminuted left tripod malar fracture is visualized on Waters' view. A step deformity of the orbital rim can be anticipated on physical examination. Note the opacity of the left maxillary sinus.

Surgical reduction of the isolated zygomatic arch fracture can be done either intraorally or extraorally. Extraorally, an incision is made either in the lateral eyebrow or in the temporal portion of the scalp behind the hairline. The fracture is reduced by passing an instrument beneath the temporal muscle fascia to a point behind the zygomatic arch and popping the depressed segment into place. If the fracture's reduction is unstable, a circumferential wire is passed percutaneously around the zygomatic arch and tied over a metal eye shield to maintain reduction for three weeks. At the end of the three-week period the wire is removed in the office.

Treatment of displaced tripod malar fractures may be accomplished by closed or open reduction. Closed reduction consists of inserting a bone hook at the base of the zygoma and reducing the fracture with the opposite malar prominence as a reference point. However, the incidence of late complications of diplopia,

malunion, and facial deformity are relatively high. Most surgeons prefer an open reduction of zygoma fractures. After reduction of the bone fragments, the position is maintained by interosseous fixation and/or a transnasal pin, or maxillary antral packing. If reduction is performed within three weeks of injury and is stable, the use of a transnasal pin is most efficacious. However, an unstable reduction would require both interosseous fixation at the zygomaticofrontal and the zygomaticomaxillary suture lines, in addition to the transnasal pinning. Rarely is packing of the maxillary sinus needed to maintain the malar reduction. The orbital floor should be examined before and after reduction of the zygoma fracture. A defect in the orbital floor may increase with satisfactory malar reduction and require reconstruction with either synthetic implant or bone graft.

Postoperatively, antibiotic coverage is continued for a week. A light dressing may be applied over the ipsilateral eye, but it is removed on the first postoperative day. The patient is followed up weekly in the office in order to monitor both malar symmetry and extraocular muscle function. The transnasal pin is removed without difficulty four weeks after reduction with the patient under local anesthesia.

Complications secondary to zygoma fractures are unusual, but would include infection, malunion, and nonunion. Infection usually occurs in those cases requiring orbital floor reconstruction with an implant, especially if the maxillary sinus has also been packed. The infection may develop early or late with respect to the repair of the fracture and requires removal of the implant as well as antibiotics administered for systemic effect. Malunion of the zygoma may cause facial asymmetry and interference with mandibular function. Correction can be achieved by osteotomies at the zygomaticofrontal and zygomaticomaxillary suture line, elevation of the zygoma, bone grafting, and fixation with Kirschner wires. Nonunions will necessitate bone grafting and Kirschner wire fixation for an extended period. Any residual contour deformity may be corrected at a later date with the use of onlay bone or cartilage grafts.

BLOW-OUT FRACTURES

Strictly speaking, the term "blow-out" fracture should be restricted to fractures of the orbital floor without involvement of the orbital rim. Blow-out fractures result from the transmission of a sudden increased intraocular pressure through the weakest point of the orbital floor, most commonly near the infraorbital nerve canal. A second common site of fracture is the medial orbital wall.

The most frequent cause of blow-out fractures is the automobile accident. A third of the cases usually result from blunt trauma secondary to fist blows, ball injuries, falls, and other forms of assault. Although the orbital rim protects the eyeball itself against direct injury from objects greater than 5 cm in size, ocular injury must be ruled out in all blow-out fractures. Direct ocular injury is more common in low-velocity injuries (14%) than in auto accidents (0.6%), resulting in either blindness or decreased vision.

During examination, the patient may volunteer the presence of diplopia, infraorbital nerve numbness, and, possibly, decreased vision. Clinically, periorbital edema and ecchymosis may handicap the initial examination. However, the eyelids usually can be pried open to allow a gross examination of vision and light perception. Diplopia may occur as a result of limitation of superior gaze (Fig 17–10). As the periorbital edema resolves, diplopia may lessen in severity. If the periorbital edema is minimal, enophthalmos may be present.

The most common cause of diplopia in blow-out fractures is the entrapment of the inferior rectus muscle in the orbital floor defect. Other causes of immediate diplopia include injury to the cranial nerves III, IV, and VI; direct injury or hemorrhage into the extraocular muscles; or displacement of the eyeball into the maxillary sinus. The "traction test" will simplify the differential diagnosis. Topical anesthesia is applied to the conjunctiva. The eyeball is pinched with a fine forceps at the insertion of the inferior rectus muscle and rotated. If rotation of the eyeball cannot be accomplished, entrapment of the inferior rectus muscle is demonstrated. If rotation of the eyeball is achieved, then the diplopia is due to one of the other causes.

Enophthalmos may be evident on the initial examination or masked by the periorbital edema. With subsequent resolution of the edema, enophthalmos will become more apparent. The mechanism of enophthalmos includes herniation of the orbital fat into the maxillary sinus, posterior position of the ocular globe due to entrapment of the inferior rectus muscle, or the downward displacement of the ocular globe through a large orbital floor fracture. Additionally, enophthalmos may develop as a result of orbital fat necrosis secondary to the injury, to pressure from an orbital hematoma, or to a low-grade inflammatory process.

The most pertinent roentgenographic

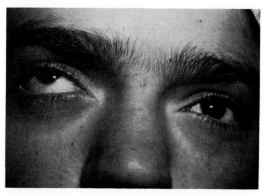

Fig 17–10. — Impairment of superior gaze occurred after blow to left eye. A traction test confirmed entrapment of the inferior rectus muscle.

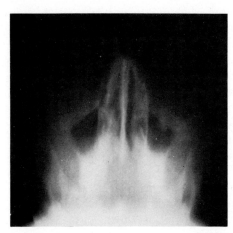

Fig 17–11.—A tomogram of the left orbital floor shows herniation of the orbital fat into the maxillary sinus of the patient shown in Figure 17 – 10.

studies are a Waters' view initially, followed by orbital floor tomograms after resolution of edema. Abnormal findings would include lowering of the orbital floor, orbital fat entrapment in the maxillary sinus (Fig 17 – 11), or massive orbital contents displacement into the maxillary sinus.

Treatment of blow-out fracture is twofold. If definite ocular injury is demonstrated on initial examination, an opthalmologic consultation must be obtained immediately for evaluation. If no ocular injury is present, surgical considerations are postponed until the resolution of periorbital edema. The two primary indications for surgical correction of a blow-out fracture include diplopia demonstrated by a positive traction test or enophthalmos. Usually, roentgenographic evidence will support the diagnosis of a blow-out fracture, but a normal study should not postpone surgery if there is a positive traction test or enophthalmos present.

The surgical procedure should be performed within one week after injury since the incarcerated contents become more difficult to release after this period. If surgery is postponed more than two or three weeks, motility problems and enophthalmos may appear as late complications. The surgical procedure consists of exploration of the orbital floor through a lower eyelid incision, release of the entrapped inferior rectus muscle, retrieval of the herniated orbital contents, and reconstruction of the orbital floor with either a synthetic implant or bone graft.

Antibiotics are recommended both preoperatively and postoperatively due to the involvement with the maxillary sinus. A light dressing is usually applied at the completion of the operation and removed on the first postoperative day. The patient is followed up as an outpatient for persistence of either diplopia or enophthalmos. Useful binocular vision at the end of three months commonly occurs. However, if diplopia is not improved by that time, an ophthalmology consultation will be required for further evaluation and possible prescription of glass prisms to allow useful vision. After six months, extraocular muscle surgery may be necessary to correct the persistent diplopia. The persistence of enophthalmos presents a very difficult problem. At the present time, there is not a reliable surgical treatment. Surgical treatment for this complication and all efforts should be directed toward correcting enophthalmos at the time of initial surgery.

NASAL FRACTURES

Fractures of the nasal bones are the most common of all facial bone fractures. Early treatment will allow easy reduction with satisfactory postoperative results. Neglect of treatment, however, may produce both a physiologic and a cosmetic deformity much more difficult to correct.

The types of nasal fracture may vary from a simple displacement of the nasal pyramid to a more complex comminuted fracture with a resultant "smashed" nose appearance. Associated injuries include fractures extending through the cribiform plate, medial canthal ligament displacement, or lacrimal gland or duct injuries. Sequelae of the comminuted nasal fracture include traumatic telecanthus, dacryocystitis, and epiphora.

Clinical evaluation plays the most important role in making an accurate diagnosis. The presence of preexisting disease, nasal deformity, or a previous nasal operation should be investigated at the time of the initial examination. On physical examination, nasal and periorbital edema are common. Nasal obstruction may be present secondary to either edema, clots, or displaced nasal bone fractures. Movement of the nasal bone fragments may be elicited by palpation. Subcutaneous emphysema may be present. The possibility of a telescoping-type injury should be considered, if the nasolabial angle is greater than 100° (especially, in a man) or if a step deformity is noted dorsally at the junction of the nasal bone with the septum.

The importance of identifying a hematoma of the septum at the time of the initial examination cannot be stressed too strongly. If overlooked, a septal hematoma can progress either to a partial nasal obstruction or to a septal perforation. Topical application of 10% cocaine will shrink the nasal mucosa and allow examination of the nasal passageways by speculum. The presence of a septal hematoma should be treated immediately by incision and drainage.

Very often, the posteroanterior and lateral roentgenographic views of the nasal bones are not very helpful in supporting the clinical impression of a nasal fracture. A Waters' view may better demonstrate fractures of either the nasal septum or the bony pyramid. However, the clinical impression is much more meaningful as regards to this fracture.

Ideally, the treatment of a nasal fracture should be done when initially seen. Usually, however, the presence of nasal edema does not permit immediate reduction. At the end of three to five days, the edema will resolve sufficiently to allow satisfactory reduction of the nasal fracture. Although the procedure can be performed with the patient under either general anesthesia or a combination of local and topical anesthesia, general anesthesia is recommended to protect the airway from posterior nasal bleeding. After satisfactory reduction, the nasal speculum should be used to demonstrate the patency of the airways and to evaluate the position of the nasal septum. A displaced septum should be returned to its position in the vomerine groove. Nasal packing consisting of 2.5-cm plain gauze saturated with tetracycline ointment is inserted to maintain the nasal bone reduction. A nasal splint is applied for further stabilization.

Postoperatively, the nasal packing will be left in place for approximately five days and the nasal splint for seven. During the second week, the nasal splint is usually worn only at night. Any activity that would endanger the nasal reduction (for example, contact sports) should be avoided for six weeks. During the interval of packing, nasal decongestants and antibiotics are used.

Late complications of nasal fracture include nasal deformity or airway obstruction. The nasal deformity may be secondary to malunion of the nasal bones or to a septal injury. Malunion usually occurs as a result of the patient's failure to seek early medical attention. Correcting a nasal fracture after fourteen days after the injury is rarely successful and will require a rhinoplasty to correct the deformity. Persistent nasal deformity or airway obstruction may be due to a septal injury and will also require a rhinoplasty and possible submucous cartilage resection for correction. In the pediatric age group, rhinoplasties are normally postponed until the age of fifteen to avoid any possible growth disturbances with the development of the nose. In the adult, a rhinoplasty can be performed after satisfactory wound healing has occurred, usually about three months after the injury.

FRONTAL SINUS FRACTURES

Frontal sinus fractures are not common (6%), but they do warrant special considerations. Such injuries are usually accompanied by fractures of other facial bones and may be associated with an intracranial injury.

On clinical examination, anesthesia of the forehead and scalp may be present as a result of soft tissue injury to the supratrochlear and supraorbital nerves. If a depressed supraorbital ridge fracture is present, diplopia will be demonstrated as a result of dysfunction of the superior rectus and superior oblique muscles. Periorbital ecchymosis and edema will be present, which may mask the frontal depression secondary to the fracture. Tenderness and crepitation to palpation may be elicited. Rhinorrhea may also be noted.

Roentgenographic studies should include a skull series and a Waters' view of the facial bones. Occasionally, there may be difficulty in demonstrating a frontal sinus fracture since fractures of the posterior wall are difficult to see, roentgenographically, even with good tomographic studies. However, the presence of an intracranial aerocele is pathognomonic for a dura tear and would implicate a fracture of the posterior wall of the frontal sinus.

Treatment of a frontal sinus fracture depends on the extent of the fracture and the amount of fragmentation present. Antibiotic coverage should begin on the day of injury. Surgical treatment of the fracture itself is divided between simple elevation and interosseous wiring of the bony fragments versus ablation of the frontal sinus with late reconstruction by bone graft or plastic implants. In the presence of a dura tear, a transfrontal craniotomy with repair of the dura should be done in conjunction with the reduction of the fracture.

Potential complications of frontal sinus fractures can be life-threatening. A posterior wall fracture with a dura tear may develop either a retrograde meningitis or brain abscess. Frontal sinus infections may also extend into the orbital cavities. The frontal sinus duct may be obstructed with the subsequent development of a mucocele.

FACIAL FRACTURES IN THE PEDIATRIC PATIENT

The incidence of facial fractures in the pediatric age group varies in reported series from 1.4% to 10%. Most fractures are greenstick in nature due to the resiliency of the facial bones in this age. Although the principles outlined for treatment of facial fractures do not change with age, several important considerations should be noted.

Clinical and roentgenographic evaluation may be more difficult to obtain. The child may not understand or answer questions about his injury. Cooperation in the physical examination may be difficult to obtain, but tenderness to palpation usually can be elicited. Roentgenographic studies may require sedation to insure films of good detail. The presence of unerupted teeth may mask the site of a fracture.

In general, the treatment of maxillofacial injuries in the child is basically similar to the treatment described in the previous pages. Difficulty sometimes arises in maintaining intermaxillary fixation since the ligation of arch bars to the short roots of deciduous teeth is difficult and precarious. Care also must be used to avoid injury to the unerupted teeth with application of the arch bars by wire ligatures.

Late complications of a facial fracture would also include the loss, delay, or maleruption of developing teeth; malocclusion; and facial deformity. Facial deformity may be the result of abnormal development secondary to a growth center disturbance at the time of injury. Consequently, the parents should be alerted to this possibility and the child should be observed throughout adolescence for any evidence of growth abnormality.

BIBLIOGRAPHY

Converse, J. M., and Dingman, R. O.: Facial Injuries in Children, in Converse, J. M. (ed.): *Reconstructive Plastic Surgery* (2d ed.; Philadelphia: W. B. Saunders Co., 1977).

Converse, J. M., Smith, B., and Wood-Smith, D.: Orbital and Naso-orbital Fractures, in Converse, J. M. (ed.): *Reconstructive Plastic Surgery* (2d ed.; Philadelphia: W. B. Saunders Co., 1977).

Dingman, R. O., and Converse, J. M.: Clinical Management of Facial Injuries and Fractures of Facial Bones, in Converse, J. M. (ed.): *Reconstructive Plastic Surgery* (2d ed.; Philadelphia: W. B. Saunders Co., 1977).

Dingman, R. O., and Natvig, P.: *Surgery of Facial Fractures* (Philadelphia: W. B. Saunders Co., 1964).

Luce, E. A., Tubb, T. D., and Moore, A. M.: Review of 1,000 major fractures and associated injuries, Plast. Reconstr. Surg. 63:26, 1979.

McCoy, F. J., et al.: An analysis of facial fractures and their complications, Plast. Reconstr. Surg. 29:381, 1962.

Milaukas, A. T., and Fueger, G. F.: Serious ocular complications associated with blowout fractures of the orbit, Am. J. Ophthal. 62:670, 1966.

Natvig, P., and Dootzbach, R. K.: Facial Bone Fractures, in Grabb, W. C., and Smith, J. W. (eds.): *Plastic Surgery* (2d ed.; Boston: Little, Brown, & Co., 1973).

Schneider, R. C., and Thompson, J. M.: Chronic and delayed cerebrospinal rhinorrhea as a source of recurrent attacks of meningitis, Am. J. Surg. 145:517, 1957.

Schultz, R. C.: Facial injuries from automobile accidents: A study of 400 consecutive cases, Plast. Reconstr. Surg. 40:45, 1967.

Schultz, R. C.: Supraorbital and glabellar fractures, Plast. Reconstr. Surg. 45:227, 1970.

Index